Handbook

Obstetric Medicine

FOURTH EDITION

Catherine Nelson-Piercy MA FRCP FRCOG
Consultant Obstetric Physician
Guy's & St Thomas' NHS Foundation Trust,
Imperial College Healthcare NHS Trust,
and Professor of Obstetric Medicine, King's College London,
London, UK

informa
healthcare

New York   London

First published in the United Kingdom in 1997 by Martin Dunitz.
This edition published in the United Kingdom in 2010 by Informa Healthcare, Telephone House,
69-77 Paul Street, London EC2A 4LQ, UK.
Simultaneously published in the USA by Informa Healthcare, 52 Vanderbilt Avenue, 7th Floor, New
York, NY 10017, USA.

A CIP record for this book is available from the British Library.

ISBN-13: 978-1-84184-737-5

Orders may be sent to: Informa Healthcare, Sheepen Place, Colchester, Essex CO3 3LP, UK
Telephone: +44 (0)20 7017 5540
Email: CSDhealthcarebooks@informa.com
Website: http://informahealthcarebooks.com/

For corporate sales please contact: CorporateBooksIHC@informa.com
For foreign rights please contact: RightsIHC@informa.com
For reprint permissions please contact: PermissionsIHC@informa.com

Typeset by Aptara, Delhi, India
Printed and bound in the United Kingdom

Handbook of

Obstetric Medicine

DATE

Contents

Preface to the fourth edition

Women with pre-existing or new-onset medical problems in pregnancy are encountered in every antenatal clinic and on every delivery suite in every country. The prevalence of medical disorders in pregnancy is increasing and these conditions are becoming more important as causes of maternal death. In developed countries, women are delaying pregnancy until they are older and more likely to have medical disorders, and, in addition, advances in medicine and surgery have resulted in women with complex medical histories now presenting either pregnant or requesting assisted reproductive therapies. Every clinician caring for pregnant women therefore needs to understand the interaction between medical disorders and pregnancy and needs to be able to counsel women about these interactions as well as about the safety of investigations and drug therapy during pregnancy and while breastfeeding. The explosion in the numbers of multidisciplinary, joint antenatal medical clinics is a welcome advance in care but this is only one aspect. All obstetricians need to be confident in the diagnosis of new-onset medical problems that may face them with increasing frequency.

This Handbook is designed as a pragmatic, easy-to-use, ready reference guide. In the fourth edition, I have again retained the same basic format of two sections. Section A is divided into chapters by systems, and each chapter describes the incidence, clinical features, pathogenesis, diagnosis and the effect of pregnancy and management of each condition. 'Points to remember' boxes serve as summaries and revision. Section B describes the differential diagnosis of common symptoms, signs and abnormal investigations encountered in pregnancy. All the chapters have been updated and revised to reflect current understanding and evidence to support management strategies for medical disorders in pregnancy. The suggestions for further reading include relevant guidelines where appropriate. Readers are also reminded about other resources such as the website of the International Society of Obstetric Medicine at http://www.isomnet.org and the new journal of the Society *'Obstetric Medicine: The Medicine of Pregnancy'* also available online at http://obmed.rsmjournals.com.

I am delighted that this Handbook continues to be used by trainees to help them revise for and pass examinations, but more importantly that it fuels an interest and thirst for knowledge in the exciting field of Obstetric Medicine. I am hugely grateful to all those doctors and midwives that have provided such useful feedback and comments about the Handbook over the years. I am also indebted to my many colleagues and patients who have taught me so much. To practise Obstetric Medicine remains an enormous privilege.

Catherine Nelson-Piercy

Glossary

ABG	Arterial blood gases
aCL	Anticardiolipin antibodies
ACTH	Adrenocorticotrophic hormone
AFLP	Acute fatty liver of pregnancy
ALP	Alkaline phosphatase
ANA	Anti-nuclear antibodies
APS	Antiphospholipid syndrome
APTT	Activated partial thromboplastin time
AVM	Arteriovenous malformation
CMV	Cytomegalovirus
CSF	Cerebrospinal fluid
CT	Computerised tomography
CTG	Cardiotocography
CVP	Central venous pressure
CXR	Chest X-ray
DIC	Disseminated intravascular coagulation
EBV	Epstein–Barr virus
ECG	Electrocardiogram
EEG	Electroencephalogram
FBC	Full blood count
FEV_1	Forced expiratory volume in one second
FFP	Fresh frozen plasma
FGR	Fetal growth restriction
GH	Growth hormone
HELLP	Haemolysis, Elevated Liver enzymes, and Low Platelets (syndrome)
HPL	Human placental lactogen
HUS	Haemolytic uraemic syndrome
HVS	High vaginal swab
IGT	Impaired glucose tolerance
ILD	Interstitial lung disease
kDa	Kilo Dalton
LFTs	Liver function tests
LMP	Last menstrual period
LSCS	Lower segment caesarean section

Glossary

MAP	Mean arterial (blood) pressure $= D + 1/3\ (S - D)$, where $D =$ diastolic blood pressure and $S =$ systolic blood pressure
$MgSO_4$	Magnesium sulphate
MRI	Magnetic resonance imaging
MSU	Mid-stream urine specimen
OGTT	Oral glucose tolerance test
PEFR	Peak expiratory flow rate
PNMR	Perinatal mortality rate
RDS	Respiratory distress syndrome
SLE	Systemic lupus erythematosus
SVD	Spontaneous vaginal delivery
SVR	Systemic vascular resistance
TFTs	Thyroid function tests
TSH	Thyroid-stimulating hormone
TTP	Thrombotic thrombocytopenic purpura
U+E	Urea and electrolytes
US	Ultrasound
UTI	Urinary tract infection
VSD	Ventricular septal defect
WBC	White blood cell
ZIG	Zoster immunoglobulin

To Sophie, Emma, Rebecca and Alice

CHAPTER 1

Hypertension and pre-eclampsia

Physiological changes

- Blood pressure is directly proportional to systemic vascular resistance and cardiac output.
- Vasodilation is probably the primary change in the circulation in pregnancy (see also cardiovascular adaptation to pregnancy, p. 19).
- Before the increase in cardiac output can adequately compensate for the fall in systemic vascular resistance, blood pressure begins to decrease in early pregnancy. It continues to decrease in the second trimester of normal pregnancy until the nadir in systolic and diastolic blood pressure is reached by approximately 22 to 24 weeks' gestation. From then on, there is a steady rise to pre-pregnant levels until term.
- Phase V (disappearance) rather than phase IV (muffling) of Korotkoff sounds should be taken as the diastolic reading. Phase V is more reproducible, correlates better with intra-arterial measurements of diastolic blood pressure, and is more closely related to outcome.
- Blood pressure taken supine during the late second and third trimesters will be lower due to decreased venous return to the heart because of pressure from the gravid uterus. Blood pressure should be taken with the woman sitting or lying on her side with a 30° tilt. The upper arm (when using a cuff) should be at the same level as the heart. The cuff should be of the correct size, as failure to use a large cuff with a large upper arm circumference will result in an overestimation of the blood pressure.
- Blood pressure usually falls immediately after delivery, although it tends to rise subsequently, reaching a peak three to six days postpartum.
- Previously normotensive women may become transiently hypertensive following delivery. This may relate to return of normal vascular tone and a period of vasomotor instability while normal, non-pregnant vasoregulation is re-established.

Scope of the problem

- Hypertension is the commonest medical problem encountered in pregnancy, complicating 10% to 15% of all pregnancies.
- Pre-eclampsia affects 3% to 5% of pregnancies; mild pre-eclampsia affects up to 10% of primiparous women; the incidence of severe pre-eclampsia is approximately 1%.
- Eclampsia complicates approximately 1 in 3000 (0.03%) pregnancies in the United Kingdom and Europe. In some developing countries, the incidence rate reaches 1%.
- Eclampsia occurs in approximately 1% of women with pre-eclampsia in developed countries.
- Hypertensive disorders of pregnancy are a leading cause of maternal mortality and morbidity in the United Kingdom; about five to six women die each year in the United Kingdom from pre-eclampsia or eclampsia, and severe pre-eclampsia is responsible for approximately 40% of severe obstetric morbidity.
- The death rate from eclampsia in the United Kingdom is now <1%. A third of women who die from pre-eclampsia have eclamptic seizures.
- Pre-eclampsia is the commonest cause of iatrogenic prematurity.
- Hypertension accounts for 12% to 25% of all antenatal admissions.
- Antenatal care, especially in the second half of pregnancy, is largely geared towards the detection of hypertension and pre-eclampsia.

Clinical features

Hypertension in pregnancy may be divided into pre-existing hypertension, pregnancy-induced hypertension and pre-eclampsia. There are several definitions of 'hypertension' and these are discussed on p. 9.

Pre-existing hypertension

- Some women may have been diagnosed as hypertensive prior to pregnancy.
- If hypertension is noted for the first time in the first trimester, it is likely that it is a chronic, pre-existing problem, because pregnancy-induced hypertension (including pre-eclampsia) usually, but not invariably, appears in the second half of pregnancy.
- Diagnosis of pre-existing hypertension may, on occasion, only be made retrospectively, that is, three to six months after delivery when the blood pressure has not returned to normal.
- Hypertension in any young person should not be attributed to essential (idiopathic) hypertension before secondary causes such as renal or cardiac disease, and rarely Cushing's syndrome, Conn's syndrome or phaeochromocytoma have been excluded.
- Women presenting with hypertension for the first time in early pregnancy should be examined for clues to a possible secondary cause. This should include
  - examination of the femoral pulses (looking for radiofemoral delay suggesting coarctation of the aorta),
  - listening for renal bruits (possible renal artery stenosis) and
  - urinalysis (looking for proteinuria or haematuria suggesting renal disease).
- Screening investigations for secondary causes of hypertension include
  - serum creatinine and urea (to exclude chronic kidney disease (CKD)),
  - electrolytes (to exclude hypokalaemia, which may suggest Conn's syndrome),

- serum calcium (to exclude hyperparathyroidism) and
- measurement of urinary catecholamines in cases suggestive of phaeochromocytoma (see Chapter 7).
- Women with pre-existing hypertension from whatever cause are at increased risk of superimposed pre-eclampsia, small for gestational age (SGA) infants and placental abruption. Consequently, the perinatal mortality and preterm delivery rates are increased in this population.
- If a woman is sufficiently hypertensive to require treatment before pregnancy, the risk of pre-eclampsia in pregnancy is approximately doubled. For those with severe hypertension (diastolic blood pressure >110 mmHg before 20 weeks' gestation), the risk of pre-eclampsia in one study was found to be more than 46%. These women are also at particular risk of early onset pre-eclampsia.

Pregnancy-induced hypertension

- Pregnancy-induced hypertension and pre-eclampsia usually appear in the second half of pregnancy and resolve within six weeks of delivery, although blood pressure may remain elevated up to three months postpartum.
- Pregnancy-induced hypertension may be defined as hypertension occurring in the second half of pregnancy but in the absence of proteinuria or any other features of pre-eclampsia (Table 1.1). The distinction between pregnancy-induced hypertension and pre-eclampsia may be difficult, especially as many of the definitions of pre-eclampsia are based solely on hypertension.
- Differentiation between pre-existing and pregnancy-induced hypertension is not important when considering whether, how and when to institute treatment, because the drugs suitable for the treatment of hypertension in pregnancy are the same for both conditions (Table 1.2).
- The distinction between pre-eclampsia and pregnancy-induced hypertension is however important since pre-eclampsia is associated with a worse pregnancy outcome and warrants admission to hospital.
- If hypertension develops after 20 weeks, the likelihood of progression to pre-eclampsia is approximately 15%. This risk is related to the gestation at presentation of pregnancy-induced hypertension. Thus, for hypertension presenting before 30 weeks, the risk is approximately 40%, but if it presents after 38 weeks, the risk is only 7%.
- Pregnancy-induced hypertension tends to recur in subsequent pregnancies. Some women remain hypertensive following a pregnancy complicated by pregnancy-induced hypertension.

Pre-eclampsia

- Pre-eclampsia is a pregnancy-specific multi-system disorder with unpredictable, variable and widespread manifestations.
- Women with pre-eclampsia are usually asymptomatic when the disease is first manifested.
- Diffuse vascular endothelial dysfunction may cause widespread circulatory disturbances, involving the renal, hepatic, cardiovascular, central nervous and coagulation systems.
- The 'classic' signs of pre-eclampsia are hypertension, proteinuria and oedema, but their absence does not exclude the diagnosis.

Table 1.1 – Clinical features of pre-eclampsia

Symptoms
Headache/flashing lights
Epigastric/right upper quadrant pain
Nausea/vomiting
Rapidly increasing/severe swelling of face, fingers or legs
Signs
Pregnancy-induced hypertension (see p. 3)
Proteinuria (new onset)
Rapidly progressive oedema
Epigastric/right upper quadrant tenderness
Convulsions, mental disorientation
Fetal growth restriction/intrauterine death
Placental abruption
Investigations (Interpret with reference to normal values in pregnancy, Appendix 2 and inside back cover)
24-hour urinary protein excretion >0.3 g
Protein creatinine ratio >30 mg/mmol
Raised serum uric acid level
Thrombocytopenia
Prolonged clotting times
Raised serum creatinine and urea levels
Increased haematocrit and haemoglobin levels
Anaemia if haemolysis; associated with raised LDH and bilirubin
Abnormal liver function tests, particularly raised transaminases
Reduced fetal growth, oligohydramnios
Abnormal uterine artery Doppler scan (bilateral notches and increased resistance index at 24 weeks predict pre-eclampsia)
Abnormal umbilical artery Doppler scan (shows fetal compromise)

Table 1.2 – Drugs used to treat hypertension in pregnancy

Drug	Indication	Starting dose	Maximum dose	Contraindications	Safe when breast-feeding?
Methyldopa	First-line therapy	250 mg b.d.	1 g t.d.s.	Depression	Yes*
Labetalol[a]	First-line therapy	100 mg b.d.	500 mg q.d.s.	Asthma	Yes
Nifedipine	Second-line therapy	10 mg slow-release b.d.	40 mg slow-release b.d.		Yes
Hydralazine	Second-line therapy	25 mg t.d.s.	75 mg q.d.s.		Yes
α-Blockers, e.g. doxazosin	Third-line therapy	1 mg o.d.	8 mg b.d.		No[b]
ACE inhibitors, e.g. enalapril	Not in pregnancy only postpartum	5 mg b.d.	20 mg b.d.		Yes

[a]May be used as first-line therapy in the second and third trimester.
[b]Doxazosin accumulates in breast milk; enalapril should be used instead.
* avoid postpartum.

Table 1.3 – Crises in pre-eclampsia

Eclampsia
HELLP syndrome (see Chapter 11, "Liver Disease," p. 206)
Pulmonary oedema
Placental abruption
Cerebral haemorrhage
Cortical blindness
Disseminated intravascular coagulation
Renal failure
Hepatic rupture

- Although hypertension and proteinuria are the most common manifestations of pre-eclampsia, they may be late or mild features, and the wider spectrum of the disorder should always be considered.
- Women may present with headache, visual disturbance, epigastric or right upper quadrant pain, nausea, vomiting or rapidly progressive oedema.
- The disorder is remarkably heterogeneous, with enormous variation in the severity, timing, progression and order of onset of different clinical features.
- Manifestations of pre-eclampsia (including eclampsia) may present antepartum, intrapartum or postpartum. Postpartum pre-eclampsia is more likely to be associated with symptoms.
- Effects on the kidney result in decreased glomerular filtration rate, proteinuria, a rise in serum creatinine and/or serum uric acid levels and oliguria.
- Hyperuricaemia also results from placental ischaemia, accelerating trophoblast turnover and the production of purines (substrate for xanthine oxidase).
- Other features of the syndrome include a reduced plasma volume, haemoconcentration, abnormal liver function and thrombocytopenia.
- HELLP syndrome (one severe variant of pre-eclampsia) includes **H**aemolysis, **E**levated **L**iver enzymes and **L**ow **P**latelets and may be associated with severe disseminated intravascular coagulation (see Chapter 11, p. 206).
- Several possible crises (Table 1.3) may develop.
- Hyponatraemia is usually due to fluid overload with an element of SIADH (syndrome of inappropriate antidiuretic hormone). If severe (Na < 130 mmol/L), it may cause cerebral oedema leading to confusion and convulsions. Treatment is with fluid restriction.
- The commonest causes of death in pre-eclampsia are cerebral haemorrhage, multiorgan failure and adult respiratory distress syndrome.
- The placental manifestations lead to fetal growth restriction (FGR), placental abruption and, in severe cases, intrauterine death.

Eclampsia

- Eclampsia may be defined as a tonic clonic (grand mal) seizure occurring in association with features of pre-eclampsia (although the diagnosis may be possible only in retrospect) (Table 1.1).
- Only one-third of women in the United Kingdom experiencing their first eclamptic seizure have established hypertension and proteinuria in the week before. One fifth have their first seizure prior to admission.
- Three-quarters of women with eclampsia in the United Kingdom have at least one premonitory symptom (commonly headache or visual disturbance) or sign before their first seizure.
- Convulsions may occur antepartum (45%), intrapartum (18–19%) or postpartum (36%).
- Teenagers are three times more likely than older women to suffer eclampsia.
- Although eclampsia, like pre-eclampsia, is more common in primiparous women, 18% of women with eclampsia in one U.K. study were multiparous without a history of pre-eclampsia.
- Eclampsia may be associated with ischaemic or haemorrhagic stroke with cerebral vasospasm and oedema.
- Cortical blindness (usually reversible) is a well described, although rare association of pre-eclampsia/eclampsia. Cerebral imaging with magnetic resonance imaging will usually reveal findings typical of posterior reversible encephalopathy syndrome (PRES). The typical clinical features of PRES syndrome are thought to be due to vasogenic oedema in the central nervous system leading to headache, seizure, confusion and frequent visual loss.

Pathogenesis

- This involves a genetic predisposition. The risk of pre-eclampsia is increased three-fold in women with a family history (sister or mother) of pre-eclampsia.
- Pre-eclampsia and otherwise idiopathic FGR are part of the same disease spectrum, and both relate to a problem of placentation (occurring in the first half of pregnancy) and consequent placental ischaemia. They differ with regard to the extent of the maternal response (developing in the second half of pregnancy). Pre-eclampsia can be thought of as a two-stage disorder. The first stage is abnormal perfusion of the placenta. The second is the maternal syndrome. Both placental and maternal factors can predispose to the development of pre-eclampsia.

    Stage 1—Abnormal Placentation
    - The spiral arteries in the placental bed do not undergo normal vascular remodelling, as trophoblast invasion is abnormal. The invading placenta is unable to optimise its blood supply from maternal uterine vessels. The spiral arteries fail to adapt to become high-capacitance, low-resistance vessels.
    - It is uteroplacental ischaemia, whether due to poor implantation in underlying microvascular disease or due to under-perfusion of a relatively large placenta (e.g. in a pregnancy complicated by diabetes, a multiple pregnancy or a hydropic fetus) that is the common feature in pre-eclamptic pregnancies.

Stage 2—Maternal Response
- Normal pregnancy is associated with a systemic inflammatory response, and this is exacerbated in pre-eclampsia. The maternal features of pre-eclampsia include metabolic disturbance including high levels of triglycerides and an exaggerated inflammatory response with higher levels of pro-inflammatory cytokines associated with endothelial dysfunction.
- Endothelial cell activation leads to increased capillary permeability, increased endothelial expression of cell adhesion molecules and prothrombotic factors, increased platelet activation and increased vascular tone. There is a decrease in prostacyclin synthesis and an increase in thromboxane A_2 (TXA_2) synthesis. It is thought that this reversal in prostanoid balance contributes to the platelet activation and vasoconstriction.
- These factors cause widespread microvascular damage and dysfunction that lead to the clinical manifestations of the maternal syndrome such as hypertension, proteinuria and hepatic disturbance.
- Women who already have a degree of metabolic derangement (e.g. because of obesity, dyslipidaemia or insulin resistance) causing chronic systemic inflammation are more susceptible to pre-eclampsia, thus explaining the risk factors described later.
- The precise mechanism by which the two stages of pre-eclampsia are linked and through which the ischaemic placenta leads to the widespread endothelial cell damage that characterises the maternal syndrome is not known. Theories include increased cytokine release or deportation of syncytiotrophoblast microparticles, which may trigger an exaggerated maternal response.
- Serum concentrations of the angiogenic placental growth factor (PlGF) are decreased in the early second trimester in pregnancies destined to develop pre-eclampsia, and serum concentrations of the antiangiogenic soluble fms-like tyrosine kinase (sFlt) are elevated approximately five weeks before the onset of pre-eclampsia. The sFlt/PlGF ratio may be of value in the prediction of pre-eclampsia. Near-patient testing for PlGF may develop into a diagnostic test for pre-eclampsia.

Risk factors

The risk factors include general, genetic, obstetric and medical factors.

General factors

- *Age.* Women older than 40 years have double the risk of pre-eclampsia, and this increased risk exists for primiparous and multiparous women.
- *Obesity.* Increased body mass index (BMI) pre-pregnancy or in early pregnancy increases the risk of pre-eclampsia, and obesity (BMI $\geq$ 30) is associated with an approximate doubling of the risk.

Genetic factors

- Women whose mothers had pre-eclampsia have a 20% to 25% risk of developing pre-eclampsia.
- In women with a sister with a history of pre-eclampsia, the risk may be as high as 35% to 40%.

Obstetric factors

- Primiparity (two- to three-fold risk)
- Multiple pregnancy (two-fold risk for twins)
- Previous pre-eclampsia (seven-fold risk)
- Long birth interval (two- to three-fold if 10 years)
- Hydrops with a large placenta
- Hydatidiform mole
- Triploidy [particularly association with very early onset (before 24 weeks' gestation) pre-eclampsia].

Although pre-eclampsia is more common in primiparous women, it is the multiparous women with pre-eclampsia who develop more severe disease and have higher morbidity and mortality rates.

Medical factors

- Pre-existing hypertension
- Chronic kidney disease (CKD) (even without renal impairment)
- Diabetes (pre-existing or gestational)
- Antiphospholipid antibodies (see Chapter 8)
- Connective tissue disease (see Chapter 8)

Diagnosis

- Because women with pre-eclampsia may be asymptomatic, much antenatal care is directed towards screening for this condition.
- In the first instance, this is done by measuring the blood pressure and checking the urine for protein.
- There is no diagnostic test for pre-eclampsia, but there are 'pointers' to the diagnosis (Table 1.1).
- There are several different definitions for hypertension in pregnancy, but most are based on a diastolic blood pressure >90 mmHg on two occasions or a diastolic blood pressure >110 mmHg on a single occasion.
- Because it is the rise in blood pressure that may be important, rather than the absolute value, some definitions include a rise in systolic blood pressure of 30 mmHg above the earliest recorded pregnancy reading or a diastolic increase of 15 to 25 mmHg.
- Proteinuric pre-eclampsia is defined as hypertension together with >0.3 g/24 hr proteinuria. 'Dipstick proteinuria', which is very inaccurate, or a protein creatinine ratio of >30 mg/mmol must always be confirmed with a 24-hour urinary collection.
- These definitions of pre-eclampsia are very simplistic because pre-eclampsia is a syndrome that may affect any system in the mother and indeed the fetus. In practice, the diagnosis is made when there is a constellation of recognised features (Table 1.1).
- It is the association of hypertension with these features that allows distinction of pre-eclampsia from pre-existing hypertension without superimposed pre-eclampsia and from pregnancy-induced hypertension.
- The diagnosis of pre-eclampsia is even more challenging in the presence of pre-existing hypertension and/or proteinuria. In these situations, the clinician is reliant on other clinical features as well as the degree of increase in blood pressure and proteinuria (see Chapter 10).

Management

Management of women with hypertension in pregnancy can be considered as

- screening for secondary causes of hypertension (if hypertension is present before 20 weeks gestation), see p. 2;
- screening for pre-eclampsia (regular blood tests, urinalysis; hypertension appearing >16 weeks' gestation);
- treatment of hypertension;
- fetal surveillance;
- decision regarding timing of delivery.

Mild cases, especially where there is no evidence of pre-eclampsia, may be managed as outpatients.

If there is new-onset hypertension and proteinuria, the woman should be admitted for assessment and will usually need to remain in hospital if pre-eclampsia is confirmed.

Monitoring for pre-eclampsia

- Regular checks of serum urea and creatinine, uric acid, haemoglobin, platelet count (and if thrombocytopenia is present and platelet count $<100 \times 10^9/L$, a coagulation screen) and liver function.
- Regular urinalysis, and if proteinuria ($\geq$1+) is detected, protein creatinine ratio or measurement of 24-hour protein excretion.
- Uterine artery Doppler blood flow examination at 20 to 24 weeks' gestation, looking particularly for the presence of a prediastolic 'notch'. A persistent high-resistance waveform is predictive of subsequent pre-eclampsia, FGR and placental abruption. The negative predictive value is high and such screening is useful in high-risk women, for example, those with antiphospholipid syndrome or previous severe pre-eclampsia.

Treatment of hypertension

- Hypertension should be treated in its own right regardless of the assumed underlying pathology (pre-eclampsia, pre-existing hypertension or pregnancy-induced hypertension). This is because above a mean arterial (blood) pressure (MAP) of 150, there is loss of cerebral autoregulation and the mother is at risk of cerebral haemorrhage. In one study of stroke in association with pre-eclampsia, 95% of cases had a systolic blood pressure >160 mmHg.
- $MAP = D + 1/3 (S - D)$, where D is the diastolic blood pressure and S the systolic blood pressure.
- The exact level of systolic or diastolic pressure at which to institute antihypertensive treatment is controversial depending on whether treatment is thought to be of benefit to fetal outcome; most clinicians will treat at levels >140 to 160 mmHg systolic and >90 to 110 mmHg diastolic blood pressure. Treatment is mandatory if the blood pressure is $\geq$160/110.
- The target blood pressure is disputed; overzealous control runs the risk of jeopardising the uteroplacental circulation, but MAP should be maintained at <125 mmHg, for example 150/100 mmHg.
- Treatment of pre-existing hypertension in pregnancy reduces the risk of severe hypertension (and therefore such severe complications as maternal cerebral haemorrhage), but there is no good evidence to suggest that good control of blood

pressure (although desirable) decreases the risk of superimposed proteinuric pre-eclampsia.

- In the late second trimester or early third trimester, treatment of severe hypertension associated with pre-eclampsia that would otherwise be an indication for delivery may allow prolongation of pregnancy (and therefore indirectly improve fetal outcome), but this does not actually modify the disease process.
- Later in pregnancy, treatment of hypertension may mask one of the important signs of pre-eclampsia. By treating the hypertension, clinicians are not treating but only palliating pre-eclampsia.
- Good control of blood pressure is important, but it should not preclude the definitive treatment of delivery if this is indicated for maternal (e.g. in HELLP syndrome or another crisis) or fetal (e.g. with severe growth restriction) reasons.

Fetal surveillance

- Women with either pre-existing hypertension or pre-eclampsia are at risk of FGR, and management should therefore include regular ultrasound examination of the fetus to assess growth, liquor volume and umbilical artery blood flow.
- Women developing pre-eclampsia who are likely to need delivery before 34 weeks' gestation should receive betamethasone in order to induce fetal lung maturation. However, there is accumulating evidence that repeated antenatal steroid injections might be harmful to fetal growth and lung and neurodevelopment, and these are no longer recommended.

Decision regarding timing of delivery

- The only cure for pre-eclampsia is delivery.
- This should not be attempted before adequate control of blood pressure, coagulopathy, eclamptic seizures and haemodynamic stability is achieved.
- In order to avoid neonatal deaths or long-term complications from prematurity, it is customary to try and prolong the pregnancy with 'expectant' management. This is often not possible for more than a few weeks, and in severe cases, only hours or days may be gained.
- On average most women with pre-eclampsia require delivery within two weeks from the time of diagnosis.
- Indications for delivery are shown in Table 1.4. These are not necessarily absolute and obviously depend on the gestational age and the speed of deterioration.

Drug treatment

See Table 1.2 for drugs used to treat hypertension in pregnancy.

First-line drugs

Methyldopa
Methyldopa is the drug of choice in pregnancy because it has been used for many years without any reports of serious adverse effects on the fetus or on children up to the age of seven years. Methyldopa does have side effects, including depression, sedation and postural hypotension. Patients become tolerant to the sedative effect and this is less of a problem beyond one week after starting or increasing therapy. Depression or other side effects such as liver function test abnormalities, which persist or are severe, and haemolytic anaemia necessitate a change to a second-line drug.

Table 1.4 – Indications for delivery

Inability to control blood pressure, for example maximal dose of three antihypertensive drugs
Rapidly worsening maternal biochemistry/haematology, for example falling platelet levels (<100 × 109/L), coagulopathy, deteriorating liver or renal function and falling albumin levels (<20 g/L)
Eclampsia or other crisis (see Table 1.3)
Maternal symptoms, for example severe headache, epigastric pain
Fetal distress/severe FGR/reversed umbilical artery diastolic flow

Labetalol

Some clinicians prefer labetalol, a combined α- and β-adrenergic blocker, to treat hypertension in pregnancy. However, because of the reservations outlined below concerning β-blockers, labetalol is often reserved for use in the second and third trimesters, in combination with other drugs, or in women who are intolerant of first- or second-line agents. Parenteral labetalol has an important role in the intrapartum management of acute severe hypertension (see later).

Second-line drugs

Second-line drugs used for the treatment of hypertension in pregnancy include calcium antagonists (e.g. slow-release nifedipine) and oral hydralazine. These should be used in conjunction with methyldopa in women who fail to respond to monotherapy, or be used to replace methyldopa in the minority of women who are unable to tolerate it. Side effects include headache, facial flushing and oedema and may necessitate withdrawal in some patients. α-Adrenergic blockers (e.g. doxazosin) are also safe and well tolerated and can be used as second- or third-line therapy.

Third-line drugs

β-Blockers

β-Blockers have fewer maternal side effects than does methyldopa, but their safety in the fetus is not so well established. There is concern that these drugs (and atenolol in particular) may inhibit fetal growth when used long term (and started in the first trimester) throughout pregnancy, but claims of neonatal hypotension and hypoglycaemia have not been substantiated in the randomised controlled trials performed. There is no evidence for the superiority of any one β-blocker over the others. β-Blockers should not be given to women with a history of asthma. Guidelines of the International Society for the Study of Hypertension in Pregnancy (ISSHP) do not recommend the use of oral β-blockers for treatment of mild hypertension in pregnancy.

Other antihypertensives

Diuretics

Diuretics to treat hypertension are normally avoided in pregnancy, as in pre-eclampsia they cause further depletion of a reduced intravascular volume. Their use should be reserved for the treatment of heart failure, pulmonary oedema and idiopathic intracranial hypertension (see Chapter 9, p. 168).

Angiotensin-converting enzyme inhibitors
The angiotensin-converting enzyme (ACE) inhibitors (e.g. ramipril, enalapril) should not be used in pregnancy, because they are teratogenic, increasing the risk of cardiovascular and neurological malformations, when used in the first trimester. Their use later in pregnancy may cause oligohydramnios, renal failure and hypotension in the fetus. Their use has been associated with decreased skull ossification, hypocalvaria and renal tubular dysgenesis, and there is also a risk of intrauterine death. Any woman on maintenance antihypertensive therapy with an ACE inhibitor should discontinue this prior to pregnancy (and if necessary switch to an alternative suitable for pregnancy such as amlodipine or methyldopa).

Angiotensin II receptor blockers
There are little data concerning these agents (e.g. losartan) in pregnancy, but they are similar to the ACE inhibitors and therefore should be avoided.

Treatment of acute severe hypertension/pre-eclampsia

- A protocol for the management of severe pre-eclampsia including criteria for transfer to intensive care unit should be available and agreed by obstetricians, anaesthetists, neonatologists and physicians.
- Women with severe pre-eclampsia should be managed in a high-dependency unit environment (on the delivery suite if undelivered).
- Control of hypertension is the single most important pharmacological manoeuvre.
- Automated oscillometric devices may underestimate blood pressure compared with mercury sphygmomanometers.
- Many pre-eclamptic women have a reduced intravascular volume and require pretreatment with fluid before parenteral hypotensive therapy is started.
- Volume expansion optimises cardiac pre-load and improves renal and uteroplacental blood flow. However, in the absence of blood loss, no patient should receive >500 mL of colloid without knowledge of the central venous pressure. Volume loading is usually omitted if the pre-eclampsia protocol is commenced after delivery.
- The choice of antihypertensive agent for acute control varies but is usually hydralazine (intermittent i.v. bolus, followed by infusion if required), labetalol (intermittent i.v. bolus, followed by continuous i.v. infusion) or nifedipine (orally). Sublingual nifedipine causes too rapid a fall in blood pressure and uteroplacental perfusion and therefore should not be used. All are effective but labetalol is associated with fewer side effects.
- Vasodilators (hydralazine and nifedipine) cause headache and tachycardia in many patients and are easier to use if the sympathetic nervous system is already inhibited with methyldopa.
- Nifedipine used in conjunction with magnesium sulphate may cause profound hypotension. In general, diuretic therapy should be avoided unless there is volume overload or pulmonary oedema.
- Continuous fetal heart rate monitoring is appropriate because fetal distress may be precipitated by antihypertensive therapy.
- Renal function and fluid balance must be monitored carefully. There is usually oliguria and poor tolerance to volume loading. Continuous oxygen saturation (Sao_2)

monitoring is vital, as aspiration of gastric contents and pulmonary oedema are potential risks.

■ Platelet count (and, if low, clotting studies) and liver function should also be monitored.

■ Management in the most critically ill patient must be based on haemodynamic monitoring with intra-arterial lines and occasionally central venous lines.

Management of eclampsia

■ The drug of choice for primary and secondary prophylaxis in eclampsia is magnesium sulphate. This probably acts as a cerebral vasodilator.

■ Eclampsia should be treated with i.v. magnesium sulphate followed by an infusion (for 24–48 hours after delivery or after the last seizure) to prevent further seizures.

■ Seizure prophylaxis may be given to women with pre-eclampsia (especially those who have continued signs of cerebral irritation, such as headache, agitation and clonus, or drowsiness despite good blood pressure control) as primary prophylaxis for eclampsia, but the case for routine prophylaxis in the developed world in all cases of severe pre-eclampsia is more controversial.

■ Magnesium sulphate is given as a loading dose of 4 g (diluted to 40 mL) over 5 to 10 minutes, followed by a maintenance infusion of 1 g/hr.

■ Recurrent seizures should be treated by a further bolus of 2 g.

■ Side effects of parenteral magnesium sulphate include neuromuscular blockade and loss of tendon reflexes, double vision and slurred speech, respiratory depression and cardiac arrest. Its use necessitates close monitoring of the respiratory rate, oxygen saturation and tendon reflexes.

■ If the woman is oliguric, has liver or renal impairment or has a further convulsion, serum magnesium levels should be monitored (therapeutic range 2–4 mmol/L).

Management of delivery

■ Women with pre-eclampsia are encouraged to have regional analgesia/anaesthesia in labour or for caesarean section.

■ This helps control of hypertension by reduction of pre- and after-load and by providing adequate analgesia. It also avoids the fluctuations in blood pressure associated with general anaesthesia and intubation.

■ In the presence of thrombocytopenia, regional blockade may not be deemed safe, and general anaesthesia becomes necessary for caesarean section. Most obstetric anaesthetists use a cut-off of 60 to 80×10^9/L for the platelet count.

■ Ergometrine should be avoided, as it may produce an acute rise in blood pressure.

Postpartum management

■ Although delivery removes the cause of pre-eclampsia, the manifestations, particularly hypertension, may take many weeks to resolve. There is often transient deterioration in the clinical state following delivery.

■ Therefore, women require intensive monitoring following delivery with attention to blood pressure control, fluid balance, haematology and biochemistry.

■ Diuresis usually occurs spontaneously but is often preceded by a period of oliguria.

■ Non-steroidal anti-inflammatory drugs should be avoided in women with pre-eclampsia because of the risk of renal impairment, especially in volume-depleted patients.

Oliguria

■ Oliguria is a normal feature of pre-eclampsia, especially following operative delivery or after induction of labour with oxytocin (Syntocinon).
■ The risk of pulmonary oedema from fluid overload continues postpartum, and it is safer to err on the side of volume depletion and mild renal impairment than to treat immediate postpartum oliguria with aggressive volume replacement. This is an example of the need for a different strategy from that used in other causes of oliguria presenting to intensive care units.
■ If an infusion of oxytocin is deemed necessary, this may be administered in a more concentrated form (e.g. through a syringe driver) to avoid excess fluid.
■ Diuretics are usually inappropriate in the management of postpartum oliguria, unless there are obvious signs of fluid overload or pulmonary oedema.
■ There is no demonstrable long-term benefit from the use of dopamine in this setting.
■ The proteinuria also resolves spontaneously unless there is underlying renal pathology, but may take several weeks or months to do so.

Hypertension

■ Postpartum hypertension is common and often not anticipated. The blood pressure rises after normal pregnancy, often not reaching a peak until three to six days postpartum. Consequently, although normotensive immediately following delivery, women with hypertension during pregnancy may become hypertensive again within the first week postpartum. This is often apparent prior to planned discharge and may prolong the stay in hospital until the hypertension is brought under control.
■ Methyldopa should be avoided postpartum because of its tendency to cause depression.
■ β-Blockers (e.g. atenolol 50–100 mg o.d.), with the addition of a calcium antagonist (e.g. slow-release nifedipine 10–20 mg b.d.) and/or an ACE inhibitor (e.g. enalapril 5–10 mg b.d.), if required, are appropriate for the treatment of postpartum hypertension.
■ In women who develop hypertension during pregnancy, it is usually possible to stop antihypertensive medication within six weeks postpartum.
■ All the drugs discussed earlier, including the ACE inhibitors, are safe to use in a woman who is breast-feeding.
■ However, diuretics are usually avoided in breast-feeding mothers because of the associated side effect of increased maternal thirst.
■ For women with pre-existing hypertension, it is usual to switch from methyldopa to the patient's previous antihypertensive regime after delivery.

Prophylaxis

Low-dose aspirin

■ The rationale for the use of low-dose aspirin is that it inhibits platelet cyclo-oxygenase and therefore TXA_2 synthesis.
■ Meta-analysis of all trials of antiplatelet therapy for the prophylaxis of pre-eclampsia shows a 15% reduction in the incidence of pre-eclampsia in women taking

antiplatelet therapy. However, 90 women need to be treated with low-dose aspirin to prevent one case of pre-eclampsia.

■ The results of individual large randomised trials such as the MRC Collaborative Low-dose Aspirin Study in Pregnancy (CLASP) trial suggest that aspirin may be effective in reducing the risk of early onset pre-eclampsia (i.e. that necessitating delivery before 32 weeks' gestation).

■ Importantly, there is good evidence for the safety of low-dose aspirin use in pregnancy. It would therefore seem reasonable to prescribe prophylactic aspirin (75 mg/day) for women with the following conditions that are associated with a significantly increased risk of pre-eclampsia:
  – Hypertension
  – Chronic kidney disease
  – Diabetes
  – Women at high risk of pre-eclampsia and in particular early onset pre-eclampsia (see section risk factors)
  – Women who have had recurrent, severe or early onset pre-eclampsia in previous pregnancies.

■ There is evidence that aspirin reduces the incidence of pre-eclampsia and other adverse pregnancy outcomes in women with acquired thrombophilia (antiphospholipid syndrome).

■ If aspirin is used, therapy should commence before 12 weeks' gestation and be continued throughout pregnancy.

Calcium

Meta-analysis of 12 randomised trials comparing at least 1 g of calcium daily during pregnancy with placebo showed a >50% reduction in the risk of pre-eclampsia. The effect was greatest for high-risk women where the reduction was 80% and for those with low baseline calcium intake.

Antioxidants

■ The rationale for the use of antioxidants is that they are free radical scavengers. Free radicals and oxidative stress contribute to the pathogenesis of pre-eclampsia (see earlier).

■ Randomised, placebo-controlled multi-centre trials of supplementation with vitamin C and vitamin E in high-risk (including history of pre-eclampsia or abnormal uterine artery Doppler scan) populations do not demonstrate a reduction in the incidence of pre-eclampsia.

Recurrence/pre-pregnancy counselling

■ Women who have pre-eclampsia in their first pregnancy have approximately 15% risk (or seven-fold increased risk compared to women who have not had previous pre-eclampsia) of developing pre-eclampsia in their second pregnancy.

■ This risk is increased if they have an underlying medical risk factor such as pre-existing hypertension, renal disease or antiphospholipid syndrome.

■ The recurrence risk is also higher in women who had early onset pre-eclampsia (see Table 1.5) or HELLP syndrome.

■ Pre-eclampsia increases the risk of subsequent hypertension (three- to four-fold), ischaemic heart disease (two-fold) and cerebrovascular disease.

Table 1.5 – Recurrence risk of pre-eclampsia

Delivery due to pre-eclampsia in preceding pregnancy	Recurrence risk (%)
20–28 wk	40
29–32 wk	30
33–36 wk	20
37+ wk	10

- These risks also are higher with early onset pre-eclampsia and FGR.
- Pre-eclampsia and cardiovascular disease (CVD) share many of the same risk factors and pathological changes including widespread endothelial damage and dysfunction and an increased systemic inflammatory response. Thus, these women may in the future be candidates for CVD risk screening and possible intervention.

Hypertensive disorders in pregnancy—points to remember

- Hypertension is the commonest medical problem in pregnancy.
- Pre-eclampsia remains a common direct cause of maternal death and a significant cause of maternal morbidity in the United Kingdom.
- Pre-eclampsia is a heterogeneous multi-system endothelial disorder that causes widespread effects, more than just hypertension and proteinuria.
- Methyldopa is the drug of choice for treatment of hypertension in pregnancy.
- Eclampsia may pre-date hypertension and proteinuria.
- Women with pre-eclampsia require close monitoring, with particular regard to symptoms, blood pressure, renal and liver function, platelet count and fetal well-being.
- Delivery is the only cure for pre-eclampsia and this may be indicated for fetal or maternal reasons.
- Women with hypertension in pregnancy often require treatment with postpartum antihypertensives, but methyldopa should be avoided because of the risk of depression.
- Oliguria is a normal feature in the immediate postpartum period and should not be treated with large volumes of i.v. fluids, except if there is objective evidence of volume depletion.
- Normal maintenance antihypertensive therapy for women with pre-existing hypertension can replace methyldopa therapy after delivery, and these drugs are safe to use when breast-feeding.
- Women who have had a pregnancy complicated by pre-eclampsia are significantly more likely to develop hypertension, ischaemic heart disease and cerebrovascular disease in later life.

Further reading

Bellamy L, Casas JP, Hingorani AD, et al. Pre-eclampsia and risk of cardiovascular disease and cancer in later life: systematic review and meta-analysis. BMJ 2007; 335:974.

Confidential Enquiries into Maternal and Child Health (CEMACH). Saving mothers' lives: reviewing maternal deaths to make motherhood safer 2003–2005. The Seventh Report on Confidential Enquiries into Maternal Deaths in the UK. London, UK: CEMACH; December 2007.

Critchley H, MacLean A, Poston L, et al., eds. Pre-eclampsia. London, UK: RCOG Press; 2003.

Duckitt K, Harrington D. Risk factors for pre-eclampsia at antenatal booking: systematic review of controlled studies. BMJ 2005; 330:565–567.

Duley L, Henderson-Smart DJ, Meher S, et al. Antiplatelet agents for preventing pre-eclampsia and its complications. Cochrane Database Syst Rev 2007; (2). Art. No.: CD004659. doi: 10.1002/14651858.CD004659.pub2.

Duley L. Meher S. Abalos E. Management of pre-eclampsia. BMJ 2006; 332:463–468.

Hofmeyr GJ, Atallah AN, Duley L. Calcium supplementation during pregnancy for preventing hypertensive disorders and related problems. Cochrane Database Syst Rev 2006; (3):CD001059.

Knight M; on behalf of UKOSS. Eclampsia in the United Kingdom 2005. BJOG 2007; 114:1072–1078.

Magee LA, Cham C, Waterman EJ, et al. Hydralazine for treatment of severe hypertension in pregnancy: meta-analysis. BMJ 2003; 327;955–960.

McCowan LME, Buist RG, North RA, et al. Perinatal morbidity in chronic hypertension. Br J Obstet Gynaecol 1996; 103;123–129.

RCOG. The management of severe pre-eclampsia/eclampsia. RCOG Green Top Guideline No. 10 (A), March 2006. http://www.rcog.org.uk/index.asp?PageID=1542. Accessed January 2010.

Redman CWG, Roberts JM. Management of pre-eclampsia. Lancet 1993; 341:1451–1454.

Sattar N, Greer I. Maternal response to pregnancy and future cardiovascular risk. BMJ 2002; 325:157–160.

Saudan P, Brown MA, Buddle ML, et al. Does gestational hypertension become pre-eclampsia. Br J Obstet Gynaecol 1998; 105:1177–1184.

The Magpie Trial Collaborating Group. Do women with pre-eclampsia, and their babies, benefit from magnesium sulphate? The Magpie trial: a randomized placebo-controlled trial. Lancet 2002; 359:1877–1890.

Waterstone M, Bewley S, Wolfe C. Incidence and predictors of severe obstetric morbidity: case-control study. BMJ 2001; 322:1089–1093.

CHAPTER 2

Heart disease

Cardiovascular adaptation to pregnancy

- The primary event is probably peripheral vasodilatation. This is mediated by endothelium-dependent factors, including nitric oxide synthesis upregulated by oestradiol and possibly vasodilatory prostaglandins.
- Peripheral vasodilation leads to a fall in systemic vascular resistance (SVR) (Table 2.1) and to compensate for this, the cardiac output increases by approximately 40% during pregnancy. This is achieved predominantly by an increase in stroke volume and by a lesser increase in heart rate.
- These changes begin early in pregnancy and by 8 weeks' gestation the cardiac output has already increased by 20%.
- The maximum cardiac output is found at about 20 to 28 weeks' gestation. There is a minimal fall at term. An increase in stroke volume is possible due to the early increase in ventricular wall muscle mass and end-diastolic volume (but not end-diastolic pressure) seen in pregnancy. The heart is physiologically dilated and myocardial contractility is increased.
- Although stroke volume declines towards the term, the increase in maternal heart rate [10–20 beats per minute (bpm)] is maintained, thus preserving the increased cardiac output.
- There is a profound effect of maternal position towards term upon the haemodynamic profile of both the mother and the fetus. In the supine position, pressure of the gravid uterus on the inferior vena cava (IVC) causes a reduction in venous return to the heart and a consequent fall in stroke volume and cardiac output. Turning from the lateral to the supine position may result in a 25% reduction in cardiac output. Pregnant women should therefore be nursed in the left or right lateral position wherever possible. If the woman has to be kept on her back, the pelvis should be rotated so that the uterus drops to the side and off the IVC and cardiac output and uteroplacental blood flow are optimised.

Table 2.1 – Cardiovascular adaptation to pregnancy

Physiological variable	Direction of change	Degree/timing of change
Cardiac output	↑	40%
Stroke volume	↑	
Heart rate	↑	10–20 bpm
Blood pressure	↓	First and second trimesters
	↑	Third trimester
Central venous pressure	→	
Pulmonary capillary wedge pressure (PCWP)	→	
Systemic vascular resistance (SVR) and pulmonary vascular resistance (PVR)	↓	25–30%
Serum colloid osmotic pressure	↓	10–15%

■ Reduced cardiac output is associated with a reduction in uterine blood flow and therefore in placental perfusion; this can compromise the fetus.
■ Although both blood volume and stroke volume increase during pregnancy, pulmonary capillary wedge pressure (PCWP) and central venous pressure do not increase significantly.
■ Pulmonary vascular resistance (PVR), like SVR, decreases significantly in normal pregnancy.
■ Although there is no increase in PCWP, serum colloid osmotic pressure is reduced. The colloid osmotic pressure/PCWP gradient is reduced by approximately 30%, making pregnant women particularly susceptible to pulmonary oedema.
■ Pulmonary oedema will be precipitated if there is an increase in cardiac pre-load (such as infusion of fluids) or pulmonary capillary permeability (such as in pre-eclampsia) or both.

Intrapartum and postpartum haemodynamic changes

■ Labour is associated with further increases in cardiac output (15% in the first stage and 50% in the second stage). Uterine contractions lead to auto-transfusion of 300 to 500 mL of blood back into the circulation, and the sympathetic response to pain and anxiety further elevate heart rate and blood pressure. Cardiac output is increased more during contractions and also between contractions.
■ Following delivery, there is an immediate rise in cardiac output due to the relief of IVC obstruction and contraction of the uterus that empties blood into the systemic circulation. Cardiac output increases by 60% to 80% followed by a rapid decline to

pre-labour values within approximately 1 hour of delivery. Transfer of fluid from the extravascular space increases venous return and stroke volume further.

- Those women with cardiovascular compromise are therefore most at risk of pulmonary oedema during the second stage of labour and the immediate postpartum period.
- Cardiac output has nearly returned to normal (pre-pregnancy values) two weeks after delivery, although some pathological changes (e.g., hypertension in pre-eclampsia) may take much longer (see Chapter 1).

Normal findings on examination of cardiovascular system in pregnancy

Normal findings on examination of cardiovascular system in pregnancy may include the following:

- Bounding/collapsing pulse
- Ejection systolic murmur (present in more than 90% of pregnant women; may be quite loud and audible all over the precordium)
- Loud first heart sound
- Third heart sound
- Relative sinus tachycardia
- Ectopic beats
- Peripheral oedema.

Normal findings on electrocardiogram (ECG) in pregnancy

These are partly related to changes in the position of the heart and may include the following:

- Atrial and ventricular ectopics
- Q-wave (small) and inverted T-wave in lead III
- ST segment depression and T-wave inversion inferior and lateral leads
- QRS axis leftward shift.

General considerations

Ideally, pre-pregnancy counselling of women with heart disease will allow detailed assessment of cardiac status and any potential risk to be explained before conception. But although most women with heart defects are aware of the diagnosis, many pregnancies are not planned, and increasingly, migrant women who may never have had a medical check-up present with previously undiagnosed heart disease in pregnancy.

The heart has relatively less reserve than the lungs (see p. 77). Whatever the underlying causes of cardiac insufficiency, the ability to tolerate pregnancy is related to the following:

- Presence of pulmonary hypertension
- Haemodynamic significance of any lesion
- Functional class (New York Heart Association) (Table 2.2)
- Presence of cyanosis (arterial oxygen saturation < 80%).

Table 2.2 – New York heart association functional classification

Class I	No breathlessness/uncompromised
Class II	Breathlessness on severe exertion/slightly compromised
Class III	Breathlessness on mild exertion/moderately compromised
Class IV	Breathlessness at rest/severely compromised

Other predictors of cardiac events in pregnant women with heart disease include the following:

- History of transient ischaemic attacks or arrhythmias
- History of heart failure
- Left heart obstruction [mitral valve area <2 cm^2, aortic valve area <1.5 cm^2, aortic valve gradient (mean non-pregnant) >30 mmHg]
- Myocardial dysfunction (left ventricular ejection fraction <40%)

Cyanosis alone may not be as important in predicting poor outcome as the association of cyanosis with pulmonary hypertension typically in Eisenmenger's syndrome, poor functional class, or both.

Poor pregnancy outcome is more likely if the woman has a poor functional status (NYHA class III or IV) regardless of the specific lesion. Conversely, those in functional classes I or II are likely to do well in pregnancy. Each case must be assessed individually, but those that require special consideration (even if asymptomatic) are women with the following conditions:

- Mitral stenosis (risk of pulmonary oedema)
- Marfan syndrome (risk of aortic dissection or rupture)
- Pulmonary hypertension

Detailed assessment by a cardiologist, obstetrician and obstetric anaesthetist with an agreed and documented plan for delivery is crucial. Any woman with any of the aforementioned features should be referred to a specialist unit for counselling and management during pregnancy.

Women advised against pregnancy should be given appropriate contraceptive advice, and guidelines are available.

Pulmonary hypertension

Women with pulmonary hypertension from whatever cause are at increased risk during pregnancy (see also later under "Eisenmenger's syndrome," p. 26). The maternal mortality rate was 40%, but more recent data suggest that this may have fallen to approximately 25%. Pulmonary hypertension in the pregnant woman may be due to the following:

- Lung disease, for example, cystic fibrosis
- Connective tissue disease, for example, scleroderma
- Primary (idiopathic) pulmonary arterial hypertension

- Pulmonary veno-occlusive disease
- Eisenmenger's syndrome (usually an atrial septal defect/ventricular septal defect with pulmonary hypertension and a reversed shunt, i.e., right to left).

Review of the literature between 1997 and 2007 showed maternal death rates of 17% in idiopathic pulmonary arterial hypertension, 28% in congenital heart disease–associated pulmonary hypertension and 33% in other forms.

Fixed PVR (in contrast to the normal fall in pregnancy) means that these women cannot increase pulmonary blood flow to match the increased cardiac output and they tolerate pregnancy poorly. Therefore, such women should be actively advised against pregnancy and adequate contraception recommended such as the subdermal progestogen-only implant (Implanon®). If they do become pregnant, termination should be offered. Termination itself is associated with maternal mortality in up to 7% but this is less than that associated with such a pregnancy allowed to progress.

- Pulmonary hypertension is defined as a non-pregnant elevation of mean (not systolic) pulmonary artery pressure ≥ 25 mmHg at rest or 30 mmHg on exercise in the absence of a left-to-right shunt.
- Pulmonary artery systolic (not mean) pressure is usually estimated by using Doppler ultrasound to measure the regurgitant jet velocity (Vm/s) across the tricuspid valve. The right ventricular systolic pressure (RVSP) can then be derived by using the equation RVSP $= 4V^2 + $JVP (jugular venous pressure). This should be considered a screening test. There is no agreed relation between the mean pulmonary pressure and the estimated systolic pulmonary pressure.
- If there is pulmonary hypertension in the presence of a left-to-right shunt, the diagnosis of pulmonary vascular disease is particularly difficult and further investigation including cardiac catheterisation to calculate PVR is likely to be necessary.
- Pulmonary hypertension as defined by Doppler studies may also occur in mitral stenosis and with large left-to-right shunts that have not reversed.
- Women with pulmonary hypertension who still have predominant left-to-right shunts are at lesser risk and may do well during pregnancy, but although such women may not have pulmonary vascular disease and a fixed PVR (or this may not have been established prior to pregnancy), they have the potential to develop it and require very careful monitoring with serial echocardiograms.

Congenital heart disease

The incidence of congenital heart disease in pregnancy is increasing as women with more severe defects, who underwent corrective surgery as children, are now able to have children themselves. The most common congenital heart diseases in pregnancy are patent ductus arteriosus (PDA), atrial septal defect (ASD) and ventricular septal defect (VSD). Together, these account for approximately 60% of cases.

Simple acyanotic defects and uncomplicated left-to-right shunts pose little problem, and women with defects of minimal haemodynamic significance do well in pregnancy. The more common defects will be considered individually.

Patent ductus arteriosus

- Most cases encountered in pregnancy nowadays have undergone surgical correction in childhood.

- Corrected cases pose no problems in pregnancy and do not require antibiotic prophylaxis.
- Uncorrected cases usually do well but are at risk of congestive cardiac failure.
- If the woman has pulmonary hypertension, she has Eisenmenger's syndrome (see later).

Atrial septal defect

- Commonest congenital heart defect in women
- Usually well tolerated in pregnancy
- May be associated with migraine
- Potential risk of paradoxical embolism, but risk is low
- Women may deteriorate and become hypotensive if there is an increase in the left-to-right shunt following blood loss at delivery. This causes a drop in left ventricular output and coronary blood flow.
- Supraventricular arrhythmias are uncommon before the age of 40 years but may rarely complicate pregnancy.

Ventricular septal defect

- Increased volume load of left ventricle
- Usually well tolerated in pregnancy unless the woman has Eisenmenger's syndrome (see later)

Congenital aortic stenosis

- Significant obstruction results if the aortic valve area is <1 cm^2 or if the mean gradient is severe (>50 mmHg in the non-pregnant state).
- The risks with moderate to severe disease are angina, hypertension, heart failure and sudden death.
- Indicators of risk include a failure to achieve a normal increase in blood pressure in response to exercise, impaired left ventricular function, or symptoms.
- In pregnancy, symptoms (e.g., angina, dyspnoea, pre-syncope, syncope) and hypertension may be controlled with β-blockers, provided left ventricular function is good. They will increase diastolic coronary flow and left ventricular filling.
- The development of resting tachycardia may indicate a failing left ventricle, unable to maintain the increased stroke volume of pregnancy.
- It is normal for the gradient across the valve, measured via echocardiography, to increase as the cardiac output increases in pregnancy. This increase does not mean the stenosis is increasing, and failure to increase or a decrease in the gradient is a cause for concern as it indicates the left ventricle is decompensating.
- Complications mainly arise in those with severe aortic stenosis because of a restricted capacity to increase cardiac output.
- Balloon valvotomy may allow temporary relief of severe stenosis and continuation of the pregnancy in severe cases.

Coarctation of the aorta

- This most commonly affects the descending aorta, distal to the origin of the left subclavian artery.

- It is frequently associated with a bicuspid aortic valve. If diagnosed, this is usually corrected prior to pregnancy, but residual coarctation is not uncommon.
- The risks with uncorrected coarctation are angina, hypertension and congestive heart failure. Many remain hypertensive even after surgical correction. There is also an association with aortic rupture and aortic dissection.
- It is important to document the form of surgical repair undertaken (stent, subclavian flap, excision with end-to-end anastomosis, patch repair) and also to perform a magnetic resonance imaging preferably prior to pregnancy to exclude any aneurysms or post-stenotic dilatation around the site of repair.
- The risk of aortic dissection may be minimised by strict control of the blood pressure and β-blockade to decrease cardiac contractility.

Marfan syndrome

Approximately 80% of patients with Marfan syndrome have cardiac involvement, most commonly the following:

- mitral valve prolapse
- mitral regurgitation
- aortic root dilatation

In pregnancy, this syndrome carries a risk of aortic dissection and aortic rupture. Predictors for dissection and rupture include the following:

- Pre-existing or progressive aortic root dilatation (10% risk if root >4 cm)
- Positive family history of dissection or aortic rupture

Management

- Pregnancy is contraindicated if the aortic root is >4–4.5 cm.
- Patients at high risk (and particularly if root >4.5 cm) should be offered aortic root replacement prior to pregnancy.
- β-Blockers have been shown to reduce the rate of aortic dilatation and the risk of complications in patients with Marfan syndrome. They should be continued or started in pregnant patients with aortic dilatation or hypertension.
- Regular echocardiograms should be performed to assess aortic root diameter.
- Elective caesarean section is usually recommended for women with aortic roots showing progressive enlargement or >4.5 cm.

Marfan syndrome is an autosomal dominant disorder caused by a defect in the fibrillin 1 gene. Those with cardiac lesions tend to have offspring with cardiac abnormalities. The other features of Marfan syndrome include:

- Increased height
- Arm span greater than the height
- Arachnodactyly
- Joint laxity
- Depressed sternum
- Scoliosis
- High-arched palate
- Dislocation of the lens

Cyanotic congenital heart disease

Main causes encountered in adults are as follows:

- Pulmonary atresia
- Tetralogy of Fallot

Cyanosis carries significant risks for mother and fetus. Problems include the following:

- Worsening cyanosis because of increased right-to-left shunting secondary to falling peripheral vascular resistance
- Thromboembolic risk increased because of polycythaemia (secondary to hypoxaemia)
- Increased risk of fetal loss (especially if oxygen saturation <80–85%) and increased risk of fetal growth restriction. Their chance of a livebirth is <20%.
- Associated pulmonary hypertension

Pregnancy outcome is improved if:

- Resting oxygen saturation is >85%
- Haemoglobin level is <18 g/dl
- Haematocrit level is <55%

Tetralogy of Fallot

Tetralogy of Fallot is one of the commonest conditions encountered in adult congenital heart disease clinics. Most women encountered in pregnancy will have undergone surgical correction. If unoperated, those without pulmonary vascular disease may negotiate pregnancy successfully. There are two main concerns:

- Paradoxical embolism through the right-to-left shunt causing cerebrovascular accidents
- Effects of cyanosis and maternal hypoxaemia on the fetus
  - Oxygen saturation falls markedly on exercise
  - Fetal growth restriction
  - Increased risk of miscarriage
  - Increased risk of spontaneous and iatrogenic prematurity

These risks can be minimised by use of the following:

- Thromboprophylaxis
- Elective admission for bed rest and oxygen therapy to maximize oxygen saturation

Women with repaired Fallot usually tolerate pregnancy well; the main issue is right ventricular dysfunction that can deteriorate in view of the pulmonary regurgitation resulting from earlier surgery.

Eisenmenger's syndrome

If women with Eisenmenger's syndrome (25–40% maternal mortality) decline termination of pregnancy, they require the following treatment antenatally:

- Thromboprophylaxis
- Elective admission for bed rest and oxygen therapy

Most women with Eisenmenger's syndrome who die as a result of pregnancy, do so soon after delivery. There is no evidence that caesarean versus vaginal delivery or regional versus general analgesia/anaesthesia reduces this risk. The dangers relate to increasing the right-to-left shunt and escalating pulmonary hypertension, often despite intensive and appropriate care. Principles of management include the following:

- Multidisciplinary discussion and planning of elective delivery
- Management in an intensive care environment with intensivists, anaesthetists, cardiologists and obstetricians with expertise in the care of those with complicated heart disease
- Using supplemental oxygen to reduce PVR
- Avoiding hypovolaemia; maintaining pre-load
- Avoiding acidosis
- Avoiding thromboembolism; using thromboprophylaxis
- Avoiding pulmonary artery catheters (which carry a risk of potentially devastating in situ thrombosis); monitoring oxygen saturation, central venous pressure, blood pressure
- Avoiding systemic vasodilation (therefore using caution with regional anaesthesia and Syntocinon)
- Many women with pulmonary hypertension will be treated with bosentan (an endothelin antagonist) and/or sildenafil
- In addition, selective pulmonary vasodilators, for example, inhaled nitric oxide, i.v. prostacyclin, may be used.

Postoperative congenital heart disease

Detailed consideration of women with complicated congenital heart disease, who may have undergone palliative surgery, is beyond the scope of this handbook, but the following are important considerations:

- The risk of ventricular failure (particularly when the right ventricle is acting as the systemic pumping chamber)
- Any residual pulmonary hypertension

Most cases of simple defects corrected in infancy pose no problem in pregnancy.

Fontan circulation
Fontan circulation results after surgery for tricuspid atresia or transposition with pulmonary stenosis.

- The right ventricle is bypassed and the left ventricle provides the pump for both the systemic and pulmonary circulations
- Increases in venous pressure may cause hepatic congestion and oedema, but sufficient volume loading is required to ensure adequate perfusion of the pulmonary circulation
- Women are often anticoagulated outside pregnancy and treatment or high prophylactic doses of low-molecular-weight heparin (LMWH) are recommended during pregnancy.

Genetic counselling

- The risk of the fetus having a congenital heart defect is higher if the mother rather than the father has congenital heart disease. Overall, the risk is approximately 2% to 5% (i.e., well over double the risk in the general population).
- The level of risk depends on the specific lesion and is higher for left-sided outflow tract lesions. If the fetus is affected, it tends to have the same lesion.
- In women with an atrial septal defect (ASD), the risk of an ASD in the fetus is approximately 5% to 10%; for aortic stenosis, the risk is highest (18–20%).
- Both Marfan and hypertrophic cardiomyopathy (HCM) (see later) have autosomal dominant inheritance.
- Women with congenital heart disease should be referred for a detailed fetal cardiac ultrasound.

If the congenital heart defect in the parent was thought to be due to acquired abnormalities in pregnancy, for example, to congenital rubella infection, the risk to any offspring is probably not increased.

Acquired heart disease

- Worldwide, the acquired heart disease most likely to affect women wishing to have children is rheumatic heart disease. This is caused by rheumatic fever, which damages one or more of the heart valves. It is usually contracted in childhood and is now very rare in women born in the United Kingdom. It is, however, not uncommon in migrant women where it may have been diagnosed and sometimes treated/palliated prior to pregnancy.
- Rheumatic heart disease may present for the first time in pregnancy, especially in migrant women who have never been examined previously by a doctor.
- Mitral stenosis accounts for 90% of rheumatic heart disease in pregnancy.

Mitral stenosis

Particularly if undiagnosed, this may be dangerous in pregnancy. Women may have been previously treated with valvotomy or valvuloplasty, but stenosis can recur. Just because a woman is asymptomatic does not mean that she will tolerate pregnancy and delivery without complications.

Symptoms

- May be asymptomatic
- Dyspnoea, orthopnoea, paroxysmal nocturnal dyspnoea
- Cough (productive pink, frothy sputum, or haemoptysis)

Signs

- Mitral facies
- Tapping, undisplaced apex beat
- Usually in sinus rhythm, but risk of atrial flutter and fibrillation
- Loud first heart sound (S_1), loud pulmonary second sound (P_2), opening snap

- Low-pitched, mid-diastolic rumble
- Signs of pulmonary oedema—this may present with wheeze, and confusion with asthma will lead to the wrong and dangerous treatment (i.e., bronchodilators)

Effect of pregnancy on mitral stenosis

- Even if a woman is asymptomatic at the beginning of pregnancy, she can deteriorate rapidly and develop pulmonary oedema.
- This is usually precipitated by tachycardia.
- This may be as a result of intercurrent infection, exercise, pain and anxiety or may be secondary to a failure to adequately increase stroke volume.
- Tachycardia is particularly dangerous in mitral stenosis since diastolic filling of the left ventricle (which is impaired in mitral stenosis) is further decreased and there is a consequent fall in stroke volume and a rise in left atrial pressure precipitating pulmonary oedema.
- Most women who develop complications do so in the late second or third trimester or peripartum period.
- Poor prognostic features for development of pulmonary oedema include the following:
  - Severe mitral stenosis as assessed by valve area <1 cm^2
  - Presence of moderate to severe symptoms prior to pregnancy

Management

- Confirm diagnosis and assess severity with echocardiogram.
- Avoid injudicious intravenous fluid therapy.
- Avoid the supine and lithotomy positions.
- Pulmonary oedema should be treated with oxygen, diamorphine and diuretics.
- β-Blockers should be used to slow the heart rate and allow time for left atrial emptying.
- Atrial fibrillation should be treated aggressively with digoxin and β-blockers.
- In expert hands, balloon valvotomy and closed mitral valvotomy have very good results in pregnancy but are suitable only for non-calcified valves with minimal regurgitation.
- Surgical valvotomy carries higher risks, with fetal mortality rates of 5% to 15% for closed valvotomy and 15% to 33% for open valvotomy.
- If women with severe mitral stenosis attend prior to pregnancy, they should be offered surgery (open/closed/balloon mitral valvotomy or valve replacement) before embarking upon pregnancy.

Regurgitant valve disease

- Systemic vasodilation and a fall in peripheral vascular resistance reduce afterload and therefore act to reduce regurgitation.
- Both mitral and aortic regurgitation are well tolerated in pregnancy, provided there is no significant left ventricular dysfunction.
- Women with heart failure can be safely treated with diuretics, digoxin and hydralazine and/or nitrates as vasodilators to "off load" the left ventricle.

Cardiomyopathies

Hypertrophic cardiomyopathy

Approximately 70% of cases are familial with autosomal dominant inheritance. There is a broad spectrum of disease, and although previously regarded as a rare disease associated with a high risk of sudden death, it is now known to be more common and often benign. Some women may be asymptomatic, the diagnosis having been made because of screening following a diagnosis of HCM in a first-degree relative or echocardiography to investigate a heart murmur detected in pregnancy.

Clinical features

- Chest pain or syncope, caused by left ventricular outflow tract obstruction
- Double apical pulsation (palpable fourth heart sound)
- Ejection systolic murmur (left ventricular outflow obstruction)
- Pansystolic murmur (mitral regurgitation)
- Arrhythmias
- Heart failure

Effect of pregnancy on HCM

- Mostly well tolerated in pregnancy because of an increase in left ventricular cavity size and the stroke volume is usually able to increase.
- β-Blocker administration should be continued or started in pregnancy for women with symptoms.
- Care is required with regional anaesthesia/analgesia to avoid hypotension with consequent increased left ventricular outflow tract obstruction.
- Any hypovolaemia will have the same effect and should be rapidly and adequately corrected.

Peripartum cardiomyopathy

This rare condition is specific to pregnancy. It is defined as the development of heart failure in the absence of a known cause and without any heart disease prior to the last month of pregnancy. Onset is usually in the first month after delivery but may occur in the last month of pregnancy and up to 5 months postpartum.

Risk factors include the following:

- Multiple pregnancy
- Pregnancy complicated by hypertension
- Multiparity
- Advanced maternal age
- Afro-Caribbean race

Symptoms

- Dyspnoea
- Reduced exercise tolerance
- Palpitations
- Pulmonary and/or peripheral oedema
- Symptoms relating to peripheral or cerebral emboli

Signs

- Tachycardia, tachypnoea
- Pulmonary oedema
- Congestive cardiac failure
- Dysrhythmias
- Signs of pulmonary, cerebral and systemic embolisation
- Without thromboprophylaxis, systemic embolism occurs in 25% to 40% of those affected by peripartum cardiomyopathy, and ischaemic stroke in approximately 5%.

Aetiology

Aetiology is unknown, but in some series, a proportion of cases have histological evidence of myocarditis on endomyocardial biopsy. Other theories include an autoimmune response, microchimerism and increased myocyte apoptosis.

Diagnosis

- This requires echocardiography. The diagnostic criteria are as follows:
    - Left ventricular ejection fraction <45%
    - Fractional shortening <30%
    - Left ventricular end-diastolic pressure >2.7 cm/m^2
- Often, echocardiography shows that the heart is enlarged with global dilation of all four chambers and markedly reduced left ventricular function.

Management

- Elective delivery if antenatal
- Thromboprophylaxis—anticoagulants are mandatory if there is severely impaired left ventricular dysfunction, intracardiac thrombus, or arrhythmias.
- Conventional treatment for heart failure, including diuretics, vasodilators (hydralazine and/or nitrates), cardioselective β-blockers (bisoprolol) or β-blockers with arteriolar vasodilating action (carvedilol), digoxin, inotropes and, after delivery, angiotensin-converting enzyme inhibitors.
- Immunosuppressive therapy may be considered in cases with myocarditis documented by endomyocardial biopsy that fail to improve within 2 weeks of initiation of standard heart failure therapy.
- Intra-aortic balloon pumps and left ventricular assist devices may provide temporary support. Cardiac transplantation may be the only option in severe cases unresponsive to conventional and full supportive management.

Prognosis and recurrence

- Maternal mortality rate has decreased from 40% in older studies to 9% to 15% in more recent series. One study documented a 95% five-year survival. Many case fatalities occur close to presentation and cardiomyopathy causes approximately 25% of cardiac maternal deaths in the United Kingdom.
- Approximately 50% of patients make a spontaneous and full recovery.
- Prognosis depends on normalisation of left ventricular size and function within six months after delivery. Mortality is increased in those with persistent left ventricular dysfunction.

- Women should be counselled against further pregnancy if left ventricular size or function does not return to normal, since there is a significant risk of recurrence, worsening heart failure (50%) and death (25%) in subsequent pregnancies.
- Adequate contraception should be advised, such as the intrauterine progestogen-only system (Mirena®) or the subdermal progestogen-only implant (Implanon®).
- For those whose cardiomyopathy resolves, the recurrence risk is not known but appears to be lower (0–25%). However, the contractile reserve may be impaired, even if the left ventricle size and function are normal. Therefore, a stress echocardiogram using dobutamine or exercise may be appropriate pre-pregnancy.
- Subsequent pregnancies are of high risk and require collaborative care.

Artificial heart valves

If valve replacement is necessary in women of childbearing age, there are the following two main considerations:

- Mechanical heart valves require life-long anticoagulation.
- Grafted-tissue heart valves (bioprosthetic) (from pigs or humans) have the advantage that anticoagulation is not usually required, but bioprosthesis deterioration accelerates during pregnancy.

Management

- Because of the risk of valve thrombosis, women with metal prosthetic heart valves must continue full anticoagulation throughout pregnancy.
- The interests of the mother and fetus are in conflict. Continuation of warfarin affords the mother the lowest risk of thrombosis, whereas for the fetus, warfarin is associated with an increased risk of teratogenesis, miscarriage, stillbirth and intracerebral bleeding (see Chapter 3, p. 48).
- High-dose s.c. LMWH is safe for the fetus but is associated with a higher risk of thrombosis for the pregnant woman.
- The choice of anticoagulation regimen will depend on the following:
  - Position of the prosthesis (valves in the mitral position are more likely to thrombose than those in the aortic position)
  - Type of valve replacement (old-fashioned ball and cage valves, e.g., Starr–Edwards, or single-tilting disc, e.g., Bjork–Shiley, are more thrombogenic than the newer bi-leaflet valves, e.g., St Jude, carbomedics)
  - The number of mechanical valves—two valves give a higher risk of thrombosis.
  - History of embolic events or atrial fibrillation
  - The dose of warfarin required to maintain a therapeutic international normalised ratio (INR). The risks of embryopathy and fetal loss are increased in women requiring more than 5 mg.
  - Patient choice—some women are unhappy to accept any additional risk to the fetus.
- All women should be counselled thoroughly prior to pregnancy regarding potential risks to herself and her fetus. Even with the above-mentioned guidelines, advice regarding anticoagulation should be tailored to the individual woman with regard to both her medical and obstetric history.

- There are three broad anticoagulant regimens:
  - Warfarin throughout pregnancy (close monitoring; INR 2.5–3.5)
  - Therapeutic dose adjusted s.c. LMWH between 6 and 12 weeks' gestation followed by warfarin
  - Therapeutic dose adjusted s.c. LMWH throughout pregnancy
- When LMWH is used, doses should be adjusted according to anti–factor Xa levels, maintaining 4 hour peak anti–factor Xa level at 0.8–1.2 U/mL. Low-dose aspirin (75 mg/day) should be added as adjunctive antithrombotic therapy.
- All women should discontinue warfarin for 10 to 14 days prior to delivery to allow clearance of warfarin by the fetus. While awaiting delivery, full anticoagulant doses of s.c. LMWH or i.v. unfractionated heparin should be used. Heparin and LMWH do not cross the placenta.
- LMWH should be discontinued for labour and delivery. However, caution is needed if >24–48 hours elapse with no anticoagulation, and one option is to site regional analgesia after 24 hours and then give a further prophylactic dose (e.g., 40 mg enoxaparin) if delivery is not imminent. If i.v. heparin is used, the dose can be reduced to prophylactic levels (approximately 1000 U/hr).
- Full anticoagulant doses of heparin should be resumed after delivery.
- Warfarin may be restarted 3 to 7 days following delivery, but this should be delayed if the risk of bleeding is deemed to be increased.
- In the event of an urgent need to deliver a fully anticoagulated patient, warfarin may be reversed with fresh frozen plasma and vitamin K and heparin and LMWH with protamine sulphate.

Antibiotic prophylaxis

- The current U.K. recommendations from the National Institute for Clinical Excellence (2008) are that antibiotic prophylaxis against infective endocarditis (IE) is not required for childbirth.
- The British Society for Antimicrobial Chemotherapy (2006) and the American Heart Association have recommended cover only for patients deemed to be at high risk of developing IE (such as women with previous IE) and for those who have the poorest outcome if they develop IE (such as those with cyanotic congenital heart disease).
- If antibiotic prophylaxis is used, it should be with amoxicillin 2 g i.v. plus gentamicin 1.5 mg/kg i.v. at the onset of labour or ruptured membranes or prior to caesarean section, followed by amoxicillin 500 mg orally.
- For women who are penicillin-allergic, vancomycin 1 g i.v. over 1 to 2 hours can be used instead of amoxicillin.

Myocardial infarction/acute coronary syndromes

- Acute coronary syndromes (ACSs) are rare in women of childbearing age, but as women delay childbirth until their late 30s and 40s, coronary artery disease and myocardial infarction (MI) are becoming more frequent in pregnancy.
- Maternal deaths from MI are increasing. In the United States, there was a threefold increase in the incidence of MI during pregnancy from 1990 to 2000. There was a fourfold increase in maternal deaths reported in the United Kingdom from 2000–2002 to 2003–2005. The maternal death rate from acute MI is 5% to 7%.

Pathogenesis

Atherosclerosis is the predominant pathogenesis outside pregnancy, and increasingly, this holds true in pregnancy. However, in pregnancy, coronary artery dissection and embolus in the absence of atheroma are more frequent and must be remembered as causes of ACS. Causes include:

- Atheroma in ischaemic heart disease
- Coronary thrombosis without atheroma
- Coronary artery dissection
- Coronary artery aneurysm, spasm, or embolism
- Congenital coronary anomalies
- Cocaine abuse

Risk factors for ischaemic heart disease include the following:

- Smoking (most women who die from ischaemic heart disease in pregnancy are smokers)
- Diabetes
- Obesity
- Family history of ischaemic heart disease
- Hypertension
- Hypercholesterolaemia
- Multigravidas older than 35 years

- Acute MI/ACS occurs most commonly in the third trimester, peripartum and post-partum.
- The anterior wall of the left ventricle and the territory of the left anterior descending coronary artery are the commonest sites involved.
- There is often not a preceding history of angina, or symptoms may be atypical with epigastric pain or nausea, and the presentation may be acute.
- Artery dissection has a particular association with the peripartum period. This includes coronary artery dissection.

Diagnosis

Diagnosis outside pregnancy relies on a combination of history, ECG changes and cardiac enzymes. Troponin I (Tn I) and T are not altered in normal pregnancy but Tn I is increased in pre-eclampsia, pulmonary embolism, atrial fibrillation and myocarditis. Coronary angiography should not be withheld in pregnant patients.

Management

- Management for ACS is as for the non-pregnant woman, with heparin, β-blockers and nitrates.
- Low-dose aspirin (75–150 mg/day) is safe for use in pregnancy and should be continued or commenced in pregnancy for primary and secondary prophylaxis. In the acute management of ACS, 150 to 300 mg can be given.
- Thrombolytic (intravenous and intracoronary) therapy has been used successfully. It should not be withheld, but there is a significant risk of bleeding.

- Coronary angiography is usually appropriate to determine the underlying cause of the ACS and percutaneous transluminal angioplasty and stenting may be used if appropriate.
- Percutaneous coronary intervention, if available, is preferable to thrombolysis as the former is associated with less bleeding risk and also allows management of spontaneous dissections (and atheromatous stenoses) with stent deployment. Angioplasty is associated with an increased risk of coronary dissection in a vulnerable vessel.
- Both aspirin and clopidogrel are recommended acutely after the use of (bare metal and drug-eluting) stents. There is increasing experience with the use of clopidogrel in pregnancy, which seems to be safe, but it should be discontinued for delivery as there is an increased bleeding risk. For this reason bare metal stents are used in preference to drug-eluting stents (which require dual antiplatelet for longer) in pregnancy.
- Statins should be discontinued prior to pregnancy since high doses have caused skeletal malformations in rats, and in human pregnancy, there is an increased risk of central nervous system and limb defects. Discontinuation for the relatively short duration of pregnancy is unlikely to impact on long-term therapy for hyperlipidaemia.
- For those with previous MI, poor prognostic features for future pregnancy include residual left ventricular dysfunction and the presence of continuing ischaemia.

Dissection of thoracic aorta

Pregnancy increases the risk of aortic dissection, which is a common cause of death in pregnancy. Even if the diagnosis is made, the mortality rate associated with this condition is high.

Clinical features

- Aortic dissection should be considered in any pregnant woman presenting with acute severe chest pain, particularly with interscapular radiation, with jaw pain and in the presence of systolic hypertension and/or differential blood pressures in each arm.
- There may be symptoms or signs from territory supplied by the coronary, carotid, subclavian, spinal, or common iliac arteries or aortic regurgitation. Most cases in pregnancy are type A dissections involving the ascending aorta.
- Many cases are often misdiagnosed initially as pulmonary emboli.

Pathogenesis

Pregnancy predisposes to aortic dissection, possibly due to haemodynamic shear stress. Other risk factors include the following:

- Marfan syndrome
- Turner's syndrome
- Ehlers–Danlos syndrome type IV (vascular) see page 147.
- Coarctation of the aorta
- Bicuspid aortic valve

Diagnosis

- Chest radiograph is mandatory and may show mediastinal widening, but a normal chest radiograph does not exclude the diagnosis.
- Diagnosis may be confirmed with transthoracic or transoesophageal echocardiography, computed tomography, or magnetic resonance imaging.

Management

The management of type A dissection is surgical. This usually means the following:

- Careful and rapid control of blood pressure
- Expeditious delivery by caesarean section
- Cardiac surgery to replace the aortic root

Arrhythmias

- Although sinus tachycardia may be a feature of normal pregnancy, it requires investigation to exclude hyperthyroidism, respiratory or cardiac pathology and hypovolaemia or sepsis (see Section B, Table 2).
- Palpitations and dizziness are common symptoms in pregnancy.
- Investigation should include ECG. This will exclude pre-excitation from accessory pathways such as in Wolff–Parkinson–White syndrome. (Look for short PR interval or delta wave.)
- 24-Hour Holter monitoring should be performed if the history suggests frequent and troublesome arrhythmias.
- Atrial and ventricular premature beats are common in pregnancy but have no adverse effects on the mother or the fetus and require no further investigation.
- Atrial flutter and fibrillation are rare but may be encountered, particularly in the presence of mitral valve disease, congenital heart disease, or sepsis.
- Paroxysmal supraventricular tachycardia (SVT) is the commonest arrhythmia encountered in pregnancy. It usually pre-dates the pregnancy but may become more symptomatic or more frequent in pregnancy.
- If an arrhythmia is diagnosed, thyroid status must be tested and an echocardiogram performed to exclude structural heart disease.

Antiarrhythmic drugs in pregnancy

- Treatment is required only for life-threatening arrhythmias, atrial fibrillation/ flutter, or SVTs that are frequent, persistent, or symptomatic.
- Digoxin may be used for rate control in atrial fibrillation.
- It is best to use a drug used frequently in pregnancy, such as verapamil, or β-blockers (e.g., propranolol, metoprolol, sotalol or atenolol).
- Adenosine is safe to use to reveal underlying atrial flutter or terminate SVTs. If this fails, i.v. verapamil or flecainide infusions, or direct-current (DC) cardioversion may be used.
- Amiodarone should be avoided if possible.
- Flecainide is the drug of choice for tachyarrhythmias in the fetus. There is evidence for its safety when used for maternal arrhythmias in the second and third trimesters. Less information is available for first trimester use, but this may be justified if β-blockers or verapamil do not control arrhythmias.

Heart disease in pregnancy—points to remember

- It is common in pregnancy and is mostly benign.
- Pulmonary hypertension and fixed PVR are dangerous and often fatal in pregnancy.
- Other contraindications to pregnancy include a dilated aortic root >4.5 cm, severe left heart obstruction from critical mitral or aortic stenosis, and severe impairment of left ventricular function.
- Any strategy for anticoagulation for a pregnant woman with a mechanical heart valve is associated with risks to the mother and/or fetus. Careful pre-pregnancy counselling is vital.
- Peripartum cardiomyopathy should be treated with conventional heart failure therapy (including thromboprophylaxis), with the exception that angiotensin-converting enzyme inhibitors are withheld until after delivery.
- Women with significant heart disease need multidisciplinary care in a specialist centre by obstetricians, cardiologists and anaesthetists with expertise in the care of heart disease in pregnancy. Agreed management plans should be carefully documented.
- If pregnancy is contraindicated then appropriate contraceptive advice is paramount.

Further reading

Bédard E, Dimopoulos K, Gatzoulis MA. Has there been any progress made on pregnancy outcomes among women with pulmonary arterial hypertension? Eur Heart J 2009; 30:256–265.

Immer FF, Bansi AG, Immer-Bansi AS, et al. Aortic dissection in pregnancy: analysis of risk factors and outcome. Ann Thorac Surg 2003; 76:309–314.

Ladner HE, Danielsen B, Gilbert WM. Acute myocardial infarction in pregnancy and the puerperium: a population-based study. Obstet Gynecol 2005; 105:480–484.

McLintock C, McCowan LM, North RA. Maternal complications and pregnancy outcome in women with mechanical prosthetic heart valves treated with enoxaparin. BJOG 2009; 116:1585–1592.

Nelson-Piercy C. Cardiac disease. In: Lewis G, ed. Saving Mothers' Lives: Reviewing Maternal Deaths to Make Motherhood Safer 2003–2005. The Seventh Report on Confidential Enquiries into Maternal Deaths in the UK. London, England: Confidential Enquiry into Maternal and Child Health, 2007, pp. 117–130.

National Institute for Health and Clinical Excellence. Prophylaxis against infective endocarditis: antimicrobial prophylaxis against infective endocarditis in adults and children undergoing interventional procedures. http://www.nice.org.uk/nicemedia/pdf/CG64NICEguidance.pdf. Published March 2008. Accessed April 2010.

Oakley CM, Warnes CA, eds. Heart Disease in Pregnancy. 2nd ed. London, England: Wiley-Blackwell, 2007.

Oran B, Lee-Parritz A, Ansell J. Low molecular weight heparin for the prophylaxis of thromboembolism in women with prosthetic mechanical heart valves during pregnancy Thromb Haemost 2004; 92:747–751.

Pearson GD, Veille JC, Rahimtoola S, et al. Peripartum cardiomyopathy. National Heart, Lung and Blood Institute and Office of Rare Diseases (NIH). Workshop Recommendations and Review. J Am Med Assoc 2000; 283:1183–1188.

Sliwa K, Fett J, Elkayam U. Peripartum cardiomyopathy. Lancet 2006; 368:687–693.

Siu SC, Sermer M, Colman JM, et al. Prospective multicenter study of pregnancy outcomes in women with heart disease. Circulation 2001; 104:515–521.

Steer P, Gatzoulis M, Baker P, eds. Cardiac Disease in Pregnancy. London, England: Royal College of Obstetricians and Gynaecologists Press, 2007.

Thorne SA, Nelson-Piercy C, MacGregor A. Risks of contraception and pregnancy in heart disease. Heart 2006; 92:1520–1525.

Tsiaras S, Poppas A. Mitral valve disease in pregnancy: outcomes and management. Obstet Med 2009; 2:6–10.

CHAPTER 3

Thromboembolic disease

Physiological changes
Scope of the problem
Clinical features
Pathogenesis and risk
   factors

Thrombophilia
Diagnosis
Management
Prophylaxis
Cerebral vein thrombosis

Physiological changes

- Changes in the coagulation system during pregnancy produce a physiological hypercoagulable state (presumably in preparation for haemostasis following delivery).
- The concentrations of certain clotting factors, particularly VIII, IX and X are increased. Fibrinogen levels rise significantly by up to 50%.
- Fibrinolytic activity is decreased.
- Concentrations of endogenous anticoagulants such as antithrombin and protein S decrease. Thus pregnancy alters the balance within the coagulation system in favour of clotting, predisposing the pregnant and postpartum woman to venous thrombosis.
- This additional risk is present from the first trimester and for at least 6 weeks following delivery.
- The in vitro tests of coagulation [activated partial thromboplastin time (APTT), prothrombin time (PT) and thrombin time (TT)] remain normal in the absence of anticoagulants or a coagulopathy.
- Venous stasis in the lower limbs is associated with venodilation and decreased flow that is more marked on the left. This is due to compression of the left iliac vein by the right iliac artery and the ovarian artery. On the right, the iliac artery does not cross the vein.

Scope of the problem

- Thrombosis and thromboembolism are a leading direct cause of maternal mortality in the United Kingdom.
- Pulmonary thromboembolism (PTE) in pregnancy and the puerperium kills 6 to 15 women each year in the United Kingdom.

- Thromboembolism has been a leading cause of maternal mortality in the United Kingdom since the Confidential Enquiries into Maternal Deaths began.
- Pregnancy increases the risk of thromboembolism sixfold. The time of greatest risk is postpartum. Elective caesarean section doubles this risk. Emergency caesarean section is associated with a further doubling of the risk compared with elective caesarean section.
- Although the risk of PTE is higher in the puerperium, the antenatal period is longer and antepartum deaths from venous thromboembolism (VTE) occur as commonly as postpartum deaths.
- Almost half of antenatal VTE occur before 15 weeks' gestation and events in the first trimester make up a significant proportion.
- The incidence of non-fatal PTE and deep vein thrombosis (DVT) in pregnancy is approximately 0.1% in developed countries.
- The risk of DVT after caesarean section is approximately 1% to 2%.
- DVT increases the risk of further DVT and venous insufficiency in later life (65% in legs with previous DVT vs. 22% in unaffected legs).

Clinical features
Deep vein thrombosis

- There is a significant preponderance of left-sided DVT compared with right-sided DVT in pregnancy (ratio left:right = 9:1; left-sided 85% in pregnancy vs. 55% in non-pregnancy) because of relative increased venous stasis on the left (see earlier).
- Compared with the non-pregnant patient, iliofemoral thrombosis is more common than popliteofemoral (72% in pregnancy vs. 9% in non-pregnancy).
- The classical features of swelling, redness, pain and tenderness of the calf are unreliable in pregnancy and clinical assessment alone will be wrong in 30% to 50% of cases.
- Leg oedema (which may often be asymmetrical) and calf pain are common in pregnancy without DVT.

Pulmonary embolism

- A high index of suspicion is needed.
- Breathlessness and pleuritic pain, particularly of sudden onset, should always be investigated.
- Other features include cough and haemoptysis.
- Large PTE may present with central chest pain and/or collapse with shock.
- Examination may reveal tachypnoea, tachycardia, raised jugular venous pressure, a loud second heart sound and a right ventricular heave. With pulmonary infarction, a pleural rub and fever may also be present.

Pathogenesis and risk factors

Factors contributing to the increased risk of thromboembolism in pregnancy and the puerperium include the following.

Physiological changes common to all pregnant women (see earlier)

- Haemostatic factors creating a procoagulant state from early pregnancy
- Venous stasis
- Trauma to the pelvic veins at the time of delivery

Additional risk factors (see Table 3.1)

- Previous thromboembolism
- Thrombophilia (see later)
- Increased maternal age (>35 years)
- Obesity (body mass index >30)
- Increased maternal parity (three or more)
- Smoking
- Operative delivery (particularly emergency caesarean section)
- Prolonged bed rest/immobility
- Paraplegia
- Sickle cell disease
- Pre-eclampsia
- Gross varicose veins
- Inflammatory disorders, for example, active inflammatory bowel disease
- Some medical disorders, for example, nephrotic syndrome, cardiomyopathy
- Myeloproliferative disorders, for example, essential thrombocytosis, polycythaemia vera
- Intravenous drug use
- Hyperemesis/dehydration
- Surgery (at anytime in pregnancy)
- Multiple pregnancy, assisted reproductive therapies
- Ovarian hyperstimulation syndrome (particular association with internal jugular and subclavian venous thrombosis)
- Long distance travel

Thrombophilia

- Women with thrombophilia are at increased risk of recurrent thromboembolic events in pregnancy or the puerperium.
- Thrombophilia may be divided into heritable and acquired forms. The prevalence of these thrombophilias in the general population and the associated relative risks of thrombosis are summarised in Table 3.2.
- A history of recurrent, atypical (e.g., axillary vein) or unprovoked (not associated with combined oral contraceptive, pregnancy, trauma or surgery) thromboembolism should stimulate a search for thrombophilia.
- Similarly, a family history of thromboembolism is important, since it may point to a diagnosis of heritable thrombophilia.
- Deficiencies of the naturally occurring anticoagulants protein C, protein S and antithrombin (AT) are rare but are associated with high recurrence risks for thrombosis. These are approximately 12% to 17% (protein S deficiency), 22% to 26% (protein C deficiency) and 32% to 51% (AT deficiency).

Table 3.1 – Risk factors for VTE in pregnancy and the puerperium

Pre-existing		
Previous VTE	Thrombophilia	*Heritable* Antithrombin deficiency Protein C deficiency Protein S deficiency Factor V Leiden Prothrombin gene G20210A
		Acquired (Antiphospholipid syndrome) Persistent lupus anticoagulant Persistent moderate/high titre anticardiolipin antibodies or β_2-glycoprotein 1 antibodies
	Medical co-morbidities, for example, heart or lung disease; systemic lupus erythematosus; cancer; inflammatory conditions (inflammatory bowel disease or inflammatory polyarthropathy); nephrotic syndrome (proteinuria > 3 g/day), sickle cell disease, intravenous drug user	
	Age > 35 years	
	Obesity (BMI > 30 kg/m^2) either pre-pregnancy or in early pregnancy	
	Parity $\geq$ 3	
	Smoking	
	Gross varicose veins (symptomatic or above knee or with associated phlebitis, oedema/skin changes)	
	Paraplegia	
Obstetric risk factors	Multiple pregnancy, assisted reproduction therapy	
	Pre-eclampsia	
	Caesarean section	Prolonged labour, mid-cavity rotational operative delivery
	Postpartum haemorrhage (> 1 L)/ requiring transfusion	

Table 3.1 – *(Continued)*

New onset/transient		
	Surgical procedure in pregnancy or puerperium	For example, ERPC, appendectomy, postpartum sterilisation
These risk factors are potentially reversible and may develop at later stages in gestation than the initial risk assessment or may resolve and therefore what is important is an *ongoing individual risk assessment*	Hyperemesis, dehydration	
	Ovarian hyperstimulation syndrome	
	Admission or immobility ($\geq$ 3 days bed rest)	For example, symphysis pubis dysfunction restricting mobility
	Systemic infection (requiring antibiotics or admission to hospital)	For example, pneumonia, pyelonephritis, postpartum wound infection
	Long distance travel (> 4 hours)	

Abbreviations: BMI, body mass index; ERPC, evacuation of retained products of conception; VTE, venous thromboembolism.

Table 3.2 – Prevalence and risk of VTE with different thrombophilias

	Thrombophilic disorder	% of general population	Relative risk of VTE
Inherited	Antithrombin deficiency	0.07	5—20
	Protein C deficiency	0.3	2—8
	Protein S deficiency	0.2	2—6
	Factor V Leiden (heterozygous)	5–8	4—10
	Factor V Leiden (homozygous)	0.06	10—80
	Prothrombin gene mutation (heterozygous)	2–3	2—10
Acquired[a]	Antiphospholipid antibodies Lupus anticoagulant Anticardiolipin antibodies	2	9
	Acquired APC resistance without Factor V Leiden	8–11	2—4

Abbreviations: APC, activated protein C; VTE, venous thromboembolism.
[a]Antiphospholipid syndrome = lupus anticoagulant and/or anticardiolipin antibodies + thrombosis and/or recurrent miscarriage and/or fetal loss and/or delivery at or before 34 weeks' gestation due to severe pre-eclampsia/Fetal growth restriction (FGR).

- The factor V Leiden (FVL)—a single missense mutation in the factor V gene and the cause of 90% of cases of activated protein C resistance—is present in approximately 3% to 5% of the U.K. population.
- The G20210A mutation of the prothrombin gene leads to elevated levels of pro-thrombin and is present in 1% of the population. These thrombophilias are associated with a lower risk of recurrent thrombosis unless they are present in combination with other thrombophilias or the woman is homozygous for the mutation.
- Individuals heterozygous for FVL or the prothrombin gene G20210A have a fivefold increased risk of thrombosis. This risk may not manifest clinically unless there is a precipitating factor such as pregnancy, surgery or use of an oestrogen-containing oral contraceptive. The risk is higher for homozygotes.
- The prevalence of the prothrombin gene G20210A and FVL mutations in healthy subjects is dependent on the ethnicity and country of origin of the population under investigation. Low prevalence rates are found in Asians and Africans.
- The risk of thrombosis in women with thrombophilia is much higher in those with a personal history compared with those with only a family history of thrombosis, which in turn is higher than those who are not from a symptomatic kindred.
- Women with the less severe thrombophilias (e.g., FVL, prothrombin gene mutation) who have not themselves experienced a thrombosis can probably safely be managed in pregnancy with close surveillance. Prophylaxis with low-molecular-weight heparin (LMWH) in the postpartum period is justified.
- Thrombophilia may be a factor in thrombosis occurring in pregnancy and the puerperium in up to 50% of women.
- The risk of recurrent thrombosis in antiphospholipid syndrome (APS) may be as high as 70%, and some of these women will be on long-term warfarin treatment outside pregnancy (see Chapter 8, p. 143).
- Women with a history of thromboembolism should be screened for thrombophilia in the first trimester or ideally pre-pregnancy if they have had a previous non–oestrogen-related VTE provoked by a minor risk factor as this will influence man-agement and decisions regarding thromboprophylaxis antenatally.
- Women with recurrent or a prior unprovoked or oestrogen-provoked VTE should be considered for thromboprophylaxis and hence testing for heritable thrombophilia is not required.

Adverse pregnancy outcome

- Several studies have suggested an association between adverse pregnancy outcome (pre-eclampsia, placental abruption, fetal growth restriction, late fetal demise, recur-rent early miscarriage, intrauterine death and stillbirth) and heritable thrombophil-ias, and homozygosity for the thermolabile mutation of methylene tetrahydrofolate reductase causing mild hyper-homocysteinaemia. Other studies do not support this association in all populations.
- Systematic review of the literature and meta-analyses of the studies conclude that there is a significant association between most thrombophilias and differ-ent adverse pregnancy outcomes. However, the absolute risk of adverse outcomes is low.
- A beneficial effect for aspirin and/or heparin in the treatment of adverse pregnancy outcome in APS has been demonstrated, (see Chapter 8, p. 142).

Table 3.3 – Estimated radiation to the fetus associated with investigations for thromboembolism[a]

Investigation	Radiation (μGy) 1 rad = 10,000μGy
Chest radiograph	<10
Limited venography	<500
Unilateral venography without abdominal shield	3140
Perfusion lung scan (technetium-99 m)	400
Ventilation lung scan	
Xenon-133	40—190
Technetium-99 m	10—350
Computed tomographic pulmonary angiography	<10
Pulmonary angiography	
Brachial route	<500
Femoral route	2210—3740

[a]Maximum recommended exposure in pregnancy $= 50,000 \mu$Gy (5 rad).

There is a lack of controlled trials of antithrombotic intervention to prevent pregnancy complications in heritable thrombophilia.
■ Universal screening of women with poor obstetric histories for heritable thrombophilias is inappropriate until the results of further randomised intervention studies in such women with thrombophilia are known.

Diagnosis

Deep vein thrombosis

■ An objective diagnosis is vital because of the major implications in pregnancy of the:
  – Need for prolonged therapy
  – Potential need for prophylaxis in subsequent pregnancies
  – Concern regarding the future use of oestrogen-containing contraceptives
  – Subsequent use of hormone replacement therapy (HRT).
■ The gold standard remains venography, although this is rarely used now. If performed with abdominal shielding, it is associated with negligible radiation to the fetus (Table 3.3).
■ More convenient, less invasive and widely available is Doppler ultrasound. This tool is accurate in its detection of thrombi above the calf and below the inguinal ligament. Thrombi confined to the calf veins do not usually embolise and give rise to PTE. The advantage of Doppler is that it may be repeated to exclude extension

of calf vein thrombi above the knee. Three features of thrombi are detectable with Doppler ultrasound:

1. Direct imaging of the thrombus
2. Lack of compressibility of the vein
3. Absence of distal distension of the vein during a Valsalva manoeuvre

- Impedance plethysmography has been less fully evaluated in pregnancy but is safe.
- D-dimers, widely used outside pregnancy in algorithms for diagnosis of thrombosis, are not helpful in pregnancy since the false-positive rate is high. Although the false-negative rate is low, it is not zero, and the high pre-test probability in pregnancy means that even if the D-dimers are negative, if there is clinical suspicion, an objective imaging test is required.

Pulmonary embolism

- The chest radiograph is often normal but is an essential part of investigation to exclude other important causes of breathlessness, chest pain or hypoxia. In cases of PTE, it may show the following:
  - Areas of translucency in underperfused lung
  - Atelectasis
  - Wedge-shaped infarction
  - Pleural effusion
- The ECG may also be normal except for a sinus tachycardia. In cases of large PTE, there may be the following:
  - Right-axis deviation
  - Right-bundle branch block
  - Peaked P-waves in lead II due to right atrial dilation
  - The classical S1, Q3, T3 pattern is rarely seen.
- There is usually a raised white blood cell count and a polymorphonuclear leukocytosis.
- Arterial blood gases reveal hypoxaemia and hypocapnia.
- A useful screening test is to measure the oxygen saturation (using a pulse oximeter) at rest and after exercise, looking for resting hypoxia or a fall (>3–4%) after exercise.
- Diagnosis must be confirmed with a lung scan. If the chest radiograph is normal, a perfusion scan alone (technetium-99 m) may demonstrate underperfused areas. If the chest radiograph is abnormal and the cause of the abnormality is uncertain, an additional ventilation scan (xenon-133) will allow detection of ventilation/perfusion mismatch in cases of PTE. The total radiation to the fetus from a lung scan is minimal and well below the recommended total pregnancy maximal dose for radiation workers in the United States (Table 3.2).
- Computed tomographic pulmonary angiography (CTPA) and magnetic resonance imaging (MRI) are safe during pregnancy. The radiation dose to the fetus of a CTPA is minimal (less than with a lung scan) although there is significant radiation of the maternal breast. However, this investigation may be indicated if proximal PTE is suspected, if the CXR is abnormal, if lung pathology or aortic dissection is suspected.
- Transthoracic echocardiogram may aid in the diagnosis, especially in the haemodynamically unstable patient. Large PTE may be associated with a number of abnormal echo findings, including
  - right ventricular dilation;

- abnormal septal motion;
- loss of right ventricular contractility;
- elevated pulmonary artery or right ventricular pressures;
- moderate to severe tricuspid regurgitation, pulmonary regurgitation; and
- occasionally, visualisation of clot in the right ventricle or pulmonary artery.

■ Pulmonary angiography is usually reserved for severe cases where localisation of the embolus prior to surgical or medical embolectomy is required.

Management

■ High-dose s.c. LMWH is now the standard management of VTE both inside and outside pregnancy. Doses are based on weight but higher doses are required in pregnancy for some LMWHs [e.g., enoxaparin (Clexane) 1 mg/kg b.d. as opposed to the non-pregnant dose of 1.5 mg/kg o.d.] Prophylactic and treatment doses in pregnancy of the different LMWHs are shown in Table 3.4.

■ If there is a high level of clinical suspicion, treatment doses of s.c. LMWH should be commenced prior to confirmatory diagnostic tests.

Table 3.4 – Antenatal and postnatal prophylactic and therapeutic doses of different low-molecular-weight-heparins for women with different weight[a]

Weight (kg)	Enoxaparin	Dalteparin	Tinzaparin (75 U/kg/day)
<50	20 mg daily	2500 U daily	3500 U daily
50–90	40 mg daily	5000 U daily	4500 U daily
91–130	60 mg daily[b]	7500 U daily[b]	7000 U daily[b]
131–170	80 mg daily[b]	10,000 U daily[b]	9000 U daily[b]
>170	0.6 mg/kg/day[b]	75 U/kg/day[b]	75 U/kg/day[b]
High prophylactic (intermediate) dose for women weighing 50–90 kg	40 mg 12 hourly	5000 U 12 hourly	4500 U 12 hourly
Treatment dose	1 mg/kg/12 hourly antenatal 1.5 mg/kg/daily postnatal	100 U/kg/12 hourly or 200 U/kg/daily postnatal	175 U/kg/daily (antenatal and postnatal)

[a]Anti–factor Xa levels provide only a rough guide of the concentration of heparin present and levels provide little or no evidence on the efficacy in relation to prevention of thrombosis. Experience indicates that monitoring of anti–factor Xa levels is not required when LMWH is used for thromboprophylaxis, provided the woman has normal renal function. Lower doses of enoxaparin and dalteparin should be employed if the creatinine clearance is <30 mL/min. This would equate to a serum creatinine of about 200 μmol/L for a 30-year-old woman weighing 70 kg. For tinzaparin, dose reductions are required if the creatinine clearance is < 20 mL/min.
[b]May be given in two divided doses.

- Monitoring with anti–factor Xa levels is not usually required except perhaps at the extremes of weight or in the presence of renal impairment when lower doses of LMWH may be required. Peak values (3–4 hours postinjection) of 0.4 to 1.2 U/mL are the aim.
- I.v. unfractionated heparin (UH) is indicated for massive PTE or in situations where rapid reversibility may be required. Just as with LMWH, larger doses (than in the non-pregnant woman) of i.v. heparin (e.g., 40,000 U/24 hr) are required to prolong the APTT by 1.5 to 2.0 times control.
- Systematic review of the use of LMWH for treatment and prophylaxis of VTE in pregnancy confirms that the risk of heparin-induced thrombocytopenia (HIT) is negligible; and therefore, there is no need to monitor the platelet count with LMWH therapy.
- In cases of life-threatening PTE, thrombolysis, pulmonary artery catheter breakup of thrombus and embolectomy have been successfully used.
- The use of vena caval filters should be restricted to cases of recurrent PTE in the presence of demonstrable iliofemoral thrombosis, despite adequate full anticoagulation.
- Once VTE is confirmed, LMWH must be continued for the rest of the pregnancy and the puerperium. Long-term use of LMWH is associated with a lower risk of osteoporosis and bone fractures compared with UH use. If the VTE occurs early in pregnancy, it may be appropriate to decrease doses to a high prophylactic level after 6 months.
- Intra- and postpartum management is discussed later under "Prophylaxis".

Prophylaxis

The following are drugs, and their side effects, used for thromboprophylaxis.

Warfarin

- Warfarin crosses the placenta, is teratogenic and is therefore usually avoided during the first trimester.
- The teratogenic risk of chondrodysplasia punctata, nasal hypoplasia, growth restriction, short proximal limbs and other abnormalities is approximately 5%. The period of risk is between the 6th and 12th week of gestation; so, conception on warfarin therapy is not dangerous, provided the warfarin is replaced by heparin within 2 weeks of the first missed period.
- The risk of miscarriage and stillbirth is also increased.
- The association with microcephaly and neurological abnormalities when warfarin is used in the second trimester may be related to over-anticoagulation of the fetus.
- There is a significant risk of both maternal (retroplacental) and fetal (intracerebral) bleeding when used in the third trimester, and particularly after 36 weeks' gestation.
- The use of warfarin for obstetric thromboprophylaxis in the second and early third trimesters should only be under close supervision and following thorough discussion with the patient.
- The single undisputed indication for warfarin use in pregnancy is in some women with metal prosthetic heart valve replacements (see Chapter 2, p. 32), in whom the

risk of thrombosis is high, and for whom thrombosis carries a high mortality rate. These women require full anticoagulation throughout pregnancy.

Heparin and LMWH

- S.c. heparin and LMWH do not cross the placenta and therefore have no adverse effects on the fetus. LMWHs, produced by enzymatic or chemical breakdown of the heparin molecule, offer many advantages over standard UHs and are now the standard anticoagulants for treatment and prophylaxis of VTE in pregnancy in the United Kingdom.
- The most obvious advantage in obstetrics, where the timescale of prophylaxis is much longer than in surgery, is the increased bioavailability and longer half-life that together allow for once-daily administration for prophylaxis.
- Because LMWHs are composed of shorter molecules than UHs, the ratio of anti–factor Xa (antithrombotic) to anti–factor IIa activity (anticoagulant), which is inversely proportional to the molecular weight, is increased. This ensures an improved clinical benefit (antithrombosis) to risk (inadvertent anticoagulation and bleeding) ratio.
- The risk of heparin-induced osteoporosis is particularly pertinent in obstetrics: first, because heparin use may last for up to 10 months and, second, because pregnancy and breast-feeding cause reversible bone demineralisation (see Chapter 8). There have been several reports of vertebral collapse associated with UH use in pregnancy.
- The incidence of symptomatic osteoporosis associated with UH use in pregnancy may be as high as 2%, and it is this risk that must be balanced against the risk of recurrent thromboembolism. The risk with LMWH is much lower (0.04%).
- Heparin-induced osteopenia may be subclinical, and studies have shown that thromboprophylaxis with UH in pregnancy may cause a 5% reduction in bone density, equivalent to 2 years' postmenopausal bone loss. Fortunately, however, bone density improves once heparin therapy is discontinued.
- Thrombocytopenia is another rare but potentially dangerous side effect of heparin.

There are two forms of HIT as follows:

1. An immediate-onset non-idiosyncratic reaction that is of little clinical importance.
2. A later (6–10 days) idiosyncratic immune-mediated form that is more serious and associated with paradoxical thrombosis.

- There are reports of HIT in pregnancy, but in the United Kingdom, this complication of heparin therapy is very unusual.
- LMWHs have less effect on platelet aggregation and less inhibition of platelet function than those by UH, and this reduces the risk of early thrombocytopenia. LMWHs are less capable than UH of activating resting platelets to release platelet factor IV, and they bind less well to platelet factor IV, thereby decreasing the risk of late-onset immune thrombocytopenia. HIT is extremely rare with LMWH use.
- Some women (1–2%) develop a local allergic reaction to LMWH. If this occurs, women usually develop a similar localised pruritic urticarial skin eruption to all forms of UH and LMWH. In these unusual cases, heparinoids such as danaparoid have been used successfully.
- Hyperkalaemia via inhibition of aldosterone secretion may rarely complicate UH or LMWH use. Women with chronic renal failure or diabetes are more susceptible.

Fondaparinux

Fondaparinux is a synthetic pentasaccharide that specifically inhibits factor Xa via antithrombin. It is licensed in the United Kingdom for the prevention and treatment of VTE outside pregnancy, but there is very limited experience of its use in pregnancy although it has been used in the setting of heparin intolerance. It probably crosses the placenta since anti–factor Xa activity about 10% of that in maternal plasma has been found in the umbilical cord plasma in newborns of five mothers being treated with fondaparinux.

Aspirin

■ Antiplatelet therapy has been shown to be effective in reducing the risk of VTE in surgical and medical patients. In one study, low-dose aspirin reduced the risk of VTE after orthopaedic surgery by 36%, even in some patients taking concomitant heparin prophylaxis.
■ The use of aspirin as thromboprophylaxis in pregnancy has never been submitted to randomised controlled trial, but it is known that low-dose aspirin is safe in pregnancy.
■ The American College of Chest Physicians guideline on VTE in pregnancy recommends against the use of aspirin for VTE prophylaxis.

Indications for thromboprophylaxis

■ These are based on the risk factors detailed earlier (p. 42) (Table 3.1), which necessitate an individual risk assessment early in pregnancy or preferably prior to conception in those with previous VTE.
■ When assessing the need for thromboprophylaxis in pregnancy, an accurate history of previous VTE is vital, and one should determine whether a diagnosis of previous VTE was objectively confirmed.
■ A summary of the recommendations published in the Green-top clinical guideline of the Royal College of Obstetricians and Gynaecologists for thromboprophylaxis for pregnant women with previous VTE or those with identified thrombophilias is given in Table 3.5.

Very high risk

Women with recurrent VTE associated with either antithrombin deficiency or the APS (who will often be on long-term oral anticoagulation) are at very high risk.

■ These women require thromboprophylaxis with higher dose LMWH [either high prophylactic (12 hourly) or weight-adjusted (75% of treatment dose)] or full treatment doses antenatally and for 6 weeks postpartum or until converted back to warfarin after delivery. These women require specialist management by experts in haemostasis and pregnancy.

High risk

Women in whom the original VTE was unprovoked/idiopathic or related to oestrogen (oestrogen-containing contraception/pregnancy) or who have other risk factors, a family history of VTE in a first-degree relative (suggestive of thrombophilia) or a documented thrombophilia.

■ These women require thromboprophylaxis with LMWH antenatally and for 6 weeks postpartum.

Table 3.5 – Summary of the recommendations for thromboprophylaxis for pregnant women with previous VTE or those with identified thrombophilias

Very high risk	Previous VTE on long-term warfarin Antithrombin deficiency Antiphospholipid syndrome with previous VTE	Recommend antenatal high-dose LMWH and at least 6 weeks postnatal LMWH/warfarin. These women require specialist management by experts in haemostasis and pregnancy
High risk	Previous recurrent or unprovoked VTE Previous oestrogen (pill/pregnancy)– provoked VTE Previous VTE + thrombophilia Previous VTE + family history of VTE Asymptomatic thrombophilia (combined defects, homozygous FVL)	Recommend antenatal and 6 weeks postnatal prophylactic LMWH
Intermediate risk	Single previous VTE associated with transient risk factor no longer present without thrombophilia, family history or other risk factors	Consider antenatal LMWH (but not routinely recommended) Recommend 6 weeks postnatal prophylactic LMWH
	Asymptomatic thrombophilia (except antithrombin deficiency, combined defects, homozygous FVL)	Recommend 7 days (or 6 weeks if family history or other risk factors) postnatal prophylactic LMWH

Abbreviations: VTE, venous thromboembolism; FVL, factor V Leiden; LMWH, low-molecular-weight heparin.
Adapted from Royal College of Obstetricians and Gynaecologists Green-top guideline number 37, 2009.

Intermediate risk

Women in whom the original VTE was provoked by a transient major risk factor that is no longer present and who have no other risk factors are at intermediate risk. They require screening for thrombophilia because the results will influence whether they receive LMWH antenatally.

- In these women, thromboprophylaxis with LMWH can be withheld antenatally provided no additional risk factors (or thrombophilia) are present (in which case they should be offered LMWH). They require close surveillance for the development of other risk factors.
- They should be offered thromboprophylaxis with LMWH for 6 weeks postpartum.

Prophylaxis for women with thrombophilias

Very high risk

■ Women with AT deficiency, even if there is no history of thrombosis, require LMWH prophylaxis throughout pregnancy and the puerperium because of the high risk of thrombosis (see earlier).

■ Women with antiphospholipid antibodies (lupus anticoagulant or anticardiolipin antibodies) should receive low-dose aspirin antenatally for fetal reasons (see Chapter 8). If they have had a previous thromboembolic event, LMWH throughout pregnancy is mandatory. Many of these women will have been receiving maintenance doses of warfarin outside pregnancy.

High risk

■ Women with asymptomatic thrombophilia associated with a high risk of VTE including those with combined defects or those homozygous for FVL or the prothrombin gene mutation also fall into this high-risk category.

Intermediate risk

■ Women diagnosed as having a thrombophilia (FVL, prothrombin gene mutation, protein S or C deficiency) via family studies, but who themselves have no personal history of thrombosis, may be managed with close surveillance antenatally and with LMWH for at least 1 week postpartum. Such cases need constant review since, if, for example, a woman with a known thrombophilia was admitted for pre-eclampsia or bed rest, this would be an indication to "step up" the prophylaxis to LMWH.

■ Similarly, women with APS but without previous thrombosis or fetal indications for heparin are managed with antenatal low-dose aspirin but should receive postpartum LMWH for 1 to 6 weeks depending on the presence of other risk factors.

Additional risk factors

■ The Royal College of Obstetricians and Gynaecologists has published an updated Green-top guideline covering thromboprophylaxis in obstetrics. This highlights the importance of risk assessment in early pregnancy, on admission and after delivery (see Fig. 3.1).

■ Prophylaxis to cover delivery should not be limited to those undergoing caesarean section, since some women who die of pulmonary embolism following childbirth have had vaginal deliveries.

■ Women with three or more persisting risk factors (two or more if admitted) should be considered for thromboprophylaxis with LMWH in the antenatal period.

■ Women with two or more persisting risk factors should be considered for thromboprophylaxis with LMWH for at least 7 days postnatally.

■ All women with a body mass index $> 40 \text{ kg/m}^2$ should receive LMWH in appropriate (weight-based) doses for at least 7 days postpartum regardless of the mode of delivery.

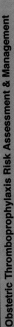
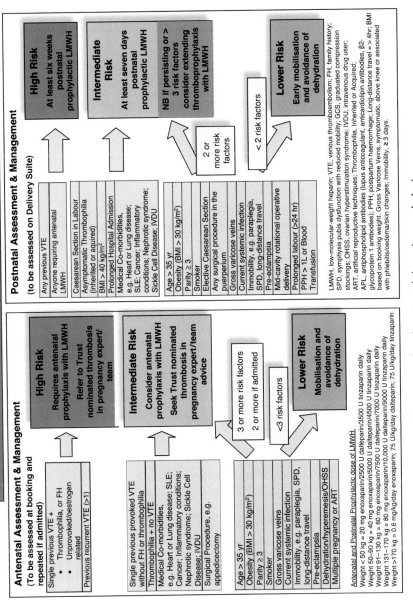

Figure 3.1 – Summary of protocol for antenatal and postnatal thromboprophylaxis.

Antenatal management

- Having decided into which risk category (Fig. 3.1 and Table 3.5) a women falls, she should be counselled appropriately. This is particularly so for women requiring LMWH prophylaxis throughout pregnancy since early presentation in pregnancy is important.
- Since the first trimester is a time of high risk for VTE, it is important that if indicated, thromboprophylaxis with LMWH is begun as soon as is practical in pregnancy.

Intrapartum management

- Because of the high risk of VTE immediately postpartum, LMWH should not be discontinued during labour for longer than is necessary to allow safe regional anaesthesia or analgesia.
- For women starting prophylaxis with LMWH postpartum, the first dose should ideally be administered as soon as possible after delivery.
- In controlled studies, at least 10,000 patients have been given the combination of LMWH in prophylactic doses and epidural/spinal anaesthesia without complications. However, following the issue of an U.S. Food and Drug Administration warning regarding the risk of epidural haematoma with LMWH use (Clexane 30 mg b.d. in mostly elderly women undergoing orthopaedic surgery in the United States), obstetric anaesthetic guidelines advise a 12-hour interval after the last LMWH injection before the siting of a regional block. LMWH can then be safely administered after about 2 hours.
- Regional anaesthesia or analgesia is usually permitted 12 hours after a prophylactic dose of LMWH, but most obstetric anaesthetists recommend a 24-hour interval between a treatment dose of LMWH and neuroaxial blockade.
- Therefore some women receiving treatment doses of LMWH may be denied regional anaesthesia, necessitating general anaesthesia if a caesarean section is required. However, with careful multidisciplinary planning of delivery, this can usually be avoided by reducing the dose of LMWH on the day prior to planned induction of labour or delivery by caesarean section. Heparin in low/prophylactic doses does not interfere with the activation of normal haemostatic mechanisms at the site of injury but only lowers the risk of spontaneous haemostatic activation.
- The most vulnerable time for epidural haematomas seems to be after removal of the epidural catheter. Therefore, this too should be in close collaboration with the obstetric anaesthetist and usually after a 12-hour period after the last LMWH injection.

Postpartum management

- Neither warfarin nor LMWH is excreted in breast milk and breast-feeding is not contraindicated with the use of these drugs.
- The important principle is that for high-risk women (Table 3.5), prophylaxis with either warfarin or s.c. LMWH should be continued for 6 weeks after delivery.
- Women in the very-high-risk category should probably switch back to warfarin before 6 weeks postpartum.
- The advantages of changing to warfarin after the first week after delivery are that:
  - Exposure to heparin is minimised
  - There is no further need for self-administered s.c. injections.

- The disadvantages relate to
  - the need for close monitoring, venepuncture and attendance at an anticoagulation clinic
  - an increased bleeding risk with warfarin versus LMWH
- Women who have suffered a VTE towards the end of their pregnancy may require longer periods (e.g., 3 months) of warfarin administration postpartum.

Cerebral vein thrombosis

- Cerebral vein thrombosis (CVT) is uncommon (incidence approximately 1 in 10,000) but associated with a high mortality rate.
- The pregnant and puerperal state account for 5% to 20% (western Europe and United States) to 60% (India) of all cases of CVT.

Clinical features

Patients usually present with the following symptoms:
- Headache
- Seizures
- Impaired consciousness
- Signs of raised intracranial pressure
- Vomiting
- Photophobia
- One-third to two-thirds of patients have focal signs such as hemiparesis. Focal signs depend on the territory of the thrombosis that may involve the cortical veins or the superior sagittal sinus
- CVT may cause fever and leukocytosis
- Venous infarction and intracerebral bleeding may result from obstruction of collateral circulation.

Pathogenesis

- This relates to the hypercoagulable postpartum state and possible trauma to the endothelial lining of cerebral sinuses and veins during labour.
  - The risk factors are very similar to those for DVT and PE, and in the 2003–2005 triennium, all the cases (4/8) where body mass indices (BMIs) were recorded were overweight or obese.
- Puerperal infection and dehydration may explain the high incidence in developing countries.
- Many cases described are associated with thrombophilia.

Diagnosis

- Differential diagnosis includes eclampsia, subarachnoid haemorrhage and herpes encephalitis.
- Diagnosis is made by CT scan to detect intracerebral bleeding, although MRI, and especially venous angiography MRI, is best able to show venous thrombosis.

Management

- This includes hydration, anticonvulsants (if seizures are a feature) and anticoagulation.

- Treatment with heparin is controversial since the risk of intracerebral bleeding may be increased, but clot formation is prevented. Evidence mainly from non-pregnant patients suggests outcome is better with heparin therapy.
- A thrombophilia screen is mandatory. This is an unusual site for venous thrombosis and thrombophilia is found in a significant proportion of cases.

Thromboembolic disease in pregnancy—points to remember

- PTE is a common direct cause of death in pregnancy and the puerperium in the United Kingdom.
- Pregnancy and especially the puerperium are associated with an increased risk of thrombosis.
- The risk of DVT and PTE in pregnancy increases with increasing maternal age and obesity.
- Although the risks are highest post emergency caesarean section, women with risk factors are at risk antenatally and after vaginal delivery.
- Objective diagnosis of DVT and PTE is vital.
- Treatment of VTE in pregnancy necessitates larger doses of some LMWHs, and warfarin is avoided.
- Following acute VTE in pregnancy, LMWH must be continued for the rest of the pregnancy and the puerperium.
- Decisions regarding thromboprophylaxis in pregnancy relate to history of VTE, the presence of detectable thrombophilia, and the other identifiable risk factors.
- Women at high risk of recurrent VTE should receive antenatal and postnatal thromboprophylaxis with LMWH. This should begin as early in pregnancy as possible.
- LMWH and warfarin are safe to use in lactating mothers.

Further reading

Confidential Enquiry into Maternal and Child Health. Saving mothers' lives: reviewing maternal deaths to make motherhood safer—2003–2005: the seventh report on confidential enquiries into maternal deaths in the United Kingdom. London, United Kingdom: Confidential Enquiry into Maternal and Child Health, 2007.

Greer IA. The challenge of thrombophilia in maternal fetal medicine. N Engl J Med 2000; 342:424–425.

Greer IA, Nelson-Piercy C. Low-molecular-weight heparins for thromboprophylaxis and treatment of venous thromboembolism in pregnancy: a systematic review of safety and efficacy. Blood 2005; 106:401–407.

Robertson L, Wu O, Langhorne P, et al. Thrombophilia in pregnancy: a systematic review. Br J Haematol 2006; 132:171–196.

Royal College of Obstetricians and Gynaecologists. Reducing the Risks of Thrombosis and Embolism During Pregnancy and the Puerperium: Guideline No 37. London, United Kingdom: Royal College of Obstetricians and Gynaecologists Press, 2009.

Royal College of Obstetricians and Gynaecologists. Thromboembolic Disease in Pregnancy and the Puerperium: Acute Management: Guideline No 28. London, United Kingdom: Royal College of Obstetricians and Gynaecologists Press, 2007.

CHAPTER 4

Respiratory disease

Physiological changes	Tuberculosis
Breathlessness of pregnancy	Sarcoidosis
Asthma	Cystic fibrosis
Hay fever	Severe restrictive and interstitial
Pneumonia	lung disease

Readers should also consult Section B for discussions on breathlessness (Table 1) and chest pain (Table 3).

Physiological changes (see Table 4.1)

- There is a significant increase in oxygen demand in normal pregnancy. This is due to the increased metabolic rate and a 20% increased consumption of oxygen.
- There is a 40% to 50% increase in minute ventilation, mostly due to an increase in tidal volume rather than in respiratory rate.
- This maternal hyperventilation causes arterial pO_2 to increase and arterial pCO_2 as for pO_2 to fall, with a compensatory fall in serum bicarbonate to 18 to 22 mmol/L. A mild fully compensated respiratory alkalosis is therefore normal in pregnancy (arterial pH 7.44).
- Diaphragmatic elevation in late pregnancy results in decreased functional residual capacity, but diaphragmatic excursion, and therefore vital capacity, remains unaltered.
- Peak expiratory flow rate (PEFR) or forced expiratory volume in 1 second (FEV_1) are unaffected by pregnancy.

Breathlessness of pregnancy

- This is common, occurring in up to three-quarters of women at some time during pregnancy and a potential source of diagnostic confusion.
- It is probably a result of increased awareness of the physiological hyperventilation of pregnancy, leading to a subjective feeling of breathlessness.
- It is commonest in the third trimester but may start at any gestation. Classicially, the breathlessness is present at rest or while talking and may paradoxically improve during mild activity.

Asthma

Asthma is the commonest chronic medical illness to complicate pregnancy, affecting up to 7% of women of childbearing age. It is often undiagnosed and, when recognised,

Table 4.1 – Physiological changes in respiratory function during pregnancy

Physiological variable	Direction of change	Degree/timing of change
Oxygen consumption	↑	20%
Metabolic rate	↑	15%
Resting minute ventilation	↑	40–50%
Tidal volume	↑	
Respiratory rate	→	
Functional residual capacity	↓	Third trimester
Vital capacity	→	
FEV$_1$ and PEFR	→	
pO$_2$	↑	
pCO$_2$	↓	4.0 kPa/30 mmHg
Arterial pH	↑	7.44

Abbreviations: FEV$_1$, forced expiratory volume in 1 second; PEFR, peak expiratory flow rate; ↑, increased; ↓, decreased; →, unchanged.

may be undertreated. Pregnancy provides an opportunity to diagnose asthma and to optimise the treatment of women already known to have asthma.

Clinical features

Symptoms

- Cough
- Breathlessness
- Wheezy breathing
- Chest tightness

Symptoms are commonly worse at night and in the early morning. There may be clear provoking trigger factors, such as the following:

- Pollen
- Animal dander
- Dust
- Exercise
- Cold
- Emotion
- Upper respiratory tract infections.

58

Signs

Signs are often absent unless seen during an acute attack.

- Increased respiratory rate
- Inability to complete sentences
- Wheeze
- Use of accessory muscles
- Tachycardia

Pathogenesis

Reversible bronchoconstriction is caused by the following:

- Smooth-muscle spasm in the airway walls
- Inflammation with swelling and excessive production of mucus

Diagnosis

- This is based on the recognition of a characteristic pattern of symptoms and signs in the absence of an alternative explanation. Eliciting a careful history is the key. A personal or family history of asthma or atopy makes the diagnosis more likely.
- The degree of bronchoconstriction is measured with a PEFR or spirometry to measure FEV_1 and forced vital capacity (FVC).
- Where the history suggests a high probability of asthma, or the FEV_1/FVC ratio is < 0.7, a trial of treatment is indicated.
- A hallmark of asthma is variability and reversibility of the bronchoconstriction.

A typical feature is morning "dipping" in the peak flow. A > 20% diurnal variation in PEFR for 3 or more days a week during a 2 week PEFR diary is diagnostic.

- Other diagnostic features include the following
  - A greater than 15% improvement in FEV_1 following inhalation of a β-sympathomimetic bronchodilator.
  - A greater than 15% fall in FEV_1 following 6 minutes of exercise

Pregnancy

Effect of pregnancy on asthma

- Asthma may improve, deteriorate or remain unchanged during pregnancy.
- Women with only mild disease are unlikely to experience problems, whereas those with severe asthma are at greater risk of deterioration, particularly late in pregnancy.
- Women whose symptoms improve during the last trimester of pregnancy may experience postnatal deterioration.
- Acute asthma in labour is unlikely because of increased endogenous steroids at that time.
- Deterioration in disease control is commonly caused by reduction or even complete cessation of medication due to fears about its safety.

Effect of asthma on pregnancy

- For most women, there are no adverse effects of their asthma on pregnancy outcome.
- Severe, poorly controlled asthma, associated with chronic or intermittent maternal hypoxaemia, may adversely affect the fetus.
- Some association (mostly from retrospective, uncontrolled or small studies) between maternal asthma and the following:
  - Pregnancy-induced hypertension/pre-eclampsia
  - Preterm births and preterm labour
  - Low-birth-weight infants
  - Fetal growth restriction
  - Neonatal morbidity, for example,
    - Transient tachypnoea of the newborn
    - Neonatal hypoglycaemia
    - Neonatal seizures
    - Admission to the neonatal intensive care unit
- In general, adverse effects on pregnancy outcome are small and related to the severity and control of the asthma.
- Most of the above-mentioned associations are uncommon in clinical practice.

Management

- Women should be advised that their asthma is unlikely to adversely affect their pregnancy and that maintaining good control of asthma throughout pregnancy may minimise any small risks.
- Current emphasis in the management of asthma is on the prevention, rather than the treatment, of acute attacks.
- It is important to check the woman's inhaler technique, since failure to do this may result in unnecessary escalation of therapy. Some women require a breath-actuated inhaler.
- Management follows a stepwise approach and readers are directed to the British Thoracic Society/Scottish Intercollegiate Guidelines Network guidelines on the management of asthma.
- Mild intermittent asthma is managed with inhaled short-acting "reliever" (β_2-agonist) medication as required (step 1)
- If usage of a "reliever" (β_2-agonist) inhaler exceeds once/day, regular inhaled anti-inflammatory medication with a steroid "preventer" (e.g., beclomethasone) inhaler (200–800 μg/day) should be commenced (step 2).
- The next step up in therapy is either the addition of a long acting reliever [β_2-agonist; long-acting β-agonist (LABA); e.g., salmeterol (Serevent)] or an increase in the dose of inhaled steroid (800 μg/day) (step 3).
- Further steps involve a trial of additional therapies, for example, leukotriene receptor antagonist (see later), slow-release oral theophylline or oral β_2-agonist. Alternatively, the dose of inhaled steroid can be increased to 2000 μg/day (step 4).
- If these measures fail to achieve adequate control then continuous or frequent use of oral steroids becomes necessary. The lowest dose providing adequate control should be used, if necessary with steroid-sparing agents (step 5).
- The aim of the treatment is to achieve virtual total freedom from symptoms, such that the lifestyle of the individual is not affected. Regrettably, many people with asthma accept chronic symptoms such as wheezing or "chest tightness" on waking

as an inevitable consequence of their disease. This is inappropriate and pregnancy provides an ideal opportunity to educate women with asthma, taking into account the following guidelines:

- Women should be advised to stop smoking.
- Explanation and reassurance regarding the importance and safety of regular medication in pregnancy is essential to ensure compliance.
- Women with asthma should be encouraged to avoid known trigger factors.
- Home peak-flow monitoring and written personalised self-management plans should be encouraged.
- Use of a large volume spacer may improve drug delivery.
- Women should be counselled about indications for an increase in inhaled steroid dosage and if appropriate given an "emergency" supply of oral steroids.

■ The treatment of asthma in pregnancy is essentially no different from the treatment of asthma in non-pregnant women. All the drugs in widespread use to treat asthma, including systemic steroids, appear to be safe in pregnancy and during lactation.

■ The challenge in the management of pregnant women with asthma is to ensure adequate preconception or early pregnancy counselling so that women do not stop important anti-inflammatory inhaled therapy.

Medication

β_2-agonists

■ β_2-agonists from the systemic circulation cross the placenta rapidly, but very little of a given inhaled dose reaches the lungs and only a minute fraction of this reaches the systemic circulation.

■ Studies show no difference in perinatal mortality, congenital malformations, birth-weight, Apgar scores or delivery complications when pregnant women with asthma treated with inhaled β_2-agonists are compared with women with asthma not using β_2-agonists and non-asthmatic controls.

■ The long-acting β_2-agonists (LABA; e.g., salmeterol) are also safe in pregnancy. They should not be discontinued or withheld in those who require them for good control of asthma.

Corticosteroids

■ Use of both inhaled and oral steroids is safe in pregnancy. Only minimal amounts of inhaled corticosteroid preparations are systemically absorbed. There is no evidence for an increased incidence of congenital malformations or adverse fetal effects attributable to the use of inhaled beclomethasone (Becotide®) or budesonide (Pulmicort®). Fluticasone propionate (Flixotide®) is a longer-acting inhaled corticosteroid that may be used for those requiring high doses of inhaled steroids.

■ Combination inhalers of corticosteroids plus LABA, for example, budesonide/formoterol (Symbicort®) fluticasone/salmeterol (Seretide®), are widely available and may aid compliance, although to increase the dose of inhaled steroid without exceeding the maximum dose of LABA may necessitate changing the strength of the inhaler rather than asking the patient to take more puffs.

■ The use of systemic corticosteroids to control exacerbations of asthma is safe, and these must not be withheld if current medications are inadequate.

- Prednisolone is metabolised by the placenta, and very little (10%) active drug reaches the fetus. Although some workers have found an increased incidence of cleft palate with first trimester exposure to steroids, this finding is refuted in larger prospective case control studies. There is no evidence of an increased risk of miscarriage, stillbirth, other congenital malformations, or neonatal death attributable to maternal steroid therapy.
- There is a non-significant increase in the relative risk of pre-eclampsia in women with asthma treated with oral but not inhaled steroids. However, it is unclear whether this is an effect of steroids or asthma control and severity.
- Although suppression of the fetal hypothalamic–pituitary–adrenal axis is a theoretical possibility with maternal systemic steroid therapy, there is little evidence from clinical practice to support this.
- Long-term, high-dose steroids may increase the risk of preterm rupture of the membranes.
- There are concerns regarding the potential adverse effects of steroid exposure in utero (such as from repeated high-dose i.m. betamethasone or dexamethasone to induce fetal lung maturation) and neurodevelopmental problems in the child. It is unlikely that lower doses of prednisolone that does not cross the placenta as well as betamethasone or dexamethasones will have similar adverse effects.
- Oral steroids will increase the risk of infection and gestational diabetes and will cause deterioration in blood–glucose control in women with established diabetes in pregnancy. Blood glucose level should be checked regularly; the hyperglycaemia is amenable to treatment with diet and, if required, insulin and is reversible on cessation or reduction of steroid dose. The development of hyperglycaemia is not an indication to discontinue or decrease the dose of oral steroids, the requirement for which must be determined by the asthma.
- Oral steroids for medical disorders in the mother should not be withheld because of pregnancy.

Other therapies

No adverse fetal effects have been reported with the use of the following drugs:

- Inhaled chromoglycates [e.g., disodium cromoglycate (Intal®); nedocromil (Tilade®)]
- Inhaled anticholinergic drugs [e.g., ipratropium bromide (Atrovent®)].

Methylxanthines

- No significant association has been demonstrated between major congenital malformations or adverse perinatal outcome and exposure to methylxanthines.
- In those few women who are dependent on theophylline, alterations in dose should be guided by drug levels. Both theophylline and aminophylline readily cross the placenta and fetal theophylline levels are similar to those of the mother.

Leukotriene receptor antagonists

- These agents (e.g., montelukast and zafirlukast) block the effects of cysteinyl leukotrienes in the airways.

- There are limited data concerning their use in pregnancy, but small studies do not suggest any increased risk of congenital malformations or other adverse outcomes.
- The current recommendation is to continue them in women who have demonstrated significant improvement in asthma control with these agents where symptom control is not achievable with other medications.

Low-dose aspirin

- It is important to consider the possibility of "aspirin sensitivity" and severe bronchospasm in a minority of women with asthma.
- Low-dose aspirin may be indicated in pregnancy as prophylaxis for certain women at high risk of early-onset pre-eclampsia (see Chapter 1), antiphospholipid syndrome (See Chapter 8), or migraine prophylaxis (see Chapter 9).
- Pregnant women with asthma should be asked about a history of aspirin sensitivity before being advised to take low-dose aspirin.

Acute severe asthma

- Acute severe attacks of asthma are dangerous and should be vigorously managed in hospital.
- The treatment is no different from the emergency management of acute severe asthma in the non-pregnant patient.
- Women with severe asthma and one or more of the following adverse psychosocial factors are at risk of death:
  - Psychiatric illness
  - Drug or alcohol abuse
  - Unemployment
  - Denial
- The features of acute severe asthma are as follows:
  - PEFR 33% to 50% best/predicted
  - Respiratory rate > 25/min
  - Heart rate > 110/min
  - inability to complete sentences in one breath
- The management of acute severe asthma should include the following:
  - High flow oxygen
  - β_2-agonists [e.g., albuterol (Salbutamol) 5 mg] administered via a nebuliser driven by oxygen. Repeated doses or continuous nebulisation may be indicated for those with a poor response
  - Nebulised ipratropium bromide (0.5 mg 4–6 hourly) should be added for severe or poorly responding asthma
  - Corticosteroids [i.v. (hydrocortisone 100 mg) and/or oral (40-50 mg prednisolone for at least 5 days)
  - Intravenous rehydration is often appropriate
  - Chest radiograph should be performed if there is any clinical suspicion of pneumonia or pneumothorax or if the woman fails to improve
- If the PEFR does not improve to >75% predicted, the woman should be admitted to hospital. If she is discharged, this must be with a course of oral steroids and arrangements for review.

- Steroids are more likely to be withheld from pregnant than non-pregnant women with asthma presenting via emergency departments. This is inappropriate and leads to an increase in ongoing exacerbation of asthma.
- Life-threatening clinical features are as follows:
  - PEFR < 33% predicted
  - Oxygen saturation < 92%
  - $pO_2 < 8$ kPa
  - Normal or raised $pCO_2 > 4.6$ kPa
  - Silent chest, cyanosis, feeble respiratory effort
  - Bradycardia, arrythmia, hypotension
  - Exhaustion, confusion, coma
- Management of life-threatening or acute severe asthma that fails to respond should involve consultation with the critical care team and consideration should be given to the following:
  - i.v. β_2-agonists
  - i.v. magnesium sulphate 1.2 to 2 g infusion over 20 minutes
  - i.v. aminophylline

Intrapartum management

- Asthma attacks in labour are exceedingly rare because of endogenous steroid production. Women should not discontinue their inhalers during labour, and there is no evidence to suggest that β_2-agonists given via the inhaled route impair uterine contraction or delay the onset of labour.
- Women receiving oral steroids (prednisolone > 7.5 mg/day for >2 weeks prior to delivery), should receive parenteral hydrocortisone (50–100 mg three or four times/day) to cover the stress of labour and until oral medication is restarted.
- Prostaglandin E2, used to induce labour, to ripen the cervix, or for early termination of pregnancy, is a bronchodilator and is safe to use.
- The use of prostaglandin F2α to treat life-threatening postpartum haemorrhage may be unavoidable, but it can cause bronchospasm and should be used with caution in women with asthma.
- All forms of pain relief in labour, including epidural analgesia and Entonox can be used safely by women with asthma, although in the unlikely event of an acute severe asthmatic attack, opiates for pain relief should only be used with extreme caution. Regional, rather than general anaesthesia, is preferable because of the decreased risk of chest infection and atelectasis.
- Ergometrine has been reported to cause bronchospasm, in particular in association with general anaesthesia, but this does not seem to be a practical problem when Syntometrine® (oxytocin and ergometrine) is used for the prophylaxis of postpartum haemorrhage.

Breast-feeding

- The risk of atopic disease developing in the child of a woman with asthma is about 1 in 10, or 1 in 3 if both parents are atopic. There is some evidence that breast-feeding may reduce this risk. This may be a result of the delay in the introduction of cows' milk protein.
- All the drugs discussed earlier, including oral steroids, are safe to use in breast-feeding mothers.

■ Prednisolone is secreted in breast milk, but there have been no reported adverse clinical effects in infants breast-fed by mothers receiving prednisolone. Concerns regarding neonatal adrenal function are unwarranted with doses less than 30 mg/day.

Asthma—points to remember

■ Pregnancy itself does not usually influence the severity of asthma.
■ For the majority of women, asthma has no adverse effect on pregnancy outcome, and women should be reassured accordingly.
■ Poorly controlled severe asthma presents more of a risk to the pregnancy than the medication used to prevent or treat it. This small risk is minimised with good control.
■ Education and reassurance, ideally prior to pregnancy, concerning the safety of asthma medications during pregnancy, are integral parts of management.
■ Decreasing or stopping inhaled anti-inflammatory therapy during pregnancy is a frequent cause of potentially dangerous deterioration in disease control.
■ Inhaled, oral and i.v. steroids and inhaled, nebulised and i.v. β_2-agonists are safe to use in pregnancy and while breast-feeding.
■ Treatment of asthma in pregnancy differs little from the management in the non-pregnant patient. Effective control of the disease process and its accompanying symptoms is a priority.
■ An increase in the dose or frequency of inhaled steroids should be the first step if symptoms are not optimally controlled on the current dose of inhaled steroids and the inhaler technique is good.

Hay fever

■ Pregnant women should be reassured that there is no evidence to suggest that drugs used to treat hay fever and allergic rhinitis are harmful in pregnancy.
■ Intranasal beclomethasone (Beconase®) is safe.
■ Chlorpheniramine (Piriton®) is a sedating antihistamine but the only antihistamine that does not list pregnancy as a contraindication.
■ The manufacturers of the non-sedating antihistamines including cetirizine and loratadine advise avoidance in pregnancy although high doses of loratadine are not teratogenic in animals. Systematic review does not suggest evidence of adverse outcome with use of cetirazine or loratadine in pregnancy. Use is probably justified during pregnancy if required for control of symptoms.

Pneumonia

■ Bacterial pneumonia is no more common in pregnant than in non-pregnant women of the same age, matched for smoking status.
■ The reduction in cell-mediated immunity renders pregnant women more susceptible to viral pneumonia, for example, influenza pneumonia. In each influenza pandemic (including influenza A H_1N_1), pregnant women have had increased mortality and more virulent disease.
■ Pregnant women are also particularly susceptible to varicella zoster (chicken pox) pneumonia.

Clinical features

Symptoms

- Cough (often dry at first)
- Fever
- Rigors
- Breathlessness
- Pleuritic pain

Signs

- Fever
- Purulent sputum
- Coarse crackles on auscultation
- Signs of consolidation

Pathogenesis

Bacterial

- *Streptococcus pneumoniae* (causative organism in >50% cases)
- *Haemophilus influenzae* (more common in chronic bronchitis)
- *Staphylococcus* (associated with influenza, i.v. drug abuse)
- *Legionella* (institutional outbreaks)

Viral

- Influenza A virus
- Varicella zoster

Other

- *Mycoplasma pneumoniae* (community-acquired, more common during community outbreaks)
- *Pneumocystis carinii* [in association with human immunodeficiency virus (HIV].

Diagnosis

- Diagnosis may be delayed if there is reluctance to perform a chest radiograph.
- The estimated radiation to the fetus from a chest radiograph is less than 0.01 mGy, a fraction of the maximum recommended exposure in pregnancy, that is, 5 rad.
- If a chest radiograph is clinically indicated, this investigation must not be withheld.
- Blood and sputum cultures should be taken especially in those with severe pneumonia.
- Pneumococcal and legionella urine antigen tests should be performed in women with severe pneumonia.
- Bacterial pneumonia is associated with an elevated white blood cell (WBC) count and raised C reactive protein (CRP).
- Mycoplasma pneumonia does not usually cause an elevated WBC count but is associated with cold agglutinins in 50% of cases and may be diagnosed by a rising antibody titre.

- If the patient is breathless, an analysis of arterial blood gases should be performed. Profound hypoxia out of proportion to the chest radiograph findings should alert the clinician to the possibility of *Pneumocystis* infection.
- If the woman fails to respond to conventional antibiotics, a search for non-bacterial causes of pneumonia should be made. Serological assays are the mainstay of diagnosis for atypical and viral respiratory pathogens including *Mycoplasma*. Bronchoscopy may occasionally be indicated, for example if a diagnosis of *Pneumocystis* infection is suspected.

Management

The principles are as follows:

- Maintain adequate oxygenation. Monitor with oximetry and administer oxygen if hypoxic.
- Maintain adequate hydration. The woman is likely to be dehydrated, especially if there is fever.
- Administer physiotherapy to help clear secretions.
- Direct antibiotic therapy at the causative organism:
- Management of bacterial pneumonia in pregnancy should follow the guidelines for treatment in the non-pregnant woman:
  - For most cases of community-acquired pneumonia admitted to hospital (especially if previously treated), oral amoxicillin (500 mg–1 g p.o. tds) and clarithromycin (500 mg b.d.) are the appropriate antibiotics.
  - For severe community-acquired and hospital-acquired pneumonia, i.v. cefuroxime (1.5 g tds) and clarithromycin (500 mg b.d.) should be used. When transferred to oral therapy, this can be with amoxycillin rather than an oral cephalopsporin.
  - Duration of therapy should be for 7 days in uncomplicated cases
  - Tetracyclines should be avoided after about 20 weeks' gestation since they can cause discoloration of the teeth in the fetus.
  - Adverse clinical features include the following:
- Respiratory rate $\geq$ 30/min
- Hypoxaemia; oxygen saturation < 92%, pO_2 < 8 kPa
- Hypotension; systolic blood pressure < 90 mmHg
- Acidosis
- Bilateral or multilobe involvement on chest radiograph

Varicella

- Chicken pox is highly infectious and most children become infected.
- The incubation period is 14 to 21 days and the period of infectivity is from 1 day prior to eruption of the rash to 6 days after the rash disappears.
- Chicken pox is more severe in adults, and pregnant women are particularly susceptible to varicella pneumonia, for which the maternal and fetal mortality rates are high.
- Infection occurs in 0.05% to 0.07% of pregnancies and about 10% to 20% of infected women develop varicella pneumonia.

- A history of previous infection and therefore likely immunity is usually reliable in the case of chicken pox since the clinical features are so unique. Serology can be checked.
- A live attenuated vaccine is available in the United States and should be offered to non-immune women pre-pregnancy.
- Because of the substantial risk accompanying chicken pox infection in pregnancy, non-immune pregnant women exposed to varicella should be given varicella zoster immunoglobulin (VZIG).
- Women should be asked about previous chicken pox infection before they are prescribed steroids in pregnancy, and those found not to be immune should be given VZIG.
- Those women who do develop clinical varicella should be treated with aciclovir and i.v. therapy may be necessary.
- Anyone with varicella should be examined at a distance from the antenatal clinic and ward to minimise exposure to other pregnant women.
- Maternal and neonatal morbidity and mortality in cases of maternal varicella pneumonia justifies the use of i.v. aciclovir.
- A study has suggested that later gestational age (perhaps because of increased immunosuppression) at the onset of varicella pneumonia is a significant risk factor for maternal mortality.
- The fetus is at risk of congenital varicella with maternal infection in the first 12 to 16 weeks of pregnancy. The risk of teratogenicity is approximately 2%.
- Detailed ultrasound scanning should be offered at 16 to 20 weeks' gestation or 5 weeks after infection, whichever is sooner. The most common abnormalities are dermatomal skin scarring, eye defects, limb hypoplasia, and neurological abnormalities.
- There is a risk of neonatal varicella if infection occurs within 10 days of delivery. If practical, delivery should be delayed until 5 to 7 days after the onset of maternal illness to allow passive transfer of antibodies. If delivery occurs within 5 days of maternal infection or if the mother develops chicken pox within 2 days of giving birth, the neonate should receive VZIG. This does not prevent all cases of neonatal infection, which may be fatal (30% mortality rate).

Pneumocystis carinii pneumonia

- The increasing number of women of childbearing age who are seropositive for HIV has contributed to the increased incidence of pneumonia in pregnancy.
- The most common opportunistic infection in patients progressing to acquired immune deficiency syndrome (AIDS) is pneumocystis carinii pneumonia (PCP).
- PCP is associated with adverse obstetric outcome, particularly if the diagnosis is not suspected.
- PCP should be treated with high-dose trimethoprim-sulphamethoxazole [co-trimoxazole (Septrin)] with or without pentamidine.
- Despite the theoretical risks of neonatal kernicterus or haemolysis from sulfonamides given at term, there is increasing evidence that co-trimoxazole use is safe in pregnancy. Indeed, PCP is one of the remaining indications for the use of co-trimoxazole. In practice, it is only long-acting sulphonamides such as sulphadimidine that have ever been shown to affect the binding of bilirubin in the fetus or neonate.

- Because PCP is an important cause of AIDS-related maternal mortality, HIV-infected pregnant women with a history of this opportunistic infection or with a CD4+ cell count of <200 cells/μL should receive prophylaxis with either co-trimoxazole or nebulised pentamidine.

(See also HIV Infection in Pregnancy, Chapter 15).

Pneumonia—points to remember

- Chest radiographs are safe to use in pregnancy.
- Most antibiotics are safe to use in pregnancy and during lactation; caution is required with aminoglycosides and tetracycline.
- A higher dose (500 mg t.d.s.) of amoxycillin is required in pregnancy.
- Varicella and influenza A pneumonia may be fatal in pregnancy and active steps must be taken to prevent chicken pox infection in pregnancy.
- Non-immune pregnant women exposed to varicella or prescribed steroids in pregnancy should be given VZIG.
- If a pregnant woman does contract chicken pox, she should be treated with aciclovir as soon as possible.

Tuberculosis

- Incidence rates of tuberculosis (TB) are increasing in the United Kingdom, Europe, the United States, and developing countries.
- This recent resurgence is partly due to the susceptibility of HIV-infected patients to TB infection.
- In the United Kingdom and the United States, there are reports of increasing rates among the homeless and in inner-city populations. In New York, the United States, rates of pulmonary TB in pregnant women increased almost eightfold between 1985 and 1992.
- A recent cohort study from the United Kingdom showed that TB in pregnancy is limited to ethnic minority women, most commonly those recently arrived from Asia and Africa.
- Recent studies also suggest that among women with TB in pregnancy, there is a high prevalence (50%) of extrapulmonary TB.

Clinical features

Symptoms

The onset is usually insidious, and symptoms include the following:

- Cough
- Haemoptysis
- Weight loss (or failure to gain weight)
- Night sweats

Signs

- TB can cause almost any chest signs.
- It most typically affects the upper lobes, with coarse crackles, dullness on percussion over the clavicle, or in advanced or old cases, signs of fibrosis with deviation of the trachea towards the side of the infection.
- Signs of associated lymphadenopathy, and erythema nodosum (see also p. 232).
- Extrapulmonary sites include the following:
  - Lymph nodes
  - Bone
  - Liver and spleen
  - Bone marrow
  - Caecum
  - Central nervous system (CNS)
  - Eye (choroidal tubercles)

Pathogenesis

- Causative organism is *Mycobacterium tuberculosis* (MBTB).
- *Mycobacterium avium-intracellulare* is an important cause of pulmonary infection in HIV patients.

Diagnosis

- This is suggested by the typical appearances on a chest radiograph.
- Diagnosis is confirmed by sputum examination for acid-fast bacilli (Ziehl–Neelsen stain).
- Culture of the organism takes approximately 6 weeks.
- If there is no sputum, washings from bronchoscopy must be obtained.
- The Mantoux test (0.1 mL of 10 tuberculin units of purified protein derivative of MBTB) is not affected by pregnancy.
- Newer diagnostic blood tests include interferon-γ release assays such as the enzyme-linked immunospot (ELISPOT) assays and QuantiFERON–TB. These blood tests can distinguish latent TB from bacille Calmette-Guérin (BCG). They have greater specificity for diagnosing latent rather than active TB.

Pregnancy

Effect of pregnancy on TB

- There is little evidence to suggest that TB has a detrimental effect on pregnancy or that pregnancy adversely affects disease progression in patients receiving, or who have received, effective anti-TB therapy.
- Congenital TB with infection via the umbilical vein or amniotic fluid is rare. Neonatal TB via airborne inoculation from the infected mother with active but undiagnosed or untreated TB is important in developing countries.

Management

- The principles of management are similar in pregnant and non-pregnant patients.
- Untreated TB represents a greater hazard to pregnant women and their fetuses than the treatment itself.

- The advice of a respiratory physician must be sought and pregnant mothers with TB should be treated without delay.
- Active disease should be treated with a prolonged supervised course of more than one drug to which the organism is sensitive. Before sensitivities are available, most patients are given triple/quadruple therapy with the following:
  - Rifampicin
  - Isoniazid
  - Pyrazinamide and/or ethambutol

Liver function should be monitored monthly because of the risk of isoniazid- or rifampicin-related hepatotoxicity.

In the event that the transaminase levels more than double, all anti-TB chemotherapy should be temporarily withdrawn and then individual agents introduced in a step-wise fashion while liver function tests are monitored closely.

Potential risk to the fetus of anti-TB chemotherapy

- Rifampicin, isoniazid, ethambutol and pyrazinamide are safe to use in pregnancy, but all patients taking isoniazid should also be prescribed pyridoxine 50 mg/day to reduce the risk of peripheral neuritis
- Streptomycin has been associated with a high (>10%) incidence of eighth nerve damage and should therefore be avoided throughout pregnancy.
- Since rifampicin induces the enzyme cytochrome P450, vitamin K should be given to the mother in the same way it is given to mothers receiving enzyme-inducing antiepileptic drugs (see page 156).

Postnatal care

- The mother usually becomes non-infectious within 2 weeks of beginning treatment.
- If the mother is sputum-positive for TB, the risk of the neonate developing active TB is high unless prophylactic treatment with isoniazid (assuming the mother's organism is isoniazid sensitive) is given.
- The baby should also be given BCG vaccination. As isoniazid does not impair the immunogenicity of the BCG vaccine, there is no benefit of using isoniazid-resistant strains of BCG for combined prophylaxis.
- The amounts of anti-TB drugs excreted in breast milk are only a fraction of the usual therapeutic dose and are not sufficient to dissuade women from breast-feeding.

Tuberculosis—points to remember

- TB is particularly common in Asian and African immigrants.
- Perform a chest radiograph if TB is suspected.
- Seek the advice of a respiratory physician.
- Diagnosis must be confirmed bacteriologically, which may necessitate bronchoscopy. New blood tests using interferon-γ release assays are available.
- Give BCG to the neonate and isoniazid in high-risk cases.

Sarcoidosis

Sarcoidosis is uncommon in pregnancy, perhaps affecting 0.05% of all pregnancies in the United Kingdom.

Clinical features

- There may be chest symptoms, but the patient is often asymptomatic. Common symptoms include breathlessness and cough.
- Extrapulmonary manifestations include the following:
  - Erythema nodosum (may also occur as an isolated finding in pregnancy without evidence of an underlying associated cause) (see also Chapter 13, p. 232)
  - Anterior uveitis
  - Hypercalcaemia
  - Arthropathy
  - Fever
  - CNS involvement.

Pathogenesis

- Sarcoidosis is a multi-system granulomatous disorder of unknown aetiology.
- Unlike TB, the granulomata are non-caseating.

Diagnosis

- Chest radiograph. The commonest feature is bilateral hilar lymphadenopathy. There may be upper lobe or extensive pulmonary infiltration progressing to fibrosis.
- Although there may be no obvious infiltration in the lung fields, the lung parenchyma is usually involved with interstitial lung disease (ILD) and diagnosis is made by high-resolution computed tomography, bronchoalveolar lavage and transbronchial biopsy.
- Lung function may be affected and the transfer factor or diffusing capacity for carbon monoxide (KCO) reduced. Transfer factor is reduced in patients with ILD secondary to thickening of the alveolar-capillary barrier which impairs gas exchange. This measurement is not affected by pregnancy and can be used to monitor disease activity.
- Serum levels of angiotensin-converting enzyme (ACE) may be altered in normal pregnancy and cannot therefore be used to help diagnosis or monitor disease activity as in the non-pregnant patient.

Effect of pregnancy on sarcoidosis

- The course of the disease may be unaffected or improved by pregnancy.
- Those with active disease may have resolution of their radiograph changes during pregnancy and there is a tendency for sarcoidosis to relapse in the puerperium.
- Any improvement that is seen antenatally may be due to the increased levels of endogenous cortisol present in pregnancy.

Management

■ Sarcoidosis often resolves spontaneously, but indications for steroid treatment include the following:
  – Extrapulmonary, especially CNS, disease
  – Functional respiratory impairment.
■ The safety of steroids in pregnancy has been discussed earlier (see under "Asthma," p. 61), and they should be continued or started in pregnancy if clinically indicated.
■ As with asthma, women receiving maintenance steroids, should be covered in labour and delivery with parenteral hydrocortisone if they are taking >7.5 mg daily prednisolone (see p. 64).
■ Azathioprine is also safe in pregnancy and should be continued (see Chapter 8, p. 132).
■ Women should be advised not to take supplemental vitamin D, unless there is proven vitamin D deficiency, since it may precipitate hypercalcaemia in patients with sarcoidosis.

Sarcoidosis—points to remember

■ Erythema nodosum may occur in a normal pregnancy.
■ The course of sarcoidosis is unaltered or improved by pregnancy.
■ Use systemic steroids and azathioprine if indicated.
■ Consider a prophylactic increase in steroid dose postpartum.
■ Serum ACE is not useful in pregnancy.
■ Avoid vitamin D unless there is proven vitamin D deficiency.

Cystic fibrosis

Increasing numbers of children with cystic fibrosis (CF) are surviving into adulthood. Males are usually sterile, but although female fertility may be impaired in the malnourished or due to tenacious cervical mucus, it is usually normal.

Clinical features

■ Early, repeated, and persistent lung infection, bronchiectasis, and respiratory failure
■ Pancreatic insufficiency leading to malnutrition and diabetes
■ The median age at death for CF patients is now more than 30 years.

Pathogenesis

■ CF is due to a dysfunction of all exocrine glands with abnormal mucus production and high sweat sodium level.
■ It is the commonest autosomal recessive disorder in the United Kingdom, with a carrier rate of 1 in 25 in Caucasians.
■ Although a specific mutation on chromosome 7 has been identified, only two-third cases have the deletion and patients with CF are heterogeneous and include different genetic errors or altered penetration.
■ CF is caused by abnormalities in the CF transmembrane conductance regulator (CFTR) protein, a transmembranous chloride channel, causing impaired movement

73

of water and electrolytes across epithelial surfaces. This leads to impaired hydration of secretions in glandular organs, thick mucus and increased sweat sodium level.

■ Gene therapy offers the potential of a more effective approach to the treatment of CF, but although clinical trials are in progress, this has yet to become a routine option in CF patients.

■ Lung or heart lung transplantation may offer prolonged survival.

Pregnancy

Effect of pregnancy on CF

■ Most patients with CF die in early adult life, but with few exceptions (see later), pregnancy does not increase this risk.

■ Maternal mortality is significantly increased compared with normal pregnant women.

■ Maternal mortality is not significantly greater than non-pregnant age-matched women with CF.

■ Pregnancy is well tolerated by most mothers with CF (perhaps because those who survive and become pregnant have a less severe form of the disease).

■ Mortality is increased in women with moderate to severe lung disease ($FEV_1 < 60\%$ predicted) at the onset of pregnancy and maternal survival is positively correlated with pre-pregnancy percentage predicted FEV_1.

■ Other adverse factors on maternal disease are similar to those that adversely affect fetal morbidity and mortality (see later), namely maternal pulmonary hypertension, cyanosis and hypoxaemia.

■ Women may deteriorate and die while the child is still young and it is important that such issues are discussed with women and their partners prior to pregnancy.

The main maternal morbidities in CF pregnancies are as follows:

■ Poor maternal weight gain. Even those without pancreatic insufficiency are often underweight at the onset of pregnancy and have difficulty gaining weight during pregnancy.

■ Deterioration in lung function with worsening dyspnoea, exercise tolerance and oxygen saturation. Although there is usually loss of lung function during pregnancy, this is regained following delivery.

■ Pulmonary infective exacerbations

■ Congestive cardiac failure

Effect of CF on pregnancy

■ The rate of spontaneous miscarriage is not increased in CF pregnancies.

■ Despite the frequent use of high doses of antibiotics in these women, the rate of congenital abnormalities is not increased.

■ Factors predicting a poor obstetric outcome include the following:
 – Pulmonary hypertension
 – Cyanosis
 – Arterial hypoxaemia (oxygen saturation <90%)
 – Moderate to severe lung disease (FEV_1 <60% predicted)
 – Poor maternal nutrition.

The commonest complications during pregnancy are

- Prematurity [the preterm (<37 weeks) delivery rate is 20–50%]
- Fetal growth restriction, chronic hypoxia (oxygen saturation <90%) and/or cyanosis increase the risk of small-for-gestational-age infants. Birth-weight is positively correlated with pre-pregnancy lung function (probably related to longer gestations).
- Women with preserved pancreatic function have improved pregnancy outcome. Poor maternal weight gain is predictive of both preterm delivery and stillbirth.

Pre-pregnancy counselling

- This is essential. Pregnancy is safe in mild disease with FEV_1 > 70% to 80% predicted but the following are contraindications to pregnancy:
  - Pulmonary hypertension
  - Cor pulmonale
  - FEV_1 < 30% to 40% predicted
- Since *Burkholderia cepacia* may be associated with rapid deterioration in lung function, recent acquisition or declining lung function in the presence of this organism may also be a contraindication to pregnancy.
- Screening for diabetes should be undertaken.
- Since all women with CF are homozygous, all offspring will be carriers of the CF gene.
- Determination of the carrier status of the partner. The risk of a child being born with CF is 2% to 2.5% if the carrier status of the father is unknown (based on a carrier rate in the general U.K. population of about 1 in 25) and 50% if the father is heterozygous for the gene.

Management

During pregnancy, women with CF should be jointly managed by a CF centre and a specialist obstetric unit with experience in the management of such women.

Medical management during pregnancy should include attention to the following:

- Adequate maternal nutrition
- Control of pulmonary infection
- Avoidance of prolonged hypoxia
- Regular assessment of fetal growth

Nutrition

- Of adult CF patients, more than 90% have pancreatic insufficiency and require enzyme supplements. Fat-soluble vitamin supplements should be continued. High-calorie dietary supplements may be required to maintain maternal weight, since patients with CF (even without malabsorption) have high energy requirements that will be further increased by pregnancy.
- Of adult CF patients, 20% have diabetes and a further 15% have impaired glucose tolerance (IGT). Insulin requirements increase in pregnancy and those with IGT will be at risk of gestational diabetes (see p. 89).

Control of pulmonary infection

- Obsessional adherence to chest physiotherapy regimes must be encouraged. Some women decrease their physiotherapy due to fears concerning the fetus. These fears should be allayed.
- Most of the older, more established antibiotics (e.g., cefuroxime) used to treat pulmonary infective exacerbations in CF have a good safety record in pregnancy. Appropriate caution is needed when considering the use of newer drugs (e.g., imipenem) for which there are fewer data in pregnancy. The risks to the fetus from poor maternal health probably outweigh the risks to the fetus from transplacental passage of drugs.
- Some patients may be taking prophylactic antibiotics either orally or via a nebuliser. Except in the case of tetracycline, which is contraindicated in pregnancy because of the effects on fetal teeth and skeleton, these should usually be continued throughout pregnancy.
- Infective exacerbations should be treated aggressively and this is likely to require admission and i.v. penicillins and aminoglycosides, or cephalosporins in cases of resistant *Pseudomonas*.
- Antibiotic therapy must be dictated by the results of sputum cultures.
- Caution is needed when using i.v. aminoglycosides in pregnancy and regular monitoring of drug levels is required.

Some patients with CF exhibit reversibility in response to bronchodilators, and women should be reassured that inhaled and nebulised corticosteroids are safe for use in pregnancy (see p. 61).

Inhaled dornase alfa (recombinant human deoxyribonuclease) hydrolyzes the DNA in the sputum, reducing the viscosity, and is probably safe and should be continued in pregnancy.

Avoidance of prolonged hypoxia and timing of delivery

- Towards the middle and end of the third trimester, women with CF often become increasingly breathless, often without any obvious infective exacerbation.
- If there is resting hypoxia, and especially if oxygen saturation (%) is in the 80s or low 90s, admission for bed rest and oxygen therapy is advised.
- In some women, symptom deterioration warrants early delivery.
- The fetus is at risk of growth restriction; and therefore, the mother should be offered growth scans throughout pregnancy.
- If the growth rate slows, it may sometimes be improved by admission of the mother for bed rest, nutritional supplements and oxygen.
- In most cases, CF women deliver vaginally at term.
- Caesarean section is necessary only for obstetric indications and general anaesthesia should be avoided if possible.
- Instrumental delivery may be indicated to avoid a prolonged second stage.
- Patients with CF are particularly prone to pneumothoraces, which may be precipitated by prolonged attempts at pushing and repeated Valsalva manoeuvres in the second stage of labour.
- Breast-feeding should usually be encouraged, although the mother may continue to require nutritional supplements in the puerperium, especially if she is breast-feeding. Most of the drugs used will be secreted into the breast milk, but this is

rarely a contraindication to breast-feeding. Analysis of breast milk of women with CF has shown normal content of sodium and protein.

Cystic fibrosis—points to remember

- Joint care should be maintained with a CF centre.
- Outcome is related to pre-pregnancy lung function.
- Perinatal outcome is usually good.
- Preterm delivery rates are high.
- Maternal outcome is variable and worse in the presence of cor pulmonale/ pulmonary hypertension.
- Specialist dietary advice with additional energy supplements should be given.
- Infective exacerbations should be treated aggressively.
- There is a risk of gestational diabetes.
- Induction of labour/early delivery may be necessary for relief of maternal symptoms.

Severe restrictive and interstitial lung disease

- Patients with severe lung disease are less likely to deteriorate in pregnancy than those with severe cardiac disease; this is because there is greater reserve in respiratory function than in cardiac function. Thus, although there is a comparative (approximately 40%) increase in both cardiac output and minute ventilation in pregnancy, for minute ventilation this represents a smaller fraction of the maximum increase achievable by the body.
- It is difficult to predict with any accuracy the minimal FVC compatible with successful pregnancy outcome in patients with kyphoscoliosis, scleroderma (see Chapter 8, p. 145) and other causes of severe restrictive lung disease. Although figures such as 1 L or 50% of predicted FVC have been suggested, women with more severe impairment have had successful pregnancies.
- In women with interstitial lung disease (ILD), e.g., sarcoidosis, connective tissue disease, non-specific interstitial pneumonia, serial measurement of transfer factor is used to track progression of disease.
- Polycythaemia gives an indirect assessment of the degree of hypoxia and, in itself, is associated with an increased risk of thrombosis due to hyperviscosity.
- Women with kyphoscoliosis are often delivered prematurely due to deterioration in respiratory function in the third trimester and by caesarean section because of associated abnormalities of the bony pelvis and of abnormal presentations of the fetus.
- Each case must be assessed individually. Whatever the underlying cause of respiratory insufficiency, significant reduction in transfer factor, hypercapnia or hypoxia and pulmonary hypertension and cor pulmonale are associated with less favourable pregnancy outcomes.

Management

This should start with pre-pregnancy counselling.

Multidisciplinary care and delivery planning is essential, especially with respiratory physicians for those with nocturnal hypoxia or hypercapnia who may require non-invasive ventilation.

Liaison with obstetric anaesthetists is important. Regional analgesia/anaesthesia where the block is high may be dangerous in a woman with limited respiratory reserve. In addition, some women have had Harrington rods inserted that may preclude regional anaesthesia.

Severe restrictive lung disease—points to remember

- Women with severe lung disease are better able to tolerate pregnancy than women with severe cardiac insufficiency.
- If the FVC is >1l, a successful pregnancy is usually possible, but individual assessment is necessary.
- Respiratory diseases complicated by pulmonary hypertension and cor pulmonale have a poor prognosis in pregnancy.

Further reading

British Thoracic Society, Scottish Intercollegiate Guidelines Network. British guideline in asthma management. Thorax 2008; 63(suppl IV):iv1–iv121. http://www.sign.ac.uk/guidelines/fulltext/101/index.html. Published May 2008. Revised June 2009. Accessed March 2010.

British Thoracic Society: Guidelines for the management of community acquired pneumonia. Thorax 2001; 56(suppl IV) and 2004; 59:364–366 (update). http://www.brit-thoracic.org.uk/c2/uploads/MACAPrevisedApr04.pdf. Accessed March 2010.

Edenborough FP, Borgo G, Knoop C, et al. Guidelines for the management of pregnancy in women with cystic fibrosis [published online ahead of print November 19, 2007]. J Cyst Fibros 2008; 7(suppl 1):S2–S32.

Knight M, Kurinczuk JJ, Nelson-Piercy C, et al. Tuberculosis in pregnancy in the UK. BJOG 2009; 116:584–588.

Royal College of Obstetricians and Gynaecologists. Chicken Pox in Pregnancy: Green Top Guideline No 13. London, England: Royal College of Obstetricians and Gynaecologists. http://www.rcog.org.uk/files/rcog-corp/uploaded-files/GT13ChickenpoxinPregnancy2007.pdf. Accessed March 2010.

Schatz M, Dombrowski MP. Asthma in pregnancy. N Engl J Med 2009; 360(18):1862–1869.

CHAPTER 5

Diabetes mellitus

Physiological changes	Gestational diabetes mellitus
Pre-existing diabetes mellitus	

Physiological changes

- Pregnancy, especially the last trimester, is a state of physiological insulin resistance and relative glucose intolerance.
- Glucose handling is significantly altered in pregnancy; fasting levels of glucose are decreased and serum levels following a meal or glucose load are increased compared with the non-pregnant state.
- Glucose tolerance decreases progressively with increasing gestation; this is largely due to the anti-insulin hormones secreted by the placenta in normal pregnancy, particularly human placental lactogen, glucagons and cortisol.
- Normal women show an approximate doubling of insulin production from the end of the first trimester to the third trimester.
- These physiological changes are likely to underlie the increased insulin requirements of women with established diabetes and the development of abnormal glucose tolerance in gestational diabetes, where there is insufficient insulin secretion to compensate for the insulin resistance.
- The diagnosis of gestational diabetes mellitus (GDM) is arbitrary depending on where the "cut-off" is placed on the normal spectrum of glucose tolerance in pregnancy.
- The renal tubular threshold for glucose falls during pregnancy. There is a tendency for glycosuria to increase as pregnancy advances, and if all urine samples are tested, most pregnant women will have glycosuria at some time. Glycosuria is not a reliable diagnostic tool for impaired glucose tolerance or diabetes in pregnancy.
- In normal pregnancy, starvation results in early breakdown of triglyceride, resulting in the liberation of fatty acids and ketone bodies.

Pre-existing diabetes mellitus

Pre-existing diabetes (Fig. 5.1) may be divided into types 1 and 2:

- Type 1, insulin-dependent diabetes mellitus—juvenile-onset.
- Type 2, non–insulin-dependent diabetes mellitus—maturity-onset.

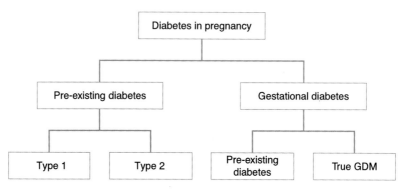

Figure 5.1 – Classification of diabetes in pregnancy.

Incidence

In the United Kingdom, the prevalence of type 1 is approximately 0.5% and that of type 2 is approximately 3% to 4% (lower in women of childbearing age but higher in Afro-Caribbean and 10% in Asian immigrants).

The prevalence of pre-existing diabetes in pregnancy in the United Kingdom is approximately 0.4%.

Clinical features

Type 1

- Patients usually present as children or young adults (age 11–14 years).
- Most commonly affects Europeans who are not usually overweight.
- The clinical features relate to absolute insulin deficiency that, if untreated, causes thirst, polyuria, blurred vision, weight loss and ketoacidosis (Table 5.1).

Type 2

- Patients are usually older and often overweight.
- All racial groups are affected, but in the United Kingdom, it is more common in Asian, Afro-Caribbean and Middle Eastern immigrants.
- It is becoming more common in pregnancy as the prevalence of obesity and older age increases in pregnancy.
- Type 2 diabetes is caused by peripheral insulin resistance and a state in which the body is unable to compensate for this by increasing insulin secretion.
- Individuals with type 2 diabetes can have hyperglycaemia for a long period without clinical symptoms. It is therefore important to screen for possible occult long-term complications of the condition at the time of diagnosis.
- Although insulin is sometimes required to treat these patients, they do not become ketotic if it is withdrawn.

Diabetes (both type 1 and type 2) may present with the classical features mentioned earlier or with complications such as the following:

- *Candida* infection (pruritus vulvae)

Table 5.1 – Complications of pregnancy in pre-existing diabetes

Maternal	Fetal
Increased insulin requirements	Congenital abnormalities
Hypoglycaemia	Increased neonatal mortality
Infection	Increased perinatal mortality
Ketoacidosis	Macrosomia
Deterioration in retinopathy	Late stillbirth
Increased proteinuria and oedema	Preterm delivery (partly iatrogenic)
Miscarriage	Neonatal hypoglycaemia
Polyhydramnios	Polycythaemia
Shoulder dystocia	Jaundice
Pre-eclampsia	Respiratory distress syndrome
Increased caesarean section rate	

- Staphylococcal skin infections
- Macrovascular arterial disease (coronary artery disease, cerebrovascular disease, peripheral vascular disease)
- Microvascular disease (diabetic retinopathy, diabetic nephropathy, diabetic neuropathy).

Women with diabetes have a reduced life expectancy related to accelerated arterial disease (twofold risk of stroke, fourfold risk of myocardial infarction) and microangiopathy.

Pathogenesis

Type 1

This is an organ-specific autoimmune disease associated with serological evidence of autoimmune destruction of the pancreas and islet-cell antibodies. There is a genetic component and a strong association with the human leukocyte antigens HLA-DR3 and DR4. A possible viral component to the aetiology is thought to explain the seasonal incidence (spring and autumn).

Type 2

There is no evidence of immune pathogenesis in contrast to type 1. The genetic component is much stronger than in type 1. The incidence increases with age and the degree of obesity.

Diagnosis of diabetes mellitus (in non-pregnant women)

One of the following criteria must be confirmed by repeated testing on a subsequent day unless the patient is symptomatic (i.e., polyuria, polydipsia and unexplained weight loss) in which case, a single abnormal value suffices:

- a random venous plasma glucose concentration ≥ 11.1 mmol/L *or*
- a fasting plasma glucose concentration ≥ 7.0 mmol/L (whole blood ≥ 6.1 mmol/L) *or*
- 2-hour plasma glucose concentration ≥ 11.1 mmol/L 2 hours after 75 g anhydrous glucose in an oral glucose tolerance test (OGTT).

Diagnosis of impaired glucose tolerance

Impaired glucose tolerance (IGT) is a stage of impaired glucose regulation (fasting plasma glucose < 7.0 mmol/L and OGTT 2-hour value ≥ 7.8 mmol/L but < 11.1 mmol/L).

Pregnancy

Effect of pregnancy on diabetes

- Since normal pregnancy is associated with an increase in insulin production and insulin resistance, women with type 1 diabetes require increasing doses of insulin as pregnancy progresses. Maximum requirements at term usually reach at least twofold pre-pregnancy doses. Women with type 2 diabetes often need the addition of insulin to their therapy or increasing doses of insulin. Rapid increases in insulin requirements occur particularly between approximately 28 and 32 weeks' gestation, when the fetus is growing rapidly.
- Women with diabetic nephropathy may experience deterioration during pregnancy in both renal function but particularly the degree of proteinuria. Deterioration in renal function (that may be irreversible) is more likely in those with moderate and severe renal impairment (creatinine > 125 μmol/L pre-pregnancy) and those with hypertension (see Chapter 10). In contrast, any deterioration in those with mild renal impairment is usually reversed following delivery, and there is no long-term detrimental effect of pregnancy on renal function.
- There is a twofold risk of progression of diabetic retinopathy during pregnancy and women with diabetes may develop retinopathy for the first time in pregnancy. The worsening retinopathy is often related to the rapid improvement in glycaemic control, which is a feature of early pregnancy, and to the increase in retinal blood flow. The risk is higher for those with type 1 than for those with type 2 diabetes and is increased with poor metabolic control, diastolic hypertension, renal disease, anaemia, and severity of baseline retinopathy.
- Hypoglycaemia is more common in pregnancy (largely related to intensified diabetic control) and may be associated with relative "hypoglycaemia unawareness." Most maternal deaths in the United Kingdom caused by diabetes are due to hypoglycaemia.
- For every 1% fall in glycated haemoglobin (HbA_{1C}) level, there is a 33% increase in hypoglycaemic attacks.

■ Diabetic ketoacidosis is rare in pregnancy, probably in part related to the close supervision, but is a risk in the presence of hyperemesis, infection, tocolytic therapy with β-sympathomimetics or corticosteroid therapy.

■ Women with autonomic neuropathy and gastric paresis often experience deterioration of their symptoms in pregnancy.

Effect of pre-existing diabetes on pregnancy

Maternal considerations

■ Women with poorly controlled diabetes have an increased risk of miscarriage.

■ Women with diabetes have a threefold to fourfold increased risk of pre-eclampsia. This risk is further increased if there is pre-existing hypertension or renal disease (the risk is approximately 30% if nephropathy and hypertension are present).

■ The risk of pre-eclampsia also relates to glycaemic control at conception and in the first half of pregnancy. Each 1% increment in first trimester HbA_{1C} level increases the risk of pre-eclampsia by 60%, and each 1% fall in HbA_{1C} achieved < 20 weeks reduces the risk by 40%.

■ Pregnancies in women with diabetic nephropathy are often complicated by severe oedema related to proteinuria and hypoalbuminaemia, and a normochromic normocytic anaemia that may only respond to treatment with recombinant erythropoietin.

■ Diabetes greatly increases the risk of infection during pregnancy, particularly urinary tract, respiratory, endometrial and wound infections. Vaginal candidiasis is very common in pregnant women with diabetes.

■ The caesarean section rate is increased to approximately 65%. This is at least partly related to early induction of labour.

Fetal considerations

■ There is an increased risk of congenital abnormalities. In the Confidential Enquiry into Maternal and Child Health (CEMACH) study of pre-existing diabetes, the overall rate was 4% (double background) with a threefold increase in the rates of both neural tube defects and congenital heart disease. The level of risk is directly related to the degree of glycaemic control around the time of conception and directly correlated with the HbA_{1C} level. Women with HbA_{1C} < 8% have a risk of approximately 5%, but in those with levels > 10%, the risk is as high as 25%. The risk is eliminated if normal HbA_{1C} levels are achieved. The recommendation is that the HbA_{1C} should be < 6.1% at the time of conception if this can be safely achieved.

■ The specific congenital abnormality associated with diabetes is sacral agenesis, but this is very rare. Much more common are congenital heart defects, skeletal abnormalities and neural tube defects.

■ The perinatal and neonatal mortality rates can be increased 5- to 10-fold in babies of mothers with diabetes, and these too relate to HbA_{1C} at conception and in early pregnancy. In the CEMACH study of diabetes in pregnancy in the United Kingdom, the perinatal mortality rate for both type 1 and type 2 diabetes was approximately 3%.

■ Fetuses of diabetic mothers are at risk of sudden unexplained intrauterine death (IUD). Again, this risk is inversely related to the degree of diabetic control and is highest after 36 weeks' gestation. Various factors may explain these sudden losses including chronic hypoxia (more common in macrosomic babies, see later) in the presence of hyperglycaemia and lactic acidosis. It is not possible to predict IUD from the cardiotocograph, Doppler velocimetry or biophysical profiles.

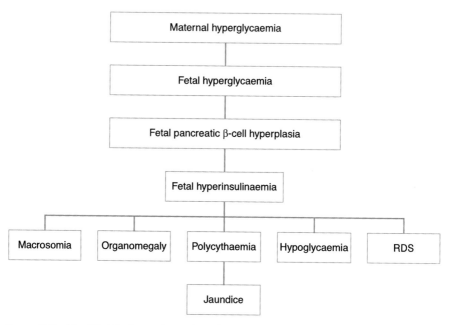

Figure 5.2 – Modified Pederson hypothesis for pathophysiology of fetal effects in diabetic pregnancy. RDS: respiratory diabetes syndrome.

- Maternal hyperglycaemia, and particularly ketoacidosis, is detrimental to the fetus, and maternal ketoacidosis is associated with a high (20–50%) fetal mortality rate.
- In contrast, maternal hypoglycaemia is well tolerated by the fetus.
- Neonatal morbidity is increased in infants of diabetic mothers. The various complications may be explained by the modified Pederson hypothesis (Fig. 5.2).
- Fetal hyperinsulinaemia may lead to chronic fetal hypoxia, which in turn stimulates extramedullary haemopoiesis, fetal polycythaemia and neonatal jaundice.
- There is an increase in respiratory distress syndrome in infants of diabetic mothers, not totally accounted for by the increased caesarean section and preterm delivery rates.
- Macrosomia has different definitions but is conventionally defined as a birth-weight > 4.5 kg or > 90th centile for gestational age. Insulin is an anabolic, growth-promoting hormone, and the macrosomic baby of the mother with diabetes is characteristically fat and plethoric, with all organs, but particularly the liver, being enlarged.
- Macrosomia is more common with poor diabetic control but may also occur in cases of excellent control. The incidence of macrosomia increases significantly when mean maternal blood glucose concentrations are > 7.2 mmol/L. In the CEMACH diabetes in pregnancy study, the incidence of birth-weight > 4 kg was 21% and the incidence of shoulder dystocia was 8%.
- In the presence of fetal hyperinsulinaemia, when the cord is clamped, the neonate is "cut-off" from its supply of glucose from the mother and is at risk of neonatal hypoglycaemia.

■ Macrosomia is often associated with polyhydramnios (related to fetal polyuria), which carries the risk of premature rupture of the membranes and cord prolapse. Macrosomia increases the risk of traumatic delivery, particularly shoulder dystocia.

Management

■ Women with diabetes who are planning a pregnancy should be referred for specialist pre-pregnancy counselling (see later, p. 88).
■ Pregnant women with diabetes should be managed in joint pregnancy diabetic clinics by obstetricians and physicians with expertise in the care of such women. Such multidisciplinary clinics should be attended by specialist dieticians, nurses and midwives who are experienced in the care of pregnant women with diabetes.
■ There is evidence that outcomes can be improved with such tertiary level care.

Medical management

■ The most important goal of management is to achieve maternal near-normoglycaemia as so many adverse perinatal outcomes are related to the degree of maternal diabetic control.
■ To achieve the desired level of control, pregnant women with diabetes will need to increase the frequency of home blood-glucose monitoring (HBGM), using glucose oxidase strips and preferably glucose meters.
■ This is especially so in early pregnancy, when control is first tightened and during periods when insulin doses are altered. HBGM also gives the woman the independence to adjust her own insulin dosages, and this is to be encouraged.
■ Target capillary blood glucose concentrations are 3.5 to 5.9 mmol/L fasting and < 7.8 mmol/L 1 hour postprandial (these targets are the same for type 1, type 2 and gestational diabetes).
■ Outcomes such as birth-weight and neonatal hypoglycaemia correlate better with postprandial than with preprandial glucose levels.
■ Using postprandial targets also leads to better improvements in maternal HbA_{1C} levels.

Management of type 1 diabetes

■ Women with type 1 diabetes require increasing doses of insulin throughout pregnancy, although insulin requirements may fall in the first trimester.
■ The inevitable result of tighter control is an increased risk of hypoglycaemic attacks. Women should be warned about the risks of hypoglycaemia and hypoglycaemia unawareness particularly in the first trimester.
■ Pregnant women with diabetes will usually require a "snack" mid-morning, mid-afternoon and before retiring at night. Women should be provided with concentrated glucose solution for use in the event of hypoglycaemia. Relatives or partners may be taught how to administer i.m. glucagon injections to avert profound hypoglycaemia in situations where the woman is unable or unwilling to eat or drink. The woman should be advised that glucagon provides only temporary relief from hypoglycaemia and should always be followed by oral intake of glucose-containing food or drink.

- Four-times-daily basal bolus regimens achieve better glycaemic control compared with regimes using mixed insulins (e.g., Mixtard®).
- Rapid-acting insulin analogues (Humalog insulin lispro; Novorapid insulin aspart) are associated with fewer instances of neonatal and maternal hypoglycaemia. They are used in combination with basal isophane insulin.
- Rapid-acting insulin analogues have a shorter time (1 hour) to peak action and can therefore be taken at the same time rather than before a meal.
- Women who continue to experience disabling hypoglycaemia despite the use of rapid-acting insulin analogues may be considered for insulin pump therapy.
- Data are accumulating regarding the safety of the long-acting insulin analogues detemir and glargine in pregnancy.
- As in the non-pregnant diabetic patient, insulin should not be stopped during periods of intercurrent illness, and the dose may often need to be increased in the presence of infection.
- Insulin requirements increase with use of corticosteroids (see later).
- Women should be offered ketone testing strips and advised to test for ketonuria or ketonaemia if they become hyperglycaemic or unwell.

Management of type 2 diabetes
- Oral hypoglycaemic drugs (both sulphonylureas and biguanides) were traditionally discontinued in pregnancy because they cross the placenta and there is a theoretical risk of this causing fetal hypoglycaemia. However, the National Institute of Clinical Evidence (NICE) guideline on the management of diabetes in pregnancy states that metformin can be used in pregnancy as an adjunct or alternative to insulin
- Most women with type 2 diabetes require treatment with insulin during pregnancy, even if they are adequately controlled with diet with or without oral hypoglycaemic drugs outside pregnancy.
- Outcomes are improved in women taking oral hypoglycaemic drugs compared with those in women who refuse insulin and take no therapy.
- The newer thiazolidinediones (e.g., rosiglitazone, pioglitazone) reduce peripheral insulin resistance. They are used as second-line therapy added to either metformin or sulfonylurea when either metformin or sulfonylurea are not tolerated or contraindicated. Their use is avoided in pregnancy.
- Strict adherence to a low-sugar, low-fat, high-fibre diet is important in pregnancy, as this will aid glycaemic control. Starvation and severe calorie restriction should be avoided because of the risk of ketoacidosis.

Diabetic complications

- Women should have a detailed ophthalmological examination pre-pregnancy and in early pregnancy if their annual assessment occurred more than 6 months previously and at 28 weeks if the first assessment is normal. If diabetic retinopathy is present, the next assessment should be at 16 to 20 weeks. NICE recommends retinal assessment by digital imaging with mydriasis using tropicamide. Laser photocoagulation can be used either to treat or to prevent proliferative retinopathy in pregnancy.
- Diabetic retinopathy is not a contraindication to rapid optimisation of glycaemic control or to a vaginal delivery.
- Women with pre-proliferative diabetic retinopathy should have ophthalmological follow-up for at least 6 months postpartum.

- NICE recommends referral to a nephrologist if the serum creatinine is $\geq 120\ \mu g/L$ or the protein leak is $> 2\ g/day$. Women with diabetic nephropathy require regular monitoring of renal function (serum urea and creatinine) and quantification of proteinuria (24-hour protein excretion; protein creatinine ratio) (see Chapter 10).
- Hypertension is found in 30% of women with diabetic nephropathy, and up to 75% will develop hypertension by the end of pregnancy.
- Strict control of hypertension in pregnancy is important to prevent ongoing renal damage. Therefore, in hypertensive or nephropathic women with diabetes, a low threshold for antihypertensive therapy (e.g., 140/90) is often used.

Obstetric management

- An early dating and viability scan is recommended.
- Because of the increased risk of congenital abnormalities, women with diabetes should be offered nuchal translucency scanning at 11 to 13 weeks' gestation and detailed ultrasound of the fetus at 18 to 20 weeks' gestation, including detailed four-chambered assessment of the fetal heart.
- Full hospital care is appropriate with regular blood pressure and urinalysis checks to detect pre-eclampsia.
- Regular ultrasound assessment of fetal growth and liquor volume in the third trimester is advisable to detect or confirm macrosomia and polyhydramnios.
- β-Sympathomimetic drugs should not be used as tocolysis in women with diabetes, and women receiving corticosteroids to induce fetal lung maturation should have additional insulin prescribed and be closely monitored to avoid severe hyperglycaemia and diabetic ketoacidosis.
- Decisions regarding the timing and the mode of delivery balance the risks of preterm delivery and its associated complications with the risks of late IUD and macrosomia with its complications.
- NICE recommends delivery by induction of labour or by elective caesarean section if indicated after 38 weeks' gestation for women with a normally grown fetus.
- The rates of risk of caesarean section (both elective and emergency) are increased in women with diabetes. In the CEMACH study of pre-existing diabetes, the overall caesarean section rate was 67% with an emergency caesarean section rate of 38%. However, given the high rate of macrosomia (21% of babies in this cohort weighed more than 4 kg; 6% > 4.5 kg) this high rate may be unavoidable.

Intrapartum management

- Women with pre-existing type 1 diabetes are managed using a sliding scale. I.v. infusions of short-acting insulin and dextrose are administered throughout active labour and delivery via separate giving sets, to allow acceleration of glucose infusion and cessation of insulin in the event of hypoglycaemia.
- The capillary blood glucose level should be estimated hourly and the insulin infusion rate altered according to a sliding scale determined by the individual daily insulin requirements.
- The usual dose range is 2 to 6 U/hr. The target glucose level during labour and delivery is 4 to 7 mmol/L, the aim being to avoid hypoglycaemia.
- The dextrose infusion (5% or 10%) should provide 500 ml of fluid every 8 hours. Insulin drives extracellular potassium into the cells. It is important, therefore, to include potassium replacement with the intravenous dextrose to avoid hypokalaemia, which may otherwise result especially if glucose levels are high.

- Following delivery of the placenta, the rate of infusion of insulin is halved in women with type 1 diabetes.
- Postpartum, insulin requirements return rapidly to pre-pregnancy levels.
- Once women with type 1 diabetes are eating normally, s.c. insulin should be recommenced at either the pre-pregnancy dose or at a 25% lower dose if the women intends to breast-feed, which is associated with increased energy expenditure. Most women with established diabetes are capable of adjusting their own insulin doses and can be advised that tight glycaemic control is not as important during the postpartum period.
- Women with type 2 diabetes who are breastfeeding can resume or continue taking metformin or glibenclamide.

Pre-pregnancy counselling

- This is one of the most important features of management of the woman with diabetes in pregnancy.
- Women should be counselled that good control of diabetes and lower HbA_{1C} levels lower the risk of congenital abnormalities in the fetus and the risk of pre-eclampsia and are associated with improved pregnancy outcome.
- Women should receive pre-conception folic acid (5 mg/day).
- The risk of diabetes in the child is 2 to 3% with maternal type 1 diabetes and 4% 5% if the father has type 1 diabetes.
- Pre-pregnancy counselling allows for optimisation of diabetic control prior to conception, as well as assessment of the presence and severity of complications such as hypertension, nephropathy and retinopathy.

Pre-existing diabetes—points to remember

- The increased risk of congenital abnormalities is related to the degree of periconception diabetic control.
- Insulin requirements increase during pregnancy.
- Oral hypoglycaemics may be used in type 2 diabetes.
- Retinopathy may deteriorate during pregnancy.
- Women with diabetes, especially those with nephropathy and hypertension, have a greatly increased risk of pre-eclampsia.
- Neonatal and perinatal morbidity and mortality are increased in infants of diabetic mothers. Complications relate to the degree of maternal hyperglycaemia, fetal hyperinsulinaemia and macrosomia and may be decreased with tight diabetic control.
- Pregnant women with diabetes should be managed in joint pregnancy diabetic clinics by obstetricians and physicians with expertise in the care of such women.
- The most important goal of management is to achieve maternal near-normoglycaemia.
- Outcome is improved if four-times-daily basal bolus regimes of insulin are used and target blood glucose levels are based on postprandial capillary glucose estimations.

- The risk of pre-eclampsia is increased in the presence of microalbuminuria (30–300 mg/day) although to a lesser degree than in those with frank nephropathy (> 300 mg/day). Proteinuria should be formally documented and quantified prior to pregnancy with an albumin creatinine ratio.
- Thus, a woman can be given a more accurate estimation of the level of risk of, for example, developing pre-eclampsia.
- If necessary, proliferative retinopathy may be treated with photocoagulation prior to conception.
- Contraindications to pregnancy include ischaemic heart disease, untreated proliferative retinopathy, severe gastroparesis, and severe renal impairment (creatinine > 250µmol/L).
- Unplanned pregnancy is a risk factor for large-for-gestational-age infants in both pre-existing diabetes and GDM.

Gestational diabetes mellitus

The definition of gestational diabetes from the National Diabetes Data Group (1985) is "carbohydrate intolerance of variable severity with onset or first recognition during the present pregnancy." Thus, it includes women with pre-existing but previously unrecognised diabetes (Fig. 5.1).

Incidence

- This is hugely variable depending on the level of glucose intolerance used to define the condition (see later under "Screening and Diagnosis") and the ethnicity and other demographics of the population under study.
- Using the definition for impaired glucose tolerance in the non-pregnant woman, the incidence is approximately 3% to 6%.
- In the United Kingdom, the prevalence is increased approximately 11-fold in women from the Indian subcontinent, 8-fold in South East Asian women, 6-fold in Arab/Mediterranean women and 3-fold in Afro-Caribbean women.
- The prevalence of GDM in the United Kingdom is the lowest in areas with a predominantly white European population and highest (in inner city areas) with a high proportion of ethnic minority women.

Clinical features

- GDM is usually asymptomatic and develops in the second or third trimester, induced by maternal changes in carbohydrate metabolism and decreased insulin sensitivity.
- GDM may be diagnosed by routine biochemical screening (see later) or may be suspected in the case of a macrosomic fetus, polyhydramnios, persistent heavy glycosuria or recurrent infections.
- Occasionally, GDM may be diagnosed retrospectively (with random plasma glucose or HbA_{1c}) following an IUD or birth of a severely macrosomic infant.
- GDM is more commonly found in women with previous GDM, a family history of diabetes, previous large-for-gestational-age infants, obesity and older age at pregnancy.

■ GDM is associated with increased perinatal morbidity (Fig. 5.2) and mortality in the same way but to a much lesser degree than pre-existing diabetes. These risks relate to macrosomia, which may develop as in the infant of the diabetic mother.

■ Unlike pre-existing diabetes, there is no increase in the congenital abnormality rate, except in those women with unrecognised diabetes pre-dating the pregnancy and hyperglycaemia in the first trimester.

■ GDM is associated with an increased risk of pre-eclampsia.

Importance of GDM

The importance of diagnosing GDM relates to three factors:

1. Women identified as having GDM have a greatly increased (40–60%) risk of developing type 2 diabetes within 10–15 years.
   – The diagnosis of type 2 diabetes is often made late and 10 to 30% of those diagnosed have established eye or renal disease by the time of diagnosis.
   – Modification of diet and lifestyle with the correction or avoidance of obesity may prevent or delay the development of diabetes later in life. The relative risk of developing type 2 diabetes almost doubles for each 4.5 kg gained.
   – Even if prevention is not possible, earlier diagnosis resulting from careful follow-up (and counselling of the woman regarding the increased risk and the advisability of regular (annual) blood glucose checks and the need to seek medical advice if she feels unwell) is beneficial and may prevent the development of microvascular complications.
2. A small proportion (1 in 1000) of women identified as having GDM will in fact have had diabetes pre-dating the pregnancy. They are therefore at risk from all the features associated with pre-existing diabetes in pregnancy, including in the case of type 1 diabetes, ketoacidosis.
3. Women with GDM have a higher incidence of macrosomia and adverse pregnancy outcome than do control populations without GDM.
   – The relationship of postload glucose and fetal size exists throughout the spectrum of glucose tolerance and there is no threshold effect.
   – The controversy surrounding this issue relates almost entirely to the different diagnostic criteria used to define GDM. The more stringent the criteria, the more apparent the association.
   – The problems with many clinical studies addressing pregnancy outcome in GDM were the lack of control of confounding variables, such as maternal weight and age, and the lack of a "control" or untreated group. Thus, obese women and those with previous large babies are at risk of both GDM and macrosomic infants, and causality is difficult to establish.
   – Most cases of macrosomia are not associated with GDM and only 20–30% of infants of mothers with GDM have macrosomia.
   – Publication of the Australian Carbohydrate Intolerance Study (ACHOIS) has eliminated much of the controversy since it randomised women with impaired glucose tolerance (blood glucose 7.8 to 11.1 mmol/L 2 hours after an OGTT) to treatment (with diet, monitoring and insulin if required) or routine obstetric care. This study showed that in women with untreated GDM, the perinatal mortality and morbidity is increased compared with a treated group.

- Decreasing birth-weight across a population raises issues regarding the relationship between low birth-weight and adult hypertension and cardiovascular disease.
- Diagnosing GDM and labelling of women as "high risk" may itself adversely affect pregnancy outcome. The most obvious example is an increase in the caesarean section rate.

Screening and diagnosis

NICE advocates screening the following groups of women with an OGTT at 24 to 28 weeks' gestation:

- Family history of diabetes in a first-degree relative
- Previous macrosomic baby (> 4.5 kg)
- Obesity [body mass index(BMI) > 30 kg/m^2]
- Family origin with high prevalence of diabetes (South Asian, Caribbean and Middle Eastern)
- Women with previous GDM should be offered self-monitoring of blood glucose or be screened with an OGTT at 16 to 18 weeks and again at 28 weeks if this is negative.
- NICE does not recommend screening with random blood glucose, fasting blood glucose, urinalysis or glucose challenge tests.
- The World Health Organization (WHO) diagnostic criteria for GDM (equivalent to those for diagnosis of impaired glucose tolerance in the non-pregnant woman) should be used. Women with a test result confirming either diabetes (fasting serum glucose level $\geq$ 7.0 mmol/L or 2-hour serum glucose level $\geq$ 11.1 mmol/L) or IGT (defined as 2-hour serum glucose level 7.8 to 11.1 mmol/L and fasting serum glucose level < 7.0 mmol/L) are regarded as having GDM.

Management

As with pre-existing diabetes, close collaboration between obstetricians and physicians is essential. Women should be managed in a specialist multidisciplinary diabetes pregnancy clinic.

Medical management

- The mainstay of treatment is diet with reduced fat, increased fibre and regulation of carbohydrate intake. Carbohydrates with a low glycaemic index (resulting in slower, more even release of glucose) are advised (e.g., bran).
- NICE recommends that women with BMI > 27 kg/m^2 should be offered calorie restriction to 25 kcal/kg/day, which is not thought to increase the risk of ketonuria.
- It is often possible to identify certain elements of a woman's diet such as large quantities of high-calorie, carbonated drinks, fresh fruit juice or high-calorie snack foods that, when removed, lead to rapid improvement in blood glucose levels.
- In addition, regular exercise (30 minutes of moderate exercise daily) is encouraged.
- As with pre-existing diabetes, HBGM is an integral part of management since it allows the woman immediate feedback.
- Persistent postprandial hyperglycaemia (>7.8 mmol/L 1 hour postmeal) or fasting hyperglycaemia (>5.9 mmol/L) despite compliance with diet and lifestyle changes for 2 weeks are indications for the introduction of hypoglycaemic therapy. This should be in addition to, not instead of, dietary treatment. Women need to be

reminded of the importance of dietary modification, although adherence to dietary advice is usually good during pregnancy.

- NICE guidelines support the use of metformin and glibenclamide to treat GDM. The metformin in GDM (MIG) trial showed that there was no difference in perinatal outcomes in women treated initially with insulin or metformin. Approximately 46% of women in the metformin group required the addition of insulin to achieve glycaemic targets. Glibenclamide does not cross the placenta and may also be safely and effectively used as an alternative to insulin in GDM in women who will not accept insulin treatment.
- Insulin, if required, is given as rapid-acting insulin analogues as with pre-existing diabetes, although it may be needed only before some meals. In more severe cases, where there is fasting hyperglycaemia, intermediate-acting insulin may in addition be required at night.
- A four-times-daily basal bolus insulin regime, with adjustment according to post-prandial rather than pre-meal glucose readings, gives improved glycaemic control and improved outcomes compared to b.d. mixed insulin and adjustment based on pre-meal glucose values.

Obstetric management

- GDM is associated with an increased risk of pre-eclampsia, and women should receive full hospital care with regular checks of blood pressure and urinalysis, especially towards term.
- Regular ultrasound assessment for fetal growth is advisable as this is likely to influence the timing and mode of delivery as well as possibly the decision to start insulin treatment.
- Recommendations from NICE regarding timing and mode of delivery in GDM are the same as for pre-existing diabetes, that is, elective birth should be offered after 38 weeks by induction of labour or elective caesarean section.
- Diabetes is not a contraindication to vaginal birth after caesarean section.

Intrapartum management
- It is often possible to manage even insulin-treated women without insulin during delivery, especially those on small doses (< 20 U/day) of insulin. This is because women do not eat much during labour. Those on larger doses of insulin are managed as women with pre-existing diabetes with i.v. dextrose and an insulin sliding scale.
- Intrapartum target blood glucose levels of 4 to 7 mmol/L are the same as pre-existing diabetes.
- Following delivery of the placenta, the insulin infusion should be discontinued. All oral hypoglycaemic drugs should also be stopped.

Postnatal management
- Blood glucose level should be checked prior to transfer to community care to ensure normoglycaemia.
- NICE recommends a fasting blood glucose at 6 weeks and then annually to screen for diabetes. Formal 75 g OGTT is no longer recommended at 6 weeks following delivery.

- Women with GDM should be counselled regarding the risks of future diabetes (see p. 90) and be made aware of the symptoms of hyperglycaemia. They should receive lifestyle advice concerning exercise and diet, particularly reduced fat intake. Obese women should be encouraged to lose weight postpartum and all should be advised to avoid obesity.

Recurrence

- GDM usually recurs in subsequent pregnancies.
- Sometimes, if a woman has lost a lot of weight between pregnancies and modified her diet substantially, she may not develop GDM.
- Women should be advised of the risk of recurrent GDM and future diabetes.
- Adequate contraception and pre-pregnancy counselling are important.
- Women with previous GDM should have fasting blood glucose checked prior to conception to detect diabetes that may have developed since the last pregnancy.

Gestational diabetes—points to remember

- The prevalence of GDM depends on ethnicity and the criteria used for diagnosis. Ethnic minorities are at increased risk.
- The importance of diagnosing GDM relates to the high risk of future diabetes, the detection of pre-existing diabetes and a risk of macrosomia and adverse pregnancy outcome.
- The GDM "label" is not itself without risk; the incidence of caesarean section with its attendant risks is increased.
- Management of GDM is with diet and exercise in the first instance followed by metformin and then insulin in resistant cases.
- Pregnancy and the puerperium provide a unique opportunity for education regarding lifestyle and dietary changes.

Further reading

Alberti KG, Zimmet PZ. Definition, diagnosis and classification of diabetes mellitus and its complications, I: diagnosis and classification of diabetes mellitus provisional report of a WHO consultation. Diabet Med 1998; 15:539–553.

Casson IF, Clarke CA, Howard CV, et al. Outcomes of pregnancy in insulin dependent diabetic women: results of a five year population cohort study. Br Med J 1997; 315:275–278.

Confidential Enquiry into Maternal and Child Health. Improving the Health of Mothers, Babies and Children: A Report on Pregnancies in Women with Type 1 and Type 2 Diabetes 2002–2003: England, Wales and Northern Ireland. London, England: Confidential Enquiry into Maternal and Child Health, 2003.

Crowther CA, Hiller JE, Moss JR, et al. Australian Carbohydrate Intolerance Study in Pregnant Women (ACHOIS) Trial Group: effect of treatment of gestational diabetes mellitus on pregnancy outcomes. N Engl J Med 2005; 352:2477–2486.

de Veciana M, Major CA, Morgan MA, et al. Postprandial versus preprandial blood glucose monitoring in women with gestational diabetes mellitus requiring insulin therapy. N Engl J Med 2005; 333:1237–1241.

Garner P, Okun N, Keely E, et al. A randomised controlled trial of strict glycaemic control and tertiary level obstetric care versus routine obstetric care in the management of gestational diabetes: a pilot study. Am J Obstet Gynecol 1997; 177:190–195.

Hawthorne G, Robson S, Ryall EA, et al. Prospective population based survey of outcome of pregnancy in diabetic women: results of the Northern Diabetic Pregnancy Audit. Br Med J 1997; 315:279–281.

Kim C, Newton KM, Knopp RH. Gestational diabetes and the incidence of type 2 diabetes: a systematic review. Diabetes Care 2002; 25:1862–1868.

National Institute for Clinical Excellence. Diabetes in Pregnancy: Management of Diabetes and Its Complications from Preconception to the Postnatal Period: Guideline CG63. London, England: National Institute for Clinical Excellence, 2008.

Rowan JA, Hague WM, Gao W, et al. Metformin versus insulin for the treatment of gestational diabetes. N Engl J Med 2008; 358:2003–2015.

CHAPTER 6

Thyroid and parathyroid disease

Thyroid disease	Parathyroid disease
Physiological changes	Physiological changes
Hyperthyroidism	Hyperparathyroidism
Hypothyroidism	Hypoparathyroidism
Postpartum thyroiditis	**Vitamin D deficiency**
Thyroid nodules	

Thyroid disease

Physiological changes (see also section B, table 6)

- Hepatic synthesis of thyroid-binding globulin is increased.
- Total levels of thyroxine (T4) and tri-iodothyronine (T3) are increased to compensate for this rise.
- Levels of free T4 are altered less by pregnancy but do fall a little in the second and third trimesters (see Table of Normal Values, Appendix 2).
- Serum concentrations of thyroid-stimulating hormone (TSH) initially rise and then fall in the first trimester, and the normal range is wide.
- Hyperemesis gravidarum may be associated with a biochemical hyperthyroidism with high levels of free T4 and a suppressed TSH in up to 60% of cases. This relates to increased concentrations of human chorionic gonadotrophin (hCG) (to which TSH is structurally similar). hCG has thyrotropic (TSH-like) activity.
- In pregnancy, TSH levels increase so the upper limit of the reference range is raised (5.5 μmol/L) compared with those in the non-pregnant woman (4.0 μmol/L).
- Similarly, the normal ranges for free T4 and T3 are reduced (see Table of Normal Values, Appendix 2). Compared with outside pregnancy, free T4 has a narrower and lower range and falls throughout pregnancy.
- TSH levels used in isolation are unreliable in pregnancy for the assessment of thyroid status
- Pregnancy is associated with a state of relative iodine deficiency that has two major causes:
  1. Maternal iodine requirements increase because of active transport to the feto-placental unit.
  2. Iodine excretion in the urine is increased twofold because of increased glomerular filtration and decreased renal tubular reabsorption.

- Because the plasma level of iodine falls, the thyroid gland increases its uptake from the blood by threefold.
- If there is already dietary insufficiency of iodine, the thyroid gland hypertrophies to trap a sufficient amount of iodine.
- Biochemical assessment of thyroid function in pregnancy should include assays of free T4 and, in some cases, free T3. Immunoradiometric assays of TSH are useful but should not be used in isolation because of the variable effects of gestation.

Hyperthyroidism

Incidence

- Hyperthyroidism is more common in women than in men (ratio 10:1).
- Thyrotoxicosis complicates about 1 in 500 pregnancies.
- Approximately 50% of affected women have a positive family history of autoimmune thyroid disease.
- Most cases encountered in pregnancy have already been diagnosed and will already be on treatment.

Clinical features

- Many of the typical features are common in normal pregnancy, including heat intolerance, tachycardia, palpitations, palmar erythema, emotional lability, vomiting and goitre.
- The most discriminatory features in pregnancy are weight loss, tremor, a persistent tachycardia, lid lag and exophthalmos. The latter feature indicates thyroid disease at some time rather than active thyrotoxicosis.
- Thyroid-associated ophthalmopathy may occur before hyperthyroidism and is present in up to 50% of patients with Graves' disease.
- If thyrotoxicosis occurs for the first time in pregnancy, it usually presents late in the first or early in the second trimester.

Pathogenesis

- Approximately 95% of cases of hyperthyroidism in pregnancy are due to Graves' disease.
- Graves' disease is an autoimmune disorder caused by TSH receptor–stimulating antibodies (TRAb).
- More rarely in women of childbearing age, hyperthyroidism may be due to toxic multi-nodular goitre or toxic adenoma, or occasionally subacute thyroiditis, acute (de Quervains/viral) thyroiditis, iodine, amiodarone or lithium therapy.

Diagnosis

- This is made by finding an elevated level of free T4 or free T3. Normal pregnant ranges for each trimester must be used (see Table of Normal Values, Appendix 2; and Section B, Table 6).
- TSH is suppressed, although this may be a feature of early pregnancy.

Table 6.1 – Pregnancy specific normal ranges for thyroid function tests.

	TSH (mU/L)	Thyroxine (pmol/L)	Tri-iodothyronine (pmol/L)
Non-pregnant	0.27–4.2	12–22	3.1–6.8
First trimester	0–5.5	10–16	3–7
Second trimester	0.5–3.5	9–15.5	3–5.5
Third trimester	0.5–4	8–14.5	2.5–5.5

Abbreviation: TSH, thyroid-stimulating hormone.
From Cotzias C, et al. 2008

■ Differentiation from hyperemesis gravidarum may be difficult (see Chapter 12, page 214). Symptoms that predate the pregnancy suggest true thyrotoxicosis.

Pregnancy

Effect of pregnancy on thyrotoxicosis

■ Thyrotoxicosis often improves during pregnancy, especially in the second and third trimesters.
■ As with other autoimmune conditions, there is a state of relative immunosuppression in pregnancy, and levels of TSH receptor–stimulating antibodies (TRAb) may fall with consequent improvement in Graves' disease and a lower requirement for antithyroid treatment.
■ Exacerbations may occur in the first trimester, possibly related to hCG production, and in the puerperium (especially if there has been improvement during pregnancy) related to a reversal of the fall in antibody levels seen during pregnancy.
■ Pregnancy has no effect on Graves' ophthalmopathy.

Effect of thyrotoxicosis on pregnancy

■ If thyrotoxicosis is severe and untreated, it is associated with inhibition of ovulation and infertility.
■ Those who do become pregnant and remain untreated have an increased rate of miscarriage, fetal growth restriction (FGR), preterm labour and perinatal mortality.
■ Thyroid-stimulating antibodies (TRAb) may cause fetal or neonatal thyrotoxicosis (see later).
■ Poorly controlled thyrotoxicosis may lead to a thyroid crisis ("storm") in the mother and heart failure, particularly at the time of delivery.
■ For those with good control on antithyroid drugs or with previously treated Graves' disease in remission, the maternal and fetal outcome is usually good and unaffected by the thyrotoxicosis.
■ Rarely, retrosternal extension of a goitre may cause tracheal obstruction or dysphagia. This is a particular problem if the patient needs to be intubated.

Management

Antithyroid drugs

■ Carbimazole and propylthiouracil (PTU) are the most commonly used antithyroid drugs in the United Kingdom. Most patients are initially treated with 15 to 40 mg carbimazole (150–400 mg PTU) initially for 4 to 6 weeks. Their onset of action is delayed until the pre-formed hormones are depleted, a process which can take 3 to 4 weeks. The dose is then gradually reduced to a maintenance dose of 5 to 15 mg (50–150 mg PTU). Therapy is continued for 12 to 18 months after the initial presentation of Graves' disease, but relapse rates are high, and some women are managed with long-term antithyroid drugs.

■ Both drugs cross the placenta, PTU less than carbimazole, and in high doses may cause fetal hypothyroidism and goitre. Neither is grossly teratogenic, although carbimazole and methimazole may very occasional cause a rare condition, aplasia cutis, patches of absent skin most commonly affecting the scalp. This has not been reported in recent large studies of antithyroid drugs in pregnancy. Liver impairment is another rare side effect (1 in 10,000) of PTU, which is why it is not the first-line drug outside pregnancy or after the first trimester.

■ The aim of treatment is to control the thyrotoxicosis as rapidly as possible and maintain optimal control of thyrotoxicosis with the lowest dose of antithyroid medication. The woman should be clinically euthyroid, with a free T4 at the upper end of the normal pregnant range.

■ Newly diagnosed thyrotoxicosis in pregnancy should be aggressively treated with high doses of carbimazole (second and third trimester) or PTU (first trimester) (45–60 mg or 450–600 mg daily, respectively) for 4 to 6 weeks, after which, gradual reduction in the dose is usually possible.

■ A drug rash or urticaria occurs in 1% to 5% of patients on antithyroid drugs and should prompt a switch to a different preparation. More rarely carbimazole and PTU may cause neutropenia and agranulocytosis. Women should be asked to report any signs of infection, particularly sore throat, a full blood count requested if there is clinical evidence of infection and carbimazole should be stopped immediately if there is any clinical or laboratory evidence of neutropenia.

■ PTU is preferable for newly diagnosed cases in the first trimester of pregnancy, but women already on maintenance carbimazole prior to pregnancy need not be switched to PTU in pregnancy.

■ Women should be seen monthly in the case of newly diagnosed hyperthyroidism, but thyroid function tests (TFTs) are required less frequently in women stable on antithyroid drugs.

■ In Graves' disease, there is often a temporary worsening of control in early pregnancy due to the rising hCG levels and perhaps reduced absorption of medication secondary to vomiting. There is then an improvement with women often requiring less medication as the relative immune suppression of pregnancy results in a fall in antibody levels. Approximately 30% can stop all medication in the last weeks of pregnancy.

■ Graves' disease can flare postnatally as maternal antibody levels rise postpartum. In those having stopped medication, it is often necessary to reintroduce it at 2 to 3 months postpartum. It is important to distinguish such a flare from a true postpartum thyroiditis (see later).

■ Doses of PTU at or below 150 mg/day and carbimazole 15 mg/day are unlikely to cause problems in the fetus.

- Very little PTU is excreted in the breast milk; only 0.07% of the dose taken by the breast-feeding mother is consumed by the breast-fed baby. It is therefore safe for mothers to breast-feed while taking doses of PTU at or below 150 mg/day and carbimazole 15 mg/day (0.5% of the dose is received by the breast-fed baby).
- Thyroid function should be checked in umbilical cord blood and at regular intervals in the neonate if the mother is breast-feeding and taking high doses of antithyroid drugs.
- There is no place for "block-and-replace" regimens in the management of thyrotoxicosis in pregnancy. The high doses of antithyroid drugs required may render the fetus hypothyroid, and the T4 "replacement" does not cross the placenta in sufficiently high doses to protect the fetus.

β-blockers

- These are often used in the early management of thyrotoxicosis or during relapse to improve sympathetic symptoms of tachycardia, sweating and tremor.
- β-Blockers also reduce peripheral conversion of T4 into T3.
- They are discontinued once the antithyroid drugs take effect and there is clinical improvement, usually evident within 3 weeks.
- Doses of propranolol of 40 mg t.d.s. for such short periods are not harmful to the fetus.

Surgery

- Thyroidectomy is rarely indicated in pregnancy but, if required, is best performed in the second trimester.
- It is usually reserved for those with dysphagia or stridor related to a large goitre, those with confirmed or suspected carcinoma, and those who have allergies to both antithyroid drugs.
- Approximately 25% to 50% of patients will become hypothyroid following thyroid surgery; and therefore, close follow-up is required to ensure rapid diagnosis and treatment with replacement therapy.
- Hypocalcaemia due to removal of the parathyroid glands is also a risk, reported in 1% to 2% of cases.

Radioactive iodine

- Radioiodine therapy is contraindicated in pregnancy and breast-feeding since it is taken up by the fetal thyroid (after 10–12 weeks) with resulting thyroid ablation and hypothyroidism.
- Diagnostic radioiodine scans (as opposed to treatment) are also contraindicated in pregnancy but may be performed if a mother is breast-feeding, although mothers should stop breast-feeding for 24 hours after the procedure.
- Pregnancy should be avoided for at least 4 months after treatment with radioiodine in view of the theoretical risk of chromosomal damage and genetic abnormalities.

Neonatal/fetal thyrotoxicosis

- This results from transplacental passage of TRAbs.
- It occurs in approximately 1% of babies of mothers with a past or current history of Graves' disease but is most common in those with active disease in the third trimester, especially if poorly controlled.

- It is possible to predict babies at risk by measuring the level of TRAb. Testing in the first trimester is useful to predict fetal thyrotoxicosis. If high titres of antibodies are detected in early pregnancy or if levels have not fallen with advancing gestation, fetal thyrotoxicosis should be anticipated and obstetric ultrasound may be recommended. If antibodies are detected in late pregnancy then cord blood and neonatal TFTs should be performed.
- It is important not to forget the possibility of neonatal/fetal thyrotoxicosis in babies of mothers with previously treated Graves' disease. A particular caveat is the woman on T4 (and therefore classified as "hypothyroid") following previous thyroidectomy or radioiodine.

Clinical features

- If the condition develops in utero, it may present with fetal tachycardia, FGR or goitre. Without treatment, the mortality rate may reach 25%.
- In the neonate, the condition may be delayed for 1 day to 1 week while maternal antithyroid drugs and/or blocking antibodies are cleared.
- The most frequent neonatal clinical signs of thyrotoxicosis are weight loss or poor weight gain, tachycardia, irritability, jitteriness, poor feeding, goitre, hyperexcitability, hepatosplenomegaly, stare and eyelid retraction, and in severe untreated cases, congestive cardiac failure.
- Without treatment, the mortality rate is approximately 15%. Neonatal thyrotoxicosis resolves with the clearance of the maternal TRAb, and clinical signs usually disappear during the first 4 months of life.

Diagnosis

- Serial ultrasound to check fetal growth, heart rate and fetal neck (for goitre) is advisable, especially in those mothers with poorly controlled or newly diagnosed thyrotoxicosis, when TRAb levels may be high.
- Percutaneous fetal blood sampling for measurement of fetal thyroid function is accurate but carries an inherent risk.

Hyperthyroidism—points to remember

- Untreated thyrotoxicosis is dangerous for both the mother and her fetus.
- Graves' disease often improves during pregnancy but may flare postpartum.
- Both carbimazole and PTU cross the placenta and in high doses may cause fetal hypothyroidism and goitre.
- The lowest possible maintenance dose of antithyroid drug should be used.
- For those with good control of thyrotoxicosis on doses of carbimazole < 15 mg/day or PTU < 150 mg/day, the maternal and fetal outcome is usually good and unaffected by the thyrotoxicosis.
- Women may safely breast-feed on these doses of antithyroid drugs.
- β-Blockers are safe to use short term if required for control of thyrotoxic symptoms.
- Neonatal or fetal thyrotoxicosis, due to transplacental passage of TRAbs is rare, but dangerous.

Management

- Treatment is with antithyroid drugs. In the case of fetal thyrotoxicosis, these are given to the mother. If the woman is euthyroid, these are combined with replacement T4.
- In the neonate, treatment must begin promptly but is only needed for a few weeks, after which maternal TRAbs disappear from the circulation.

Hypothyroidism

Incidence

- Hypothyroidism is much more common in women than in men.
- It is especially common in those with a positive family history of hypothyroidism.
- The condition is present in approximately 1% of pregnancies.
- Most cases encountered in pregnancy have already been diagnosed and will be on replacement therapy.

Clinical features

- As with hyperthyroidism, many of the typical features are common in normal pregnancy.
- These include weight gain, lethargy and tiredness, hair loss, dry skin, constipation, carpal tunnel syndrome, fluid retention and goitre.
- The most discriminatory features in pregnancy are cold intolerance, slow pulse rate and delayed relaxation of the tendon (particularly the ankle) reflexes.
- Hypothyroidism is associated with other autoimmune diseases, for example pernicious anaemia, vitiligo and type 1 diabetes mellitus.

Pathogenesis

- Most cases are due to autoimmune destruction of the thyroid gland associated with microsomal autoantibodies.
- There are two principal subtypes: atrophic thyroiditis and Hashimoto thyroiditis. The latter is the name given to the combination of autoimmune thyroiditis and goitre.
- Hypothyroidism may be iatrogenic following radioiodine therapy, thyroidectomy or related to drugs (amiodarone, lithium, iodine or antithyroid drugs). Transient hypothyroidism may be found in subacute (de Quervain's) thyroiditis and in postpartum thyroiditis (see later).
- The commonest causes encountered in pregnancy are Hashimoto's thyroiditis and treated Graves' disease.

Diagnosis

- Diagnosis is made by finding a low level of free T4. Normal pregnant ranges for each trimester must be used, since the normal range for free T4 falls in the second and third trimesters (see Table of Normal Values, Appendix 2).
- The TSH level is raised, although this may be a feature of normal late pregnancy or, occasionally, early pregnancy (see Section B, Table 6).
- The finding of thyroid autoantibodies may help confirm the diagnosis, but these are present in 20% to 30% of the population and should not be used in isolation.

Pregnancy

Effect of pregnancy on hypothyroidism

- Pregnancy itself probably has no effect on hypothyroidism.
- Approximately one-fourth of women require an increase in their T4 dose in pregnancy, but routine increase in the dose is not recommended in the United Kingdom.
- Dose increases should only occur in response to abnormal TFTs interpreted with reference to normal ranges for pregnancy.
- Poor compliance may also result in a raised TSH with a normal free T4.
- If the dose does need to be increased in early pregnancy, this may be because of inadequate replacement prior to pregnancy and most do not need to decrease their dose again postpartum.

Effect of hypothyroidism on pregnancy

- If hypothyroidism is severe and untreated, it is associated with inhibition of ovulation and infertility. Patients may complain of oligomenorrhoea or menorrhagia.
- Those who do become pregnant and remain untreated have an increased rate of miscarriage, anaemia, fetal loss, pre-eclampsia and low-birth-weight infants.
- The fetus is dependent on maternal thyroid hormone until autonomous fetal thyroid function begins at around 12 weeks' gestation.
- There is an association between untreated, overt hypothyroidism in the mother (as judged by raised TSH levels or reduced free T4 levels in the late first, early second trimester) and reduced intelligent quotient and neurodevelopmental delay in the offspring. But there are no studies to show that T4 replacement in pregnancy influences intelligence of the offspring.
- Severe maternal iodine deficiency may cause permanent brain damage— neurological cretinism (deaf mutism, spastic motor disorder and hypothyroidism)— in the child.
- For those women on adequate replacement therapy and who are euthyroid at the beginning of pregnancy, the maternal and fetal outcome is usually good and unaffected by the hypothyroidism.

Management

- Most women with hypothyroidism are on maintenance doses of T4 of 100 to 200 μg/day, although the dose required varies between individuals.
- Only very small amounts of T4 cross the placenta and women should be reassured that the fetus is not at risk of thyrotoxicosis from maternal T4 replacement therapy.
- Thyroid function should be checked in women planning a pregnancy, to ensure adequate replacement prior to conception. A repeat test should be requested in early pregnancy.
- In women on adequate replacement, thyroid function should be checked once in each trimester. Following any adjustment in T4 dose, thyroid function should be checked after 4 to 6 weeks.
- Most women who are euthyroid at the beginning of pregnancy will not require any adjustment to their T4 dose during pregnancy or in the puerperium.
- Occasionally, women assumed to have permanent hypothyroidism following an episode of postpartum thyroiditis (see later, p. 104) may present in a subsequent

pregnancy without the diagnosis having been reviewed. It may be possible to discontinue T4 replacement in these women.

■ An isolated raised TSH level in the first trimester is common, and T4 doses do not need to be increased unless underreplacement is confirmed with a low free T4 level or the raised TSH level is found to be persistent despite a normal free T4 level (subclinical hypothyroidism).

■ It is not uncommon to find women who are underreplaced at the beginning of pregnancy, but any increase in dosage requirement is likely to be sustained postpartum, confirming a pre-existing undertreatment rather than an increased demand related to pregnancy itself.

■ For those with newly diagnosed hypothyroidism in pregnancy, replacement with T4 should begin immediately. Provided there is no history of heart disease, an appropriate starting dose is 100 μg/day. If there is a history of cardiovascular disease, replacement should be introduced at lower doses.

■ Occasional patients are encountered where an increased requirement of T4 is limited to pregnancy and there is then a risk that they may be rendered hyperthyroid if this dose is not decreased in the postpartum period. Therefore, it is important to check thyroid function in the puerperium in those women where dose adjustments were made during pregnancy.

Subclinical hypothyroidism

■ This is a term used to describe those with a high (> 97.5th centile) TSH and normal T4 concentration but with no specific symptoms or signs of thyroid dysfunction.

■ It affects 5% of the general population and is more common in women, particularly those who have antithyroid antibodies.

■ It may be part of a continuum of reducing thyroid reserve. Outside pregnancy in those with TSH <10 mU/L without thyroid antibodies progression to overt hypothyroidism occurs in less than 3% a year.

■ There is some evidence for adverse pregnancy outcome (increased preterm delivery, increased risk of abruption) in subclinical hypothyroidism but less evidence that treatment with T4 improves outcome.

■ Women previously known to be antibody positive or those found to have a raised TSH level, for example, as part of investigations for subfertility or previous miscarriage should have TFTs performed before or in early pregnancy. A rising TSH or reduced free T4 levels would then be an indication to commence T4 treatment. However, what concentration of TSH to use for diagnosis, what dose of T4 to commence, and what target TSH to aim for are not known.

■ There is currently insufficient evidence to support T4 treatment for pregnant women who are thyroid antibody positive with normal thyroid function.

Neonatal/fetal hypothyroidism

■ This is very rare (1 in 180,000) and thought to be due to the transplacental passage of TSH receptor–blocking antibodies. It represents only 2% of cases of congenital hypothyroidism.

■ These antibodies are more common in women with atrophic, rather than Hashimoto's, thyroiditis.

■ The diagnosis may be suspected in the presence of fetal goitre.

■ All neonates have their TSH measured as part of the Guthrie heel prick test.

Hypothyroidism—points to remember

- Untreated hypothyroidism is associated with infertility, an increased rate of miscarriage, and fetal loss.
- Pregnancy itself probably has no effect on hypothyroidism.
- For those on adequate replacement therapy, maternal and fetal outcome is usually good and unaffected by the hypothyroidism.
- Very little thyroxine crosses the placenta and the fetus is not at risk of thyrotoxicosis from maternal thyroxine replacement therapy.
- Provided a woman is euthyroid at the beginning of pregnancy, she will not usually require any adjustment to her thyroxine dose during pregnancy or in the puerperium.
- Neonatal hypothyroidism may rarely result from transplacental passage of TSH receptor–blocking antibodies, which are more common in women with atrophic rather than Hashimoto thyroiditis.

Postpartum thyroiditis

Incidence

- The incidence is variable depending on whether active steps are taken to diagnose the condition, as well as on local dietary intake of iodine.
- Estimates of incidence vary from 1% to 17%.
- It is more common in women with a family history of hypothyroidism and in those with thyroid peroxidase (antimicrosomal) antibodies, in whom about 50% will develop postpartum thyroiditis.

Clinical features

- Many cases are asymptomatic. Presentation is usually between 3 and 4 months postpartum but may be delayed to 6 months.
- Postpartum thyroiditis can be monophasic, producing transient hypo- (40%) or hyperthyroidism (40%) or biphasic (20%), producing first hyperthyroidism and then more prolonged hypothyroidism (4–8 months postpartum).
- Symptoms are often vague and attributed to the postpartum state.
- In the hyperthyroid phase, there may be fatigue or palpitations.
- In the hypothyroid phase, there may be lethargy, tiredness or depression.
- Goitre (small and painless) is present in approximately 50% of patients.
- Approximately 25% of patients have a first-degree relative with autoimmune thyroid disease.

Pathogenesis

- There is a destructive autoimmune thyroiditis causing first release of pre-formed T4 from the thyroid (rather than hyperfunction of the gland) and then hypothyroidism as the thyroid reserve is depleted.
- Fine-needle biopsy shows a lymphocytic thyroiditis (similar to Hashimoto thyroiditis).

- It is possible that postpartum thyroiditis represents an activation of a previously subclinical thyroiditis caused by rebound in levels of antimicrosomal antibodies as the immunosuppressive effects of pregnancy are reversed.

Diagnosis

- Since up to 50% of women who are positive for thyroid peroxidase antibody develop postpartum thyroiditis, some advise routine TFTs in such women at 2 to 3 months postpartum. Others argue that as many cases are asymptomatic and most resolve spontaneously, there is little value in screening.
- Postpartum thyroiditis is also more common in women with type 1 diabetes in whom screening may be justified.
- The diagnosis is often overlooked since the symptoms are vague and difficult to distinguish from the normal postpartum state.
- The diagnosis is made by biochemical testing to confirm hyper- or hypothyroidism.
- Approximately 75 to 85% of patients have positive antithyroid antibodies.
- To distinguish postpartum thyroiditis from a postpartum flare of Graves' disease, a radioactive iodine or technetium scan can be performed. This will show a low (as opposed to a high, as in Graves') uptake in the thyroid. TRAbs will be absent in postpartum thyroiditis but present in Graves' disease.
- Distinction from Graves' disease is important, as Graves' disease requires treatment with antithyroid drugs (see later).

Management

- Most patients recover spontaneously without requiring treatment.
- The need for treatment should be determined by symptoms rather than biochemical abnormality.
- If treatment of the hyperthyroid phase is required, this should be with β-blockers rather than with antithyroid drugs. Antithyroid drugs reduce T4 synthesis and the problem in postpartum thyroiditis is increased release, not synthesis.
- The hypothyroid phase is more likely to require treatment. This should be with T4 replacement.
- T4 should be withdrawn after 6 to 8 months to ascertain whether the patient has recovered spontaneously.
- In practice, many women become pregnant again while on T4 replacement and it is often difficult to differentiate between hypothyroidism due to postpartum thyroiditis and autoimmune thyroiditis. Withdrawal of T4 when the woman is pregnant again is not advisable unless the suspicion of postpartum thyroiditis is high and the TSH is very low or suppressed or the free T4 above or at the upper end of the normal pregnant range.

Recurrence/prognosis

- Only 3% to 4% of women remain permanently hypothyroid.
- Approximately 10% to 25% of women will suffer a recurrence in future pregnancies.
- Approximately 20% to 30% of women with thyroid peroxidase antibody–positive postpartum thyroiditis develop permanent hypothyroidism within 4 years. Therefore, long-term follow-up of such women with annual measurement of TFTs is advisable.

■ Postpartum depression is more common in thyroid antibody-positive women, irrespective of thyroid status.

Postpartum thyroiditis—points to remember

■ More common in women with a family history of hypothyroidism, those with thyroid peroxidase antibodies, and those with type 1 diabetes.
■ Presentation is usually between 3 and 4 months postpartum.
■ May present with symptoms of hyper- or hypothyroidism but a high index of suspicion is needed.
■ The condition is caused by a destructive autoimmune lymphocytic thyroiditis.
■ Most patients recover spontaneously and treatment is not always required.
■ Postpartum thyroiditis often recurs and is a significant predictor of future hypothyroidism.

Thyroid nodules

Incidence

■ Thyroid nodules are present in 1% to 2% of pregnant women.
■ Up to 40% of nodules discovered in pregnancy may be malignant.

Clinical features

■ Features indicating malignancy are
  – History of radiation to the neck or chest in childhood
  – Fixation of the lump
  – Rapid growth of a painless nodule
  – Lymphadenopathy
  – Voice change
  – Horner's syndrome
■ Features indicating de Quervain's (subacute) thyroiditis are
  – Clear history of sore throat and systemic upset consistent with a viral infection preceding appearance of the nodule
  – Tenderness of nodule or goitre
■ Very sudden onset of a nodule may suggest bleeding into a cystic lesion.

Diagnosis

■ TFTs and tests for thyroid antibodies should be performed to exclude a toxic nodule or Hashimoto thyroiditis.
■ A raised thyroglobulin titre (>100 µg/L) is suggestive of malignancy, as 90% of thyroid cancers secrete thyroglobulin.
■ Ultrasound is useful to distinguish cystic from solid lesions. The former are more likely to be benign, especially if <4 cm in diameter.
■ Cystic lesions can be aspirated and the fluid sent for cytology.

- Fine-needle aspiration or biopsy of solid lesions should be considered, especially if there are other features of malignancy (e.g., if rapidly enlarging or > 2 cm; see earlier).
- Radioactive iodine scans are contraindicated in pregnancy.

Management

- Most papillary and follicular cancers of the thyroid are slow-growing and surgical removal may be deferred until after pregnancy, but surgery can be performed during the second and third trimesters if necessary
- T4 should be given postoperatively in sufficient doses to suppress TSH, since any residual tumour is usually TSH dependent.
- If radioactive iodine is required for residual tumour or metastases, this should be delayed until after delivery.
- There is no adverse effect of pregnancy on the course of previously diagnosed and treated thyroid malignancies.
- In those with previously diagnosed and treated thyroid cancer, the diagnosis is usually papillary (rather than follicular) carcinoma, which affects younger patients. T4 doses should be titrated to ensure that TSH level remains suppressed throughout pregnancy.

Thyroid nodules—points to remember

- The possibility that a solitary thyroid nodule discovered in pregnancy is malignant must be considered.
- Malignancy is more likely with larger, fixed lesions, which are solid on ultrasound.
- TFTs should be performed to exclude other causes of nodules and goitre.
- Surgery may be performed during the second and third trimesters.

Parathyroid disease

Physiological changes

- Pregnancy and lactation are associated with increased demands for calcium.
- There is an increase in urinary loss of calcium.
- Both of these factors necessitate a twofold vitamin D–mediated increase in calcium absorption from the gut.
- Vitamin D requirements are increased by 50% to 100% during pregnancy.
- There is a fall in total calcium concentration and serum albumin.
- Free ionised calcium concentrations are unchanged.

Hyperparathyroidism

Incidence

- Primary hyperparathyroidism is the third commonest endocrine disorder after diabetes and thyroid disease, although it usually presents after the childbearing years.

- The incidence in women of childbearing age is about 8 per 100,000.
- It may be caused either by parathyroid adenomas or hyperplasia.

Clinical features

- Women may be asymptomatic.
- Symptoms include fatigue, thirst, hyperemesis, constipation and depression but may be attributed to normal pregnancy.
- Other features include hypertension, renal calculi and pancreatitis.

Diagnosis

- This may be difficult in pregnancy as hypercalcaemia is masked by the increased demands of pregnancy. An apparently normal total serum calcium may be found to be raised when corrected for the low albumin of pregnancy.
- Parathyroid hormone (PTH) levels are increased.
- Ultrasound can sometimes detect parathyroid adenomas but isotope studies (sestamibi scan) are contraindicated in pregnancy.
- Hyperplasia or adenomas may not be detected until surgical exploration of the neck.

Pregnancy

Effect of pregnancy on hyperparathyroidism

- Hypercalcaemia may be improved by pregnancy and the fetal demand for calcium.
- The risks to the mother are from acute pancreatitis and hypercalcaemic crisis, especially postpartum when the maternal transfer of calcium to the fetus stops abruptly.

Effect of hyperparathyroidism on pregnancy

- There is an increased risk of miscarriage, intrauterine death and preterm labour.
- The risk to the neonate is from tetany and hypocalcaemia, caused by suppression of fetal PTH by high maternal calcium levels. Fetal calcitonin levels are high to encourage bone mineralisation. Many cases of maternal hyperparathyroidism are diagnosed retrospectively following an episode of tetany or convulsions in the neonate.
- Acute neonatal hypocalcaemia usually presents at 5 to 14 days after birth but may be delayed by up to 1 month if the infant is breast-fed. There may be associated hypomagnesaemia.

Management

- The ideal treatment is surgery and this may be safely performed in pregnancy. Surgery is usually delayed until the second trimester.
- Treatment with intravenous fluids will reduce the serum calcium while awaiting surgery.
- Mild asymptomatic hyperparathyroidism can be managed conservatively.

- The mother should be advised to increase her intake of fluids during the pregnancy, and if necessary, a low-calcium diet and oral phosphate can be used in women who decline surgery in pregnancy.
- All mothers of infants presenting with late (>5 days after birth) hypocalcaemic tetany or seizures should have their serum calcium concentration checked.

Hypoparathyroidism

- This may be caused by autoimmune disease but occurs much more commonly as a complication of thyroid surgery.
- The incidence of hypoparathyroidism following thyroid surgery is approximately 1% to 2%.

Diagnosis

Diagnosis is made by finding low free serum calcium and PTH levels.

Pregnancy

Effect of pregnancy on hypoparathyroidism

Pregnancy increases the demand for vitamin D; and therefore, doses need to be increased to maintain normocalcaemia in pregnancy.

Effect of hypoparathyroidism on pregnancy

- Untreated hypocalcaemia in the mother increases the risk of second-trimester miscarriage, fetal hypocalcaemia and secondary hyperparathyroidism, bone demineralisation and neonatal rickets.
- Maternal hypocalcaemia may also be first diagnosed because of neonatal hypocalcaemic seizures.

Management

- Normocalcaemia is maintained with vitamin D and oral calcium supplements.
- The dose of vitamin D required increases two- to threefold in pregnancy.
- Maternal serum calcium and albumin should be measured approximately monthly.
- Vitamin D therapy is best given as alfacalcidol (1α-hydroxycholecalciferol) or calcitriol (1,25-dihydroxycholecalciferol), both of which have short half-lives, allowing titration of dose against maternal calcium levels.
- Excessive vitamin D treatment leads to maternal hypercalcaemia and possible over-mineralisation of fetal bones.
- The dose of vitamin D must be decreased again after delivery.

Vitamin D deficiency

Incidence

- Vitamin D deficiency is common in non-Caucasian ethnic groups in the United Kingdom. Approximately 16% of the U.K. population have severe vitamin D

deficiency during winter and spring, with the highest rates further north. Those at increased risk are women:
- with pigmented skin
- who are covered
- who adhere to a vegan diet
- with several pregnancies with a short interbirth interval
- with obesity
- with malabsorption
- taking antiepileptic drugs, highly active antiretroviral therapy (HAART), rifampicin
- with renal or liver disease

- Vitamin D levels are lower in pregnancy because requirements are increased.
- Different studies have demonstrated that the incidence of vitamin D deficiency (25(OH)-D < 25 nmol/L) in U.K. pregnant booking populations is 5% to 35% in white women, 50% in black women and up to 80% in Asian women.

Clinical features

Maternal

- Bone loss
- Hypocalcaemia
- Osteomalacia
- Myopathy

Fetal

- Maternal vitamin D insufficiency may adversely effect fetal bone health
- Reduced neonatal calcium $\pm$ tetany

Diagnosis

- Vitamin D status is determined by measuring 25-hydroxyvitamin D (25-OHD)
- Levels < 25nmol/L represent profound deficiency
- 25 to 50 nmol/L = insufficiency

Management

- The NICE antenatal care guideline does not recommend routine vitamin D supplementation
- Calcium and vitamin D levels should be checked in symptomatic women and non-Caucasian women at high risk (e.g., covered)
- Supplementation with oral calcium and vitamin D (400–800 U/day) should be offered to women with insufficient (25-OHD 25–50 nmol/L) levels
- Higher oral or intramuscular doses should be considered in those with a poor response or in those with frank deficiency (25-OHD < 25 nmol/L). For example, 300,000 units by i.m. injection or 20,000 units colecalciferol D3 capsules two tablets and repeat monthly as guided by vitamin D levels.

Further reading

Abalovich M, Amino N, Barbour LA, et al. Management of thyroid dysfunction during pregnancy and postpartum: an endocrine society clinical practice guideline. J Clin Endocrinol Metab 2007; 92:S1–S7.

Beattie GC, Ravi NR, Lewis M, et al. Rare presentation of maternal primary hyperparathyroidism. Br Med J 2000; 321:223–224.

Cotzias C, Wong SJ, Taylor E, et al. A study to establish gestation-specific reference intervals for thyroid function tests in normal singleton pregnancy. Eur J Obstet Gynecol Reprod Biol 2008; 137:61–66.

Girling JC. Thyroid disorders in pregnancy. Curr Opin Obstet Gynecol 2006; 16:7.

Haddow JE, Palomaki GE, Allen WC, et al. Maternal thyroid deficiency during pregnancy and subsequent neuropsychological development in the child. N Engl J Med 1999; 341:549–555.

Kothari A, Girling J. Hypothyroidism in pregnancy: pre-pregnancy thyroid status influences gestational thyroxine requirements [published online ahead of print October 8, 2008]. BJOG 2008; 115:1704–1708.

Kuy S, Roman SA, Desai R, et al. Outcomes following thyroid and parathyroid surgery in pregnant women. Arch Surg 2009; 144:399–406.

Mahon P, Harvey N, Crozier S, et al. Low maternal vitamin D status and fetal bone development: cohort study [published online ahead of print July 6, 2009]. J Bone Mineral Res 2010; 25(1):14–19.

Negro R, Formoso G, Mangieri T, et al. Levothyroxine treatment in euthyroid pregnant women with autoimmune thyroid disease: effects on obstetrical complications. J Clin Endocrinol Metab 2006; 91:2587–2591.

Norman J, Politz D, Politz L. Hyperparathyroidism during pregnancy and the effect of rising calcium on pregnancy loss: a call for earlier intervention [published online ahead of print December 5, 2008]. Clin Endocrinol (Oxf) 2009; 71,104–109.

O'Doherty MJ, McElhatton PR, Thomas SHL. Treating thyrotoxicosis in pregnant or potentially pregnant women. BMJ 1999; 318:5–6.

Pearce SHS, Cheetham TD. Diagnosis and management of vitamin D deficiency. BMJ 2010; 340:142–147.

Pop VJ, Kuijpens JL, van Baar AL, et al. Low maternal free thyroxine concentrations during early pregnancy are associated with impaired psychomotor development in infancy. Clin Endocrinol 1999; 50:149–155.

Stuckey BGA, Kent GN, Allen JR. The biochemical and clinical course of postpartum thyroid dysfunction: the treatment decision. Clin Endocrinol 2001; 54:377–383.

Tan GH, Gharib H, Goeller JR, et al. Management of thyroid nodules in pregnancy. Arch Intern Med 1996; 156:2317–2320.

Wemeau JL, Cao CD. Thyroid nodule, cancer and pregnancy. Ann Endocrinol 2002; 63:438–442.

Wing DA, Millar LK, Koonings PP, et al. A comparison of propylthiouracil versus methimazole in the treatment of hyperthyroidism in pregnancy. Am J Obstet Gynecol 1994; 170:90–95.

CHAPTER 7
Pituitary and adrenal disease

Physiological changes	**Adrenal disease**
Pituitary disease	Conn's syndrome
Hyperprolactinamia	Phaeochromocytomas
Diabetes insipidus	Addison's disease
Acromegaly	Congenital adrenal hyperplasia
Hypopituitarism	
Cushing's syndrome	

Physiological changes

Pituitary

- The volume of the anterior pituitary increases progressively during pregnancy by up to 35%.
- Postpartum involution is slower if the woman breast-feeds.
- Prolactin levels increase up to 10-fold during pregnancy and return to normal by 2 weeks after delivery, unless the woman breast-feeds.
- Physiological increases in prolactin begin early in the first trimester and are thought to be mediated via increases in oestrogen and progesterone and are related to the initiation and maintenance of lactation.
- Levels of luteinizing hormone (LH) and follicle-stimulating hormone (FSH) are suppressed by the high concentrations of oestrogen and progesterone and are undetectable during pregnancy.
- Basal growth hormone (GH) levels are unchanged by pregnancy, but human placental lactogen (hPL), which closely resembles GH, and a specific placental GH are secreted by the placenta.
- Levels of antidiuretic hormone (ADH) [arginine vasopressin (AVP)] are unchanged by pregnancy, but plasma osmolality falls early in gestation due to a reduction in serum sodium level. The mean osmolality falls from approximately 290 mOsm/L to 280 mOsm/L.
- Human placenta produces cystine aminopeptidase, which has both vasopressinase and oxytocinase activity. Thus the breakdown of ADH is increased.
- The placenta secretes adrenocorticotrophic hormone (ACTH) and corticotrophin-releasing hormone, but pituitary levels of ACTH are unaltered by pregnancy.

Adrenal

- Levels of both free and bound cortisol increase during pregnancy and levels of serum and urinary free cortisol increase threefold by term.
- Hepatic synthesis of cortisol-binding globulin is also increased.
- Normal pregnant women continue to exhibit diurnal variation in ACTH and cortisol levels.
- Suppression by exogenous corticosteroid administration (as in a low-dose dexamethasone test) is blunted.
- Levels of angiotensin II are increased two- to fourfold.
- Plasma renin activity is also increased two- to threefold.
- Plasma and urinary levels of aldosterone are increased 3-fold in the first trimester and 10-fold by the third trimester.
- Levels of urinary catecholamines, metanephrines and vanillylmandelic acid are unaffected by pregnancy, although they may be affected by stress and drugs, as in the non-pregnant patient.

Pituitary disease

Hyperprolactinamia

Aetiology

- Causes of hyperprolactinaemia include:
  - Normal pregnancy
  - Pituitary adenomas (prolactinomas)
  - Hypothalamic and pituitary stalk lesions (leading to removal of dopaminergic suppression of prolactin secretion)
  - Empty-sella syndrome
  - Hypothyroidism (TSH stimulates lactotrophs)
  - Chronic kidney disease
  - Seizures
  - Drugs, for example, metoclopramide
- Prolactinomas are the most commonly encountered pituitary tumours in pregnancy.
- Prolactinomas are divided into "macro" (>1 cm) and "micro" (<1 cm) prolactinomas.

Clinical features

- Prolactinomas may present with:
  - Infertility
  - Amenorrhoea
  - Gallactorrhoea
  - Frontal headache
  - Visual field defects [bitemporal hemianopia (due to compression of optic nerve)]
  - Diabetes insipidus
- In pregnancy, only the last three symptoms are discriminatory.

Diagnosis

- Outside pregnancy, diagnosis is by finding a raised serum prolactin level. Prolactin levels in normal pregnancy are raised 10-fold and are therefore unhelpful in diagnosing prolactinomas.

- Other pituitary function tests should be performed (such as thyroid function tests) if a pituitary tumour is suspected.
- Formal visual field testing should be used to confirm any suggestive symptoms or abnormality of the visual fields to confrontation.
- Diagnosis in pregnancy relies on findings of pituitary magnetic resonance imaging (MRI) or computed tomography (CT).

Pregnancy

Effect of pregnancy on prolactinomas

- Since the pituitary enlarges during pregnancy, there is a small risk that prolactinomas will enlarge to cause clinical problems.
- This risk is higher for macroprolactinomas (15%) than for microprolactinomas (1.6%) and probably highest in the third trimester.
- The risk of tumour growth is reduced (to 3–4% for macroprolactinomas) if the tumour has been diagnosed and treated prior to pregnancy.

Effect of prolactinomas on pregnancy

- Many women have received treatment (usually with bromocriptine or cabergoline) prior to pregnancy. Some require treatment with these dopamine agonists to suppress prolactin levels, permitting restoration of oestrogen levels and fertility and to allow conception.
- In the majority, these tumours do not lead to complications in pregnancy.
- There is no evidence for an increase in congenital abnormalities, miscarriage or adverse obstetric outcome.
- There is no reason why women with prolactinomas cannot, or should not, breast-feed.

Management

- Dopamine-receptor agonists (bromocriptine/cabergoline) are usually discontinued once pregnancy is confirmed.
- These drugs may be electively continued in cases of macroprolactinoma to prevent tumour expansion.
- Women should be reviewed at least once in each trimester.
- Serial prolactin levels are unhelpful to monitor tumour growth or activity in pregnancy but may reasonably be checked 2 months following cessation of breast-feeding.
- Formal visual field testing is only necessary for symptomatic women or those with macroprolactinomas.
- Features suggesting tumour expansion are persistent severe headache, visual field defects or the development of diabetes insipidus (see later).
- Any suspicion, especially in the case of macroprolactinomas, necessitates further confirmation with MRI.
- Dopamine-receptor agonists are safe for use in pregnancy and these should be reintroduced if there is concern regarding tumour expansion. Cabergoline has a more favourable side effect profile than bromocriptine, in particular causing less nausea.
- Women with macroprolactinomas should be advised that dopamine agonists are also safe to take during breast-feeding. Because they suppress lactation,

breast-feeding may be difficult or impossible unless these drugs are discontinued prior to birth.

- Rarely, pituitary surgery or radiotherapy may be used to treat prolactinomas, but this should be delayed until after delivery.

Prolactinomas—points to remember

- These are the commonest pituitary tumours encountered in pregnancy but rarely cause problems.
- Do not measure the prolactin level during pregnancy, as it is invariably raised.
- The risk of tumour enlargement during pregnancy is increased with macroprolactinomas >1 cm.
- Visual fields should be measured regularly in those with macroprolactinomas.
- If tumour enlargement is suspected, CT or MRI of the pituitary is indicated.
- Dopamine-receptor agonists are safe for use in pregnancy and during breast-feeding: these should be reintroduced if there is concern regarding tumour expansion.

Diabetes insipidus

Incidence

This is approximately the same as in the non-pregnant population, that is, 1 in 15,000.

Clinical features

- Excessive thirst and polyuria
- Affected women will drink frequently at night and pass large volumes of dilute urine.
- Plasma osmolality is increased [except in psychogenic diabetes insipidus (DI); see later] and urine osmolality decreased (i.e., there is a failure to concentrate the urine).
- Presentation may be with seizures secondary to hyponatraemia, which are said to be more common in transient DI (see later).

Pathogenesis

DI is caused by a relative deficiency of vasopressin (ADH). There are four types:

- *Central*—(cranial) due to deficient production of ADH from the posterior pituitary that may be idiopathic or caused by enlarging pituitary adenomas, craniopharyngiomas, skull trauma or postneurosurgery, tuberculosis, Sheehan's syndrome (see below), or rarely infiltration (histiocytosis X) or lymphocytic hypophysitis (see later).
- *Nephrogenic*—due to ADH resistance and most commonly associated with chronic kidney disease or more rarely hypercalcaemia or lithium therapy.
- *Transient*—due to increased vasopressinase production by the placenta or decreased vasopressinase breakdown by the liver. The latter form of DI is found in association with pre-eclampsia; haemolysis, elevated liver enzymes and low platelets (HELLP) syndrome; or acute fatty liver of pregnancy (AFLP) (see Chapter 11), and regresses after delivery.
- *Psychogenic*—resulting from compulsive water drinking and consequent polyuria.

Diagnosis

- Other causes of polyuria such as diuretics, hyperglycaemia, hypercalcaemia and hypokalaemia should be excluded.
- In the non-pregnant, diagnosis is conventionally with a fluid deprivation test, when the patient is not allowed to drink for 15 to 22 hours, during which time serial weights, paired urine and plasma osmolalities are measured. Following dehydration and a loss of 3% to 5% of body weight, ADH is stimulated and urine concentration occurs in those without DI and in those with psychogenic DI.
- In pregnancy, such dehydration is potentially hazardous and diagnosis should be attempted first by admission of the patient for observation, documentation of polyuria, and paired plasma, and urine osmolality measurements. Urine output ranges from 4 to 15 L/day.
- Confirmation of a diagnosis of DI is straightforward if the plasma osmolality (>295 mOsm/kg) or serum sodium (>145 mmol/L) is inappropriately raised in the presence of polyuria and a low urine osmolality (<300 mOsm/kg). This excludes compulsive water drinking.
- A "short" water deprivation test, for example overnight, may be all that is required to demonstrate an increasing urine osmolality (>700 mOsm/kg should be considered normal) with normal plasma osmolality and thus exclude cranial and nephrogenic DI.
- Failure to concentrate the urine in response to a rising or abnormally high plasma osmolality (>300 mOsm/kg) is diagnostic of DI.
- It is safest to initially perform a fluid deprivation test during the day when the patient may be safely observed. However, if this does not confirm a diagnosis of DI or result in a sufficient rise in urine osmolality to exclude the diagnosis, a more prolonged fluid deprivation following an overnight fast may be required.
- Administration of dDAVP (1-desamino-8-D-arginine vasopressin—a synthetic analogue of vasopressin) 10 to 20 µg intranasally may also be used to facilitate diagnosis. It will result in concentration of urine in cranial DI, transient DI and to a greater extent in normals, but not in nephrogenic DI (who remain polyuric).
- Those with central DI have low ADH levels, but those with nephrogenic DI have high levels.

Pregnancy

Effect of pregnancy on DI

- Pregnancy may unmask previously subclinical DI.
- In those with established DI, there is a tendency to deterioration during pregnancy (60%). This may be due to the following:
  - Increased glomerular filtration rate of pregnancy
  - Placental production of vasopressinase
  - Antagonism of vasopressin (ADH) by prostaglandins

Effect of DI on pregnancy

- Severe dehydration and electrolyte disturbance are risks in undiagnosed or untreated cases. Complications include maternal seizures and oligohydramnios.
- In treated cases, there is no adverse effect on pregnancy outcome. Labour proceeds normally, and there is no contraindication to breast-feeding.

Management

- A confirmed or suspected diagnosis of new onset DI in pregnancy should prompt a search for pre-eclampsia and AFLP in particular.
- dDAVP is safe for use in pregnancy for diagnosis or treatment of DI. It is relatively resistant to vasopressinase.
- For cranial DI, dDAVP is administered intranasally 10 to 20 μg b.d. or t.d.s. Serum electrolytes and plasma osmolality should be checked regularly to ensure adequate treatment and to avoid overtreatment and water intoxication. Extreme caution is required with the concomitant use of intravenous fluids or in the presence of renal impairment.
- For nephrogenic DI outside pregnancy, chlorpropamide, which increases renal responsiveness to endogenous ADH, is sometimes used. This should be avoided in pregnancy because of the risk of fetal hypoglycaemia.
- Carbamazepine is also used for nephrogenic DI and is a reasonable alternative in pregnancy, notwithstanding the teratogenic risks (see Chapter 9).
- The mainstay of treatment of nephrogenic DI in pregnancy is water restriction, but thiazide diuretics and non-steroidal anti-inflammatory drugs have also been used.

Diabetes insipidus—points to remember

- Established or subclinical DI may worsen in pregnancy.
- Extended fluid-deprivation tests should be avoided in pregnancy and close observation with paired urine and plasma osmolality measurements may be sufficient to exclude DI.
- dDAVP is safe for use in pregnancy for diagnosis or treatment of DI.
- Transient DI may occur in pregnancy and is often associated with preeclampsia, HELLP syndrome or AFLP.

Acromegaly

Incidence

This is rarely encountered in pregnancy (5 in 100,000).

Clinical Features

- Many patients are infertile because GH-secreting pituitary adenomas often co-secrete prolactin and may also cause stalk compression, leading to secondary hyper-prolactinaemia.
- Overall, about 40% of women with acromegaly have associated hyperprolactinaemia.
- The main clinical features are those of GH excess, of which altered facial appearance, macroglossia, large hands and feet may be the most obvious.
- Headaches and sweating are other common symptoms.
- There is an increased incidence of hypertension, impaired glucose tolerance and diabetes mellitus.

Diagnosis

- This may be difficult in pregnancy, because although basal levels of GH do not change, GH assays may detect hPL and placental GH.

■ Insulin growth factor-I (IGF-I) is increasingly used as a diagnostic tool outside pregnancy, but this increases in normal pregnancy and cannot therefore be used.

Pregnancy

Effect of pregnancy on acromegaly

■ GH-secreting adenomas may expand during pregnancy, but this is less common than with prolactinomas.
■ As with prolactinomas, expansion may cause visual field defects.

Effect of acromegaly on pregnancy

■ GH does not cross the placenta or adversely affect the fetus.
■ The risk of gestational diabetes and macrosomia is increased.

Management

■ Treatment prior to pregnancy is the ideal and this is usually with surgery and/or radiotherapy.
■ Bromocriptine and cabergoline are not as effective in decreasing GH levels as decreasing prolactin levels, but do work in about 50% of cases.
■ Octreotide, lanreotide and pegvisomont (somatostatin analogues) decreases GH secretion and are used increasingly in the management of acromegaly, but data regarding safety in pregnancy are limited. The manufacturer advises that they should only be used if potential benefit outweighs risk, since they cross the placenta and the fetus expresses somatostatin receptors. There have been only a handful of pregnancies reported with somatostatin analogues but no malformations or adverse outcomes are described.

Hypopituitarism

This may be caused by the following:

■ Pituitary surgery
■ Radiotherapy
■ Pituitary or hypothalamic tumours
■ Postpartum pituitary infarction (Sheehan's syndrome)
■ Lymphocytic hypophysitis

Sheehan's syndrome

This usually presents postpartum following postpartum haemorrhage and may lead to partial or complete pituitary failure.

Clinical features

■ Failure of lactation
■ Persistent amenorrhoea
■ Loss of axillary and pubic hair
■ Hypothyroidism
■ Adrenocortical insufficiency—nausea, vomiting, hypoglycaemia, hypotension

Pathogenesis

- The anterior pituitary is particularly vulnerable to hypotension in pregnancy, probably as a result of its increased size.
- Most cases (90%) of Sheehan's syndrome are preceded by an episode of postpartum haemorrhage associated with hypotension.

Lymphocytic hypophysitis

This is an uncommon autoimmune disorder, commoner in women and most common in late pregnancy and the postpartum period. Incidence is increasing as refined radiological and surgical techniques have permitted more precise diagnosis of pituitary dysfunction.

Clinical features

It presents with features suggestive of an expanding pituitary tumour:

- 60% have mass effects
  - 40% Visual field defects
  - 60% Headache
- 85% have endocrine effects
  - Panhypopituitarism
  - Hypothyroidism
  - Adrenocortical insufficiency—nausea, vomiting, hypoglycaemia, hypotension
  - DI (in approximately 18%)

Pathogenesis

There is extensive infiltration of the anterior pituitary by chronic inflammatory cells, predominantly lymphocytes, causing pituitary expansion. Various degrees of oedema and fibrosis may be present but no adenoma. Antipituitary antibodies have been described and this condition is associated with autoimmune thyroiditis or adrenalitis in 20% of cases.

Diagnosis of hypopituitarism

- Investigation reveals reduced levels of T4, thyroid-stimulating hormone (TSH), (the TSH may be at the lower end of the normal range which is inappropriate in the presence of a low free T4), cortisol, ACTH, FSH, LH and GH.
- Secretion of ACTH, GH and prolactin in response to hypoglycaemic stress (insulin stress test) is impaired.
- Any patient with hypopituitarism should undergo pituitary imaging with MRI or CT to exclude a pituitary tumour.
- In cases of lymphocytic hypophysitis, MRI shows symmetrical (in contrast to pituitary adenomas) enlargement of the pituitary, suprasellar extension with displacement of the optic chiasm, pituitary stalk enlargement (rather than deviation) and abnormal dural enhancement with gadolinium contrast.
- Definitive diagnosis of lymphocytic hypophysitis can be made only by histological examination of pituitary tissue.
- Pituitary antibodies have low sensitivity and specificity

Pregnancy

Effect of pregnancy on hypopituitarism

■ Subsequent pregnancies after Sheehan's syndrome and lymphocytic hypophysitis have been reported.
■ Pregnancy is also possible with other causes of hypopituitarism.
■ Conception may require gonadotrophin stimulation of ovulation, but once pregnancy has been achieved, the fetoplacental unit produces enough gonadotrophin, oestrogen and progesterone to sustain the pregnancy.

Effect of hypopituitarism on pregnancy

■ If the condition is diagnosed and treated with adequate hormone replacement therapy prior to pregnancy, then maternal and fetal outcome is normal.
■ Previously undiagnosed or poorly treated hypopituitarism is associated with an increased risk of miscarriage, stillbirth and maternal morbidity and mortality from hypotension and hypoglycaemia.

Management

■ The management of acute pituitary insufficiency includes i.v. fluids, dextrose and corticosteroids.
■ The need for replacement hormones is determined by pituitary function testing, but most patients require glucocorticoids and thyroxine.
■ Corticosteroids are a logical and reportedly successful treatment for lymphocytic hypophysitis, especially during pregnancy and if there is no visual disturbance (necessitating surgery). However, many cases undergo surgery because of misdiagnosis of pituitary tumour. This results in new hypopituitarism or failure of existing dysfunction to improve.
■ Cases of Sheehan's syndrome and lymphocytic hypophysitis have resolved spontaneously.
■ Unlike Addison's disease (see later) mineralocorticoid replacement is not required, because aldosterone secretion is not ACTH dependent and is consequently not impaired.
■ During subsequent pregnancy, requirements for thyroxine do not alter, but additional parenteral corticosteroids may be required (see later under "Addison's Disease").
■ Lymphocytic hypophysitis may recur in subsequent pregnancies.

Cushing's syndrome

Incidence

This is very rare in pregnancy, with only about 50 cases reported worldwide, as most cases are associated with infertility.

Clinical features

These may easily be attributed to the pregnancy:

■ Excessive weight gain
■ Extensive purple striae

- Diabetes mellitus
- Hypertension
- Easy bruising
- Headache
- Hirsutism
- Acne
- Proximal myopathy (discriminating feature in pregnancy)

Pathogenesis

- Outside pregnancy, 80% of cases of Cushing's syndrome are due to pituitary adenomas (Cushing's disease).
- In pregnancy, <50% of cases are due to pituitary disease and most are caused by adrenal adenomas (44%) or adrenal carcinomas (12%).

Diagnosis

- Pregnancy-specific ranges for plasma and urinary cortisol must be used.
- Low ACTH, with an increased cortisol level that fails to suppress with a high-dose dexamethasone suppression test, is suggestive of an adrenal cause.
- Localisation is with ultrasound, CT or MRI of the adrenals, or CT or MRI of the pituitary.

Pregnancy

Effect of Cushing's syndrome on pregnancy

- There is an increased rate of fetal loss, prematurity and perinatal mortality. The adverse outcome is only partly explained by maternal diabetes and hypertension.
- The neonate is at risk from adrenal insufficiency because high maternal cortisol levels lead to suppression of fetal/neonatal corticosteroid secretion.
- Maternal morbidity and mortality are increased and severe pre-eclampsia is common.
- Wound infection is common after caesarean section due to poor tissue healing.
- Women with previously treated Cushing's do well in pregnancy.

Management

- Surgery is the treatment of choice for both pituitary-dependent and adrenal Cushing's syndrome.
- The management of women with Cushing's has been undertaken successfully during pregnancy.
- Experience with cyproheptadine, metyrapone and ketoconazole in pregnancy is very limited, and metyrapone has been associated with severe hypertension. Ketoconazole should be avoided as it is teratogenic in animal studies.

Adrenal disease

Conn's syndrome

Hyperaldosteronism is found in 0.7% of non-pregnant patients with hypertension, but very few cases of primary hyperaldosteronism have been reported in pregnancy. This is probably due to underreporting.

Clinical features

- Hypertension
- Hypokalaemia (serum potassium <3.0 mmol/L).

Pathogenesis

Primary hyperaldosteronism may be due to the following:

- Adrenal aldosterone-secreting adenoma
- Adrenal carcinoma
- Bilateral adrenal hyperplasia.

Diagnosis

This is suggested by finding of:

- Low serum potassium level (although in pregnancy, progesterone may antagonize aldosterone and ameliorate the hypokalaemia)
- Suppressed renin activity (compared with normal pregnancy ranges)
- High plasma aldosterone level (compared with normal pregnancy ranges)

Hypertension, particularly in the absence of a positive family history, and hypokalaemia are an indication for ultrasound scanning of the adrenal glands.

Management

- Hypertension is controlled in the usual way with methyldopa, labetalol or nifedipine (see Chapter 1), and hypokalaemia is treated with potassium supplementation or potassium-sparing diuretics.
- Amiloride is safe to use in pregnancy and high doses (e.g., 20 mg daily) may be needed.
- Spironolactone, which is used as a potassium-sparing diuretic in Conn's syndrome outside pregnancy, should be avoided as it may cause feminisation of a male fetus because it is an antiandrogen.
- Surgery for adrenal adenomas can usually be safely deferred until after delivery.

Phaeochromocytomas

Incidence

- Phaeochromocytomas are found in 0.1% of non-pregnant patients with hypertension but are only rarely encountered (1 in 50,000 cases) in pregnancy.
- It is important to consider the diagnosis since, when undiagnosed, the maternal and fetal mortality rate is extremely high.

Clinical features

- Paroxysms of:
  - Hypertension (may be sustained or labile)
  - Headache
  - Palpitations

  - Sweating
  - Anxiety
  - Vomiting
  - Glucose intolerance
- Hypertension in pregnancy is common; and therefore, a high index of suspicion must be maintained to achieve an early diagnosis. The classical paroxysms of hypertension are present only in 50% of cases of phaeochromocytoma.
- Cases often mimic pre-eclampsia.
- Hypertensive pregnant women with associated unusual features such as excessive sweating, headache and palpitations should be screened.

Pathogenesis

- Phaeochromocytomas are tumours of the adrenal medulla, secreting excess catecholamines.
- 10% are bilateral.
- 10% are extra-adrenal.
- 10% are malignant.

Phaeochromocytomas may be part of a multiple endocrine neoplasia IIa syndrome and, if diagnosis is confirmed, the patient should be screened for medullary cell carcinoma of the thyroid and parathyroid adenomas.

Diagnosis

- This does not differ from that in the non-pregnant woman and is made by finding raised 24-hour urinary catecholamines and/or raised plasma catecholamines.
- Stress may cause non-significant rises in catecholamines.
- Non-specific assays may give false-positive results if the woman is taking methyldopa or labetalol and screening should ideally be performed before antihypertensive therapy is commenced.
- Once the diagnosis has been confirmed, CT, ultrasound and MRI offer the best methods of tumour localisation, although the latter two are preferable in pregnancy.
- MIBG (131I-meta-iodobenzylguanidine) scan to localize norepinephrine uptake is contraindicated in pregnancy.

Pregnancy

Effect of pregnancy on phaeochromocytomas

- Potentially fatal hypertensive crises may be precipitated by labour, vaginal or abdominal delivery, general anaesthesia or opiates.
- Attacks in pregnancy may occur whilst supine due to pressure of the gravid uterus on the tumour.

Effect of phaeochromocytomas on pregnancy

- There is a greatly increased maternal and fetal mortality rate, especially if, as in up to 50% of cases, the diagnosis is not made antepartum.
- The maternal mortality rate is about 17% in undiagnosed cases and 4% in diagnosed cases.

- The fetal mortality rate is about 26% in undiagnosed cases and 11% in diagnosed cases.
- Mothers may die of arrhythmias, cerebrovascular accidents or pulmonary oedema.

Management

- Adequate α-blockade with phenoxybenzamine or prazosin to control hypertension followed by β-blockade, if required, to control tachycardia.
- Surgical removal is the only cure, and optimal timing of tumour resection depends on the gestation at which the diagnosis is made.
- In general, if pharmacological blockade has been achieved prior to 23 weeks' gestation, then resection is performed. If the pregnancy is more than 24 weeks' gestation, then surgery becomes more hazardous and should be delayed until fetal maturity, when caesarean section with concurrent or delayed tumour removal is undertaken. There is an increasing vogue to delay tumour resection until the puerperium.
- Expert anaesthetic care is essential and both fetal and maternal mortality rates have improved significantly since the advent of α-blockade, which should be given for at least 3 days prior to surgery.
- Hypertensive crises can be precipitated by several drugs including metoclopramide, morphine, pheno-thiazines and contrast media.

Phaeochromocytomas—points to remember

- A rare but dangerous cause of hypertension in pregnancy.
- Women with hypertension associated with unusual features of palpitations, anxiety, sweating or headache should be screened.
- Adequate α-blockade for at least 3 days prior to surgery is essential.

Addison's disease

Incidence

Addison's disease is rarely encountered in pregnancy and most cases have been previously diagnosed.

Clinical features

There is adrenocortical failure, causing both glucocorticoid and mineralocorticoid deficiency. This leads to:

- Weight loss
- Vomiting
- Postural hypotension
- Lethargy
- Hyperpigmentation, particularly in the skin folds, in recent scars and in the mouth

Investigation

Investigation reveals the following:

- Hyponatraemia
- Hyperkalaemia

- Raised blood urea
- Hypoglycaemia

Pathogenesis

- Most cases in the United Kingdom are now due to autoimmune destruction of the adrenal glands caused by adrenal antibodies.
- Tuberculosis is the other main cause.
- The autoimmune form is more common in women (female preponderance 2.5:1) and may be associated in up to 40% of cases with other autoimmune conditions, such as pernicious anaemia, diabetes or thyrotoxicosis.

Diagnosis

- This is made by finding a low 9.00 a.m. cortisol level, a raised ACTH level and a loss of cortisol response to synthetic ACTH (Synacthen).
- When interpreting the results of cortisol measurements in pregnancy, it is important to remember that both the serum total and free cortisol levels are increased. An abnormally low cortisol level for pregnancy may therefore fall within the normal non-pregnant range.

Pregnancy

Effect of pregnancy on Addison's disease

- Pregnancy has no effect on Addison's disease, except possibly causing delay in diagnosis. This is because many of the clinical features may be masked by or attributed to the pregnancy.
- There are certain times during the pregnancy when women with Addison's disease may require increased doses of steroid replacement (see later).
- Unlike autoimmune thyroid disease, autoimmune adrenal disease is not more common in the puerperium, although patients with established Addison's disease may deteriorate in the puerperium (see later).

Effect of Addison's disease on pregnancy

- Prior to the advent of steroid therapy, Addison's disease was associated with a high maternal mortality rate.
- Provided Addison's disease is diagnosed and treated prior to pregnancy, there should be no adverse effect on the pregnancy.
- Adrenal antibodies do cross the placenta, but neonatal adrenal insufficiency secondary to maternal Addison's disease is rarely encountered in clinical practice.

Management

- In contrast to adrenal failure due to pituitary disease (see earlier), in Addison's disease there is a deficiency of both cortisol and aldosterone.
- Maintenance treatment with both hydrocortisone (25–30 mg/day p.o. in divided doses) and fludrocortisone (usually 0.1 mg/day) is required.
- Treatment in the acute situation may require i.v. saline.

- Maintenance steroids should be continued throughout pregnancy. The safety of steroids in pregnancy has been previously discussed (see under "Asthma," Chapter 4, p. 61).
- Pregnant patients need to increase their dose of corticosteroids or receive parenteral hydrocortisone if they develop hyperemesis, infection or undergo any stressful event (e.g., amniocentesis).
- Labour should be managed with parenteral hydrocortisone (100 mg, i.m., 6-hourly), since women with Addison's disease are unable to mount an increased output of endogenous steroids from the adrenal gland that normally accompanies labour and delivery.
- Clinical well-being and blood pressure together provide a good index of the adequacy of steroid replacement.
- Following delivery, the physiological diuresis may cause profound hypotension in women with Addison's disease. This can be treated with i.v. saline, but prevention is possible if the higher dose of steroids to cover labour is weaned gradually over a number of days rather than over 24 hours, as it would be in patients on maintenance steroids for asthma or arthritis.

Congenital adrenal hyperplasia

Incidence

- Classic congenital adrenal hyperplasia (CAH) is rare (1 in 14,000). The gene frequency is 1 in 200 to 400 and the disorder is autosomal recessive. Milder forms are more common.
- If a couple have one affected child, the risk of a subsequent child having the disorder is 1 in 4.

Clinical features

The main problems are as follows:

- Masculisation of a female fetus
- Salt-losing crisis in a male neonate due to mineralocorticoid deficiency
- Precocious puberty in a male
- Female adults with CAH are often infertile and may have psychosexual problems related to anatomical problems following corrective surgery for virilisation of the genitalia.
- Polycystic ovaries, anovulation, hirsutism and acne may occur in association with adrenal androgen excess.
- Amenorrhoea is common, and delayed menarche and premature menopause have been reported.

Pathogenesis

- All forms are caused by deficiencies of adrenal enzymes used to synthesise glucocorticoids. There is therefore increased production of cortisol precursors and androgens.
- Approximately 90% are due to 21-hydroxylase deficiency causing both reduced cortisol and aldosterone production, and increased androgen synthesis. These

individuals have both glucocorticoid and mineralocortcoid deficiency and the "salt-losing" form of CAH.

■ Deficiency of 11-β hydroxylase is found in 8% to 9% of patients with CAH. This leads to accumulation of deoxycortisol that has mineralocorticoid activity; and therefore, these women may be hypertensive.

Pregnancy

Effect of CAH on pregnancy

■ Few cases of pregnancies in women with CAH have been reported.

■ There is an increased risk of miscarriage (inadequate corpus luteum activity), pre-eclampsia and fetal growth restriction.

■ Caesarean section may be required because of an android-shaped pelvis.

Management

Pregnancy in women with CAH

■ Increased surveillance should be performed because of the risk of pre-eclampsia.

■ Steroid replacement therapy should be continued at the pre-pregnancy dose, and most women with 21-hydroxylase deficiency require no alteration in pregnancy.

■ Adequacy of corticosteroid replacement is usually monitored with androgen levels.

■ Free testosterone levels are reduced or unchanged in pregnancy.

■ 17-Hydroxyprogesterone and androstenedione levels are raised and therefore unreliable markers of androgen suppression in pregnancy.

■ If androgen levels are elevated beyond normal pregnancy levels, doses of corticosteroid should be increased.

■ Despite high maternal serum androgens, placental aromatase converts these to oestrogens, thus protecting a female fetus from masculinisation.

■ Mineralocorticoid dosage usually requires no change.

■ Increased corticosteroids are needed to cover delivery and with intercurrent stress such as infection.

Pregnancy when the fetus is at risk of CAH

■ This situation arises if a couple have had a previously affected child or if the partner of an affected woman is a carrier for the same mutation.

■ One option is termination of the pregnancy if investigation suggests an affected female fetus.

■ Alternatively, dexamethasone given to the mother will cross the placenta and suppress the fetal adrenal production, preventing masculinisation of a female fetus. This strategy is controversial.

■ High doses of dexamethasone (1–1.5 mg/day) are needed.

■ Treatment should be started preconception, or before week 5 of pregnancy, to optimise the chance of normalisation prior to differentiation of the genitalia. However, genetic diagnosis is not possible until 12 weeks' gestation (chorionic villus biopsy weeks 10–11+ a week to obtain the result) and should be performed only if a couple have had a previously affected child and each of their genetic mutations is known.

■ Only one in eight fetuses (1 in 4 risk of homozygote and 1 in 2 risk of female fetus) may benefit from these high-dose steroids, and 7 in 8 will be treated unnecessarily for 6 weeks.

- If it is thought that a female fetus is affected, treatment of the mother should continue until term to prevent late masculinisation and neuroendocrine effects of exposure to high androgen levels.
- All female neonates should receive corticosteroids, both to treat CAH and because the neonatal adrenal glands will be suppressed following long-term, high-dose dexamethasone treatment of the mother.
- Male fetuses do not need to be treated in utero.
- Unfortunately, prevention of virilisation with the regimen mentioned earlier is not always successful and the parents must be fully counselled regarding the risks and benefits of use of such high doses of steroids throughout pregnancy.

Further reading

Ahlawat SK, Jain S, Kumari S, et al. Pheochromocytoma associated with pregnancy: case report and review of the literature. Obstet Gynecol Surv 1999; 54:728–37.

Beressi N, Beressir J-P, Cohen R, et al. Lymphocytic hypophysitis. Ann Med Intern 1999; 150:327–334.

Bronstein MD, Salgado LR, de CM. Medical management of pituitary adenomas: the special case of management of the pregnant woman. Pituitary 2002; 5:99–107.

Browne I, Brady I, Hannon V, et al. Anaesthesia for phaeochromocytoma and sickle cell disease in pregnancy. Int J Obstet Anesth 2005; 14:66–69.

Cauley K, Dalal A, Olson B, et al. Lymphocytic hypophysitis. Conn Med 2005; 69:143–146.

Garner PR. Congenital adrenal hyperplasia in pregnancy. Semin Perinatol 1998; 22:446–456.

Grodski S, Jung C, Kertes P, et al. Phaeochromocytoma in pregnancy. Intern Med J 2006; 36:604–606.

Hague W. Diabetes insipidus in pregnancy. Obstet Med 2009; 2:138–141.

Lakasing L, Williamson C. Obstetric complications due to autoantibodies. Best Pract Res Clin Endocrinol Metab 2005; 19:149–175.

Sainz Bueno JA, Villarejo OP, Hidalgo AJ, et al. Transient diabetes insipidus during pregnancy: a clinical case and a review of the syndrome. Eur J Obstet Gynecol Reprod Biol 2005; 118:251–254.

CHAPTER 8

Connective-tissue disease

Physiological changes	Scleroderma
Rheumatoid arthritis	Ehlers–Danlos syndrome (EDS)
Systemic lupus erythematosus	Vasculitis
Neonatal lupus syndromes	Pregnancy-associated
Antiphospholipid syndrome	osteoporosis

Physiological changes

Pregnancy is associated with an alteration in the maternal immune system. There is a shift away from cell-mediated immunity (Th1 response) to humoral immunity (Th 2 response). This probably occurs to protect the fetus from immunological attack by the mother and these changes are reversed postpartum.

Rheumatoid arthritis

Incidence

- The adult form of the disease is more common in women (female to male ratio 3:1).
- Approximately 1 woman in every 1000 to 2000 pregnancies is affected.

Clinical features

- Rheumatoid arthritis is a chronic inflammatory disease affecting primarily the synovial joints.
- There is a deforming polyarthritis with synovitis of joint and tendon sheaths, articular cartilage loss and erosion of juxta-articular bone.
- The prominent symptoms are joint pain and morning stiffness.
- Signs include swelling, warmth and tenderness with limitation of movement.
- There is symmetrical involvement, particularly of the metacarpophalangeal, proximal interphalangeal and wrist joints.
- Deformities such as ulnar deviation of the metacarpophalangeal joints and Swan neck and Boutonniere deformities of the fingers may be apparent in the later stages of the disease.

- Rheumatoid arthritis is a systemic disorder. Extra-articular features include: fatigue, vasculitis, subcutaneous (rheumatoid) nodules, haematological abnormalities (anaemia), pulmonary granulomas, effusions and fibrosis, cardiac involvement (pericarditis) and amyloidosis.
- The eyes may be involved with scleritis, scleromalacia or most commonly (15%) secondary Sjögren's syndrome (exocrine salivary and lacrimal gland inflammation causing dry eyes and mouth).

Pathogenesis

- Rheumatoid arthritis is initiated by CD4+ T cells which are activated in response to an, as yet unknown, endogenous or exogenous antigen.
- The activated CD4+ T cells then stimulate monocytes, macrophages and synovial fibroblasts to produce cytokines and B cells to produce antibodies including rheumatoid factor.
- Immune complexes are common in the synovial fluid and circulation.
- The two main pathological characteristics are inflammation and proliferation of the synovium.
- There is progressive joint damage causing severe disability.
- There is an association with the human leukocyte antigen HLA-D4 (70%).

Diagnosis and immunology

- Approximately 80% to 90% of patients are positive for rheumatoid factor (RhF).
- Antinuclear antibodies are positive in approximately 30% of cases.
- Anaemia (normochromic, normocytic) is related to the degree of disease activity.
- The erythrocyte sedimentation rate (ESR) and C-reactive protein (CRP) are also used as markers of disease activity, but the ESR is unreliable in pregnancy as it is normally elevated.
- Sjögren's syndrome is particularly associated with anti-Ro and anti-La antibodies (see p. 138, 'Neonatal lupus syndromes'), that is, antibodies directed against extractable nuclear antigens (ENAs).
- Approximately 5% to 10% of patients with rheumatoid arthritis have antiphospholipid antibodies (see later), but antiphospholipid syndrome is unusual (see later).

Pregnancy

Effect of pregnancy on rheumatoid arthritis

- Up to 75% of women with rheumatoid arthritis experience improvement during pregnancy, although only approximately 16% enter complete remission and approximately 25% will have substantial disability during pregnancy. Disease activity in previous pregnancies may be predictive.
- Various theories have been proposed to explain the improvement, including:
  - Raised cortisol levels
  - A maternal immune response to fetal paternally inherited HLA class II gene products
  - Decrease in T-cell-mediated immunity
  - High oestrogen levels

- Pregnancy-specific proteins such as β_2-glycoprotein (PAG) (in experimental models, PAG improves arthritis)
- Removal of immune complexes by the placenta.
- Improvement usually begins during the first trimester and rheumatoid nodules may also disappear.
- Of those who experience remission, 90% suffer postpartum exacerbations. This may be related to resurgence of T-cell-mediated immunity in the puerperium.
- Postpartum flares are made worse by breastfeeding, possibly related to prolactin.
- There is an increase in the incidence of first presentation of rheumatoid arthritis in the postpartum period, particularly after the first pregnancy.

Effect of rheumatoid arthritis on pregnancy

- Unlike systemic lupus erythematosus (SLE), there seems to be no adverse effect of rheumatoid arthritis on pregnancy.
- Neither the fertility rate nor spontaneous abortion rate is significantly altered.
- Infants of women who have anti-Ro antibodies are at risk of neonatal lupus (see later).
- Atlanto-axial subluxation is a rare complication of a general anaesthetic for caesarean section, and very rarely, limitation of hip abduction is severe enough to impede vaginal delivery.
- The main concerns relate to the safety during pregnancy and lactation of the medications used to treat rheumatoid arthritis (see later).

Management

- Women, particularly those with secondary Sjögren's syndrome, should be screened for anti-Ro and anti-La antibodies (see later).
- They should be referred to an obstetric anaesthetist especially if there is known neck involvement.
- The major challenge is control of symptoms of pain, swelling and stiffness in affected joints in those women whose disease does not improve completely in pregnancy.

Simple analgesics

Paracetamol should be the first-line analgesic and there are no known adverse effects specific to pregnancy or the fetus.

Non-steroidal anti-inflammatory drugs

- Neither aspirin nor non-steroidal anti-inflammatory drugs (NSAIDs) are teratogenic.
- NSAIDs may cause infertility via 'luteinised unruptured follicle syndrome' or impairment of blastocyst implantation.
- Salicylates (in high doses) and NSAIDs may increase the risk of neonatal haemorrhage via inhibition of platelet function.
- NSAIDs may also lead to oligohydramnios via effects on the fetal kidney, and may cause premature closure of the ductus arteriosus because they are prostaglandin synthetase inhibitors. However, both constriction of the ductus arteriosus and impairment of fetal renal function are reversible after discontinuation of NSAIDs.

- The risk of premature closure of the ductus may have been exaggerated since this has not been encountered when indomethacin is used for the treatment of preterm labour.
- NSAIDs are usually avoided, especially in the third trimester.
- In occasional circumstances, and especially prior to 28 weeks' gestation, NSAIDS may be used for control of arthritic pain if there are relative contraindications to steroids (e.g. in women with osteoporosis) or if steroids are relatively ineffective (e.g. in ankylosing spondylitis).
- If NSAIDs are used during pregnancy, they should be discontinued by 32 to 34 weeks' gestation.
- The cyclo-oxygenase type-2-selective (COX-2) NSAIDs have been reported to show only minor renal and no ductal effects on the fetus when used to prevent preterm labour. Some have been withdrawn due to associated cardiovascular risk and their use is currently contraindicated in pregnancy.

Corticosteroids

- Corticosteroids may be continued during pregnancy and are preferable to NSAIDs if paracetamol is insufficient to control symptoms in the third trimester.
- Women with rheumatoid arthritis may be treated with long-acting intramuscular steroids such as depo-medrone or intra-articular steroids. These too are safe in pregnancy.
- Women—and their doctors—are often reluctant to use corticosteroids, but this concern is misplaced.
- For a discussion on safety of corticosteroids in pregnancy, see Chapter 4 under 'Asthma', p. 61.
- Pregnant women taking steroids are at increased risk of gestational diabetes and preterm rupture of the membranes.
- If a woman is on long-term maintenance steroids (>7.5 mg prednisolone for >2 weeks), parenteral steroids should be administered to cover the stress of labour and delivery, regardless of the route of delivery.

Azathioprine

- Azathioprine is the commonest cytotoxic drug used for treatment of rheumatoid arthritis and SLE and is safe to use in pregnancy. This is partly because the fetal liver lacks the enzyme that converts azathioprine to its active metabolites.
- Years of experience in women with renal transplants and women with SLE treated with azathioprine support no adverse fetal effects. It should not be discontinued in pregnancy.
- Azathioprine may be added in pregnancy and is useful as a steroid sparing agent, although its onset of action is at least three weeks.
- Although standard advice is, for women requiring azathioprine, to avoid breastfeeding, due to a theoretical risk of immunosuppression in the neonate, only very low concentrations of the active metabolites of azathioprine are found in breast milk and levels in the blood of breastfed neonates are undetectable. Therefore, women can be reassured that breastfeeding is not contraindicated if they are taking azathioprine and it could be argued that the benefits of breastfeeding outweigh a small theoretical risk not substantiated in formal studies.

Antimalarials

■ Antimalarial drugs such as hydroxychloroquine, used in rheumatoid arthritis and to prevent flares in SLE, are safe to use.

■ Pregnancies in women exposed to chloroquine and hydroxychloroquine have congenital abnormality rates no higher than background rates in the general/unexposed population.

■ There is increasing experience of hydroxychloroquine use in pregnant and lactating women with SLE and no adverse effect on the neonates has been demonstrated.

■ Cessation of hydroxychloroquine therapy in early pregnancy is illogical for two reasons. Firstly, it has a very long half-life such that the fetus remains exposed to the drug for several weeks following discontinuation of maternal therapy. Secondly, discontinuation of hydroxychloroquine is associated with a risk of lupus flare.

Mycophenolate mofetil (MMF)

■ Like azathioprine, MMF is an antiproliferative immunosuppressant. It is, however, more selective than azothioprine and is now in widespread use in SLE as well as transplantation.

■ Data concerning use of MMF in pregnancy are accumulating and standard advice is to avoid MMF, as it is teratogenic. Fetal exposure is associated with a specific embryopathy including cleft lip and palate, microtia with atresia of external auditory canal, micrognathia and hypertelorism.

■ In certain circumstances, when used to prevent rejection in renal allografts, or for severe lupus nephritis unresponsive to other immunosuppressive agents, its continuation may represent less of a risk to the pregnancy than deterioration in renal function or active connective-tissue disease.

Penicillamine

■ Penicillamine is a chelating agent used particularly in the management of the extra-articular features of rheumatoid arthritis.

■ The drug crosses the placenta and in high doses may be a teratogen associated with abnormalities of connective tissue. The risk of congenital collagen defect is approximately 5% and therefore it should be stopped pre-conception in women with rheumatic diseases.

■ However, approximately 90 reported cases of maternal penicillamine use suggest that it is relatively safe.

■ The continued use of penicillamine is crucial for successful outcome of pregnancy in Wilson's disease.

Gold salts

■ Although teratogenic in animals, there is no conclusive evidence for a teratogenic effect in humans.

■ Gold salts should be avoided if possible during pregnancy and are rarely needed, as rheumatoid arthritis usually improves.

■ For women who are stable on gold therapy, the risk of a flare may outweigh any risk to the fetus from continuation of therapy.

Sulfasalazine

- Sulfasalazine is another second-line agent that has been used extensively in the treatment of inflammatory bowel disease in pregnancy.
- It is cleaved into 5-aminosalicylic acid and sulphapyridine in the colon.
- It may be safely continued throughout pregnancy and breastfeeding.
- It is a dihydrofolate reductase inhibitor and therefore associated with an increased risk of neural tube defects, oral clefts and cardiovascular defects. Concomitant folate (5 mg/day) supplementation is recommended.

Cytotoxic drugs

- Cyclophosphamide, methotrexate and chlorambucil are all contraindicated in pregnancy.
- Cyclophosphamide and chlorambucil are alkylating agents. The risk of congenital defects (ocular, limb, palate and skeletal) in cyclophosphamide-exposed children is approximately 16% to 22%. It must be discontinued at least three months prior to conception.
- Cyclophosphamide may be used later in pregnancy for life-threatening maternal disease.
- Methotrexate, a folic acid antagonist, is a powerful teratogen, and causes miscarriage or congenital abnormalities (craniofacial, limb, central nervous system) in approximately 15–20% if administered in early pregnancy. It must be discontinued at least three months prior to conception.

Leflunemide

- This is used as a disease-modifying drug in rheumatoid arthritis. It is teratogenic in animals and is contraindicated in pregnancy.
- Leflunemide has a long half-life and conception should be delayed for two years or until the drug is eliminated with cholestyramine or active charcoal.

TNF-α antagonists

- Infliximab is a mouse–human chimeric monoclonal antibody that blocks the action of the proinflammatory TNF-α. It has a half-life of 8 to 10 days. Etanercept has a shorter half-life of 3 to 5 days.
- These biologic agents (e.g. Etanercept, infliximab, adalimumab) are now used in the management of rheumatoid arthritis, ankylosing spondylitis, inflammatory bowel disease and some skin diseases.
- They are not teratogenic in animal studies and to date there are no data to suggest that TNF-α antagonists are associated with embryotoxicity, teratogenicity or increased pregnancy loss in humans.
- There are more data for etanercept and infliximab than the newer agents. Infliximab contains a human IgG 1 constant and crosses the placenta in the second and third trimesters. It does not however cross into breast milk.
- Possible long-term effects on the neonate have not been determined and their use in pregnancy is not generally recommended. However, if their use is required for control of maternal disease then this should, if possible, be discontinued by 30 to 32 weeks to avoid the neonate being born with significant levels.

Rheumatoid arthritis—points to remember

- Up to 75% of women with rheumatoid arthritis improve during pregnancy.
- Of those who experience remission, 90% suffer postpartum exacerbations.
- There are no adverse effects of rheumatoid arthritis on pregnancy outcome.
- Infants of woman who have anti-Ro antibodies are at risk of neonatal lupus.
- Atlanto-axial subluxation is a rare complication of a general anaesthetic for caesarean section.
- Limitation of hip abduction may be severe enough to impede vaginal delivery.
- If paracetamol-based analgesics are insufficient, corticosteroids should be used in preference to NSAIDs.
- Sulphasalazine, hydroxychloroquine and azathioprine can be safely continued in pregnancy.
- If these agents fail to control symptoms then biologic anti-TNF-α agents such as etanercept and infliximab may be used in the second and third trimesters.
- Cyclophosphamide, leflunemide, methotrexate and chlorambucil are all contraindicated in pregnancy.

Systemic lupus erythematosus

Incidence

- Women are affected much more commonly than men (ratio 9:1), particularly during the child-bearing years (ratio 15:1).
- The incidence is approximately 1 in 1000 women and may be increasing.
- In the United Kingdom, it is more common in Afro-Caribbean women.

Clinical features

- SLE is a systemic connective-tissue disease characterised by periods of disease activity (flares) and remissions.
- The average age at diagnosis is approximately 30 years and approximately 6% of patients have other autoimmune disorders.
- SLE is heterogeneous with a variety of clinical and antibody patterns.
- Joint involvement is the commonest clinical feature (90%). Arthritis is non-erosive, peripheral and characterised by tenderness and swelling.
- Other features include skin involvement (80%), for example, malar rash, photosensitivity, vasculitic lesions on the fingertips and nail folds, Raynaud's phenomenon and discoid lupus.
- There may be serositis (pleuritis, pericarditis), renal involvement (glomerulonephritis with proteinuria and cellular casts) and neurological involvement (psychosis, seizures or chorea).
- Haematological manifestations include haemolytic anaemia, thrombocytopenia and lymphopenia or leukopenia.

Pathogenesis

- The cause of SLE is not known, but involves both a genetic predisposition and environmental triggers such as ultraviolet light or viral infection.

- There is polyclonal B-cell activation, impaired T-cell regulation of the immune response and failure to remove immune complexes.
- There are circulating non–organ specific autoantibodies.
- Deposition of immune complexes causes vasculitis.

Diagnosis

- Specific clinical and laboratory criteria (American Rheumatic Association) exist for the diagnosis of SLE, but many patients have a lupus-like illness without fulfilling these.
- A full blood count may show a normochromic normocytic anaemia, neutropenia and thrombocytopenia.
- The ESR is raised because of high immunoglobulin levels, the CRP is normal, and low or falling levels of the third and fourth components of complement indicate active disease.
- The most common autoantibody found in 96% of SLE patients is antinuclear antibody (ANA). Titres do not change with disease activity.
- The most specific are antibodies to double-stranded DNA (found in 78% of patients) and Smith (Sm). Glomerulonephritis occurs more frequently in women with these antibodies.
- In addition, patients may have antibodies to other ENAs, for example, anti-Ro and anti-La or to phospholipids, that is, anticardiolipin antibodies.
- The anti-Ro and/or anti-La (present in approximately 30%) and antiphospholipid antibodies (aPLs—present in approximately 40%) considered later are of particular relevance to pregnancy.

Pregnancy

Effect of pregnancy on SLE

- Pregnancy increases the likelihood of flare, from approximately 40% to 60%.
- Unlike rheumatoid arthritis, flares are not more likely immediately postpartum.
- Lupus flares, most commonly involving the skin and joints, may occur at any stage of pregnancy or the puerperium. It is not possible to predict when, or if, an individual patient will flare, although flare is more likely if disease has been active within six months of conception. The type of flare can to some extent be predicted by previous disease patterns.
- Flares may be difficult to diagnose during pregnancy since many features such as hair loss, oedema, palmar and facial erythema, fatigue, anaemia, raised ESR and musculoskeletal pain also occur in normal pregnancy.
- Flares are not prevented with prophylactic steroids or routine increases of dose, and such prophylactic therapy is not recommended either ante- or postpartum.
- In women with lupus nephritis, pregnancy does not seem to jeopardise renal function in the long term, although SLE nephropathy may manifest for the first time in pregnancy. The risk of deterioration is greater the higher the baseline serum creatinine, although women with moderate renal impairment (serum creatinine 125–200 μmol/L) may have uncomplicated pregnancies.
- The risk of renal flare is approximately 30% and is much higher if the lupus nephritis is not in remission or only in partial remission at conception.
- Women should be advised to delay pregnancy until at least six months after a lupus nephritis flare.

Effect of SLE on pregnancy

- The increased risks of spontaneous miscarriage, fetal death, pre-eclampsia, preterm delivery and fetal growth restriction (FGR) seen in SLE pregnancies are related to the presence of anticardiolipin antibodies or lupus anticoagulant (aPLs), lupus nephritis or hypertension and active disease at the time of conception or first presentation of SLE during pregnancy.
- Pregnancy outcome is particularly affected by renal disease. Even quiescent renal lupus is associated with increased risk of fetal loss, pre-eclampsia and FGR, particularly if there is hypertension or proteinuria.
- In a recent study, the risk of preterm delivery and low birth weight (<2.5 kg) in women with lupus nephritis was approximately 30%.
- For women in remission, but without hypertension, renal involvement or aPLs, the risk of pregnancy loss and pre-eclampsia is probably no higher than in the general population.
- Chorea is a very rare complication of pregnancy in women with SLE or aPLs.

Management

- Ideally this should begin with pre-conception counselling. Knowledge of the anti-Ro/La, aPLs, renal and blood pressure status allows prediction of the risks to the woman and her fetus.
- Outcome is improved if conception occurs during disease remission.
- Women with lupus nephritis and/or aPLs should be treated with low dose aspirin in pregnancy.
- Pregnancy care is best undertaken by a multidisciplinary team in combined clinics, where physicians and obstetricians can regularly monitor disease activity as well as fetal growth parameters, uterine artery Doppler blood flow examination at 20 to 24 weeks gestation and umbilical artery blood flow from 24 weeks gestation.
- It is important to establish baseline values in early pregnancy for full blood counts, urea and electrolytes, serum creatinine, uric acid, liver function, anti-DNA and complement titres and to quantify any proteinuria. Serial measurements at intervals dependent on disease severity are then recommended.
- Features suggesting disease flare include the following:
  - Symptoms (arthralgia, pleuritic pain, skin rash)
  - Rising anti-DNA antibody titre
  - Red blood cells or cellular casts in the urinary sediment
  - Fall in complement levels (elevation of complement split products, particularly Ba and Bb, often accompanies flares, so high ratios of CH50:Ba may differentiate pre-eclampsia from active lupus). A greater than 25% fall in C3 or C4 suggests active SLE.
- Disease flares must be actively managed. Corticosteroids are the drugs of choice.
- The use of azathioprine, NSAIDs and aspirin is covered in the sections on 'Rheumatoid Arthritis' (earlier) and 'Antiphospholipid Syndrome' (later).
- Hydroxychloroquine should be continued since stopping may precipitate flare.
- For control of hypertension, the drugs of choice are methyldopa, labetalol with nifedipine or hydralazine as second-line agents (see Chapter 1). Although long-term hydralazine and methyldopa use may rarely induce a SLE-like syndrome, they are not contraindicated in SLE.

Differentiation of active renal lupus from pre-eclampsia

- This is notoriously difficult, and the two conditions may be superimposed.
- Since hypertension, proteinuria, thrombocytopenia and even renal impairment are all features of pre-eclampsia, diagnosis of lupus flare requires other features, such as those listed earlier.
  - A doubling of baseline proteinuria may be expected in pregnancy but more than this would be indicative of either worsening lupus nephritis or pre-eclampsia.
  - Hyperuricaemia and abnormal liver function tests point more towards pre-eclampsia.
- The only definitive investigation to reliably differentiate a renal lupus flare from pre-eclampsia is renal biopsy, but this is rarely undertaken in pregnancy. It is more likely to be appropriate prior to fetal viability, since confirmation of active lupus nephritis allows immunosuppressive treatment of the SLE without delivery. This will usually be with increased oral prednisolone or pulsed intravenous methyl predisolone plus azathioprine. Rarely the use of cyclophosphamide or MMF may be indicated prior to delivery.
- If lupus flare and pre-eclampsia cannot be differentiated beyond 24 to 28 weeks gestation, when the fetus is viable, delivery may be the most appropriate course if the mother or her fetus is at risk. Delivery will both cure pre-eclampsia and allow administration of drugs such as cyclophosphamide for a renal flare.

Systemic lupus erythematosus—points to remember

- There is an increased rate of flare during pregnancy.
- Disease flares must be actively managed with corticosteroids.
- Adverse pregnancy outcome is related to the presence of renal involvement, hypertension, aPLs and disease activity at the time of conception.
- These factors increase the risks of spontaneous miscarriage, fetal death, pre-eclampsia, preterm delivery and FGR.
- Pregnancy care is best undertaken in combined clinics allowing close monitoring of disease activity, fetal growth and well-being.
- In Ro-positive mothers, the risk of transient neonatal cutaneous lupus is approximately 5% and the risk of congenital heart block (CHB) approximately 2%.

Neonatal lupus syndromes

- These conditions are models of passively acquired autoimmunity. Autoantibodies directed against cytoplasmic ribonucleoproteins Ro and La cross the placenta, causing immune system damage to the fetus.
- Several clinical syndromes have been described, of which cutaneous neonatal lupus is the most common, and CHB is the most serious. These syndromes rarely coexist.
- More than 90% of mothers of affected offspring have anti-Ro antibodies, and 50% to 70% have anti-La antibodies. The prevalence of anti-Ro antibodies in the general population is <1%, although anti-Ro/La antibodies are present in approximately 30% of patients with SLE, commonly associated with photosensitivity, Sjögren's syndrome, subacute lupus erythematosus and ANA-negative SLE.

- In babies of Ro/La-positive mothers, the risk of transient cutaneous lupus is approximately 5% and the risk of CHB approximately 2%.
- The risk of neonatal lupus is increased if a previous child has been affected, rising to 16% to 18% with one affected child and 50% if two children are affected; subsequent infants tend to be affected in the same way as their siblings.
- Not all Ro/La-positive mothers of neonates with CHB have SLE; some have Sjögren's syndrome, some Raynaud's phenomenon or a photosensitive rash, and a large proportion are asymptomatic, although they may subsequently develop a connective-tissue disease.
- There is no correlation between the severity of maternal disease and the incidence of neonatal lupus.

Cutaneous form of neonatal lupus

- This usually manifests in the first two weeks of life.
- The infant develops typical erythematous geographical skin lesions similar to those of adult subacute cutaneous lupus, usually of the face and scalp, which are photosensitive, appearing after exposure to the sun or other ultraviolet light (Fig. 8.1).
- The rash disappears spontaneously within four to six months, suggesting a direct antibody-mediated mechanism.
- Residual hypopigmentation or telangiectasia may persist for up to two years, but scarring is unusual.
- Sunlight and phototherapy should be avoided.

Congenital heart block

- In contrast to cutaneous neonatal lupus, CHB appears in utero, is permanent, and may be fatal (15–30% mortality).

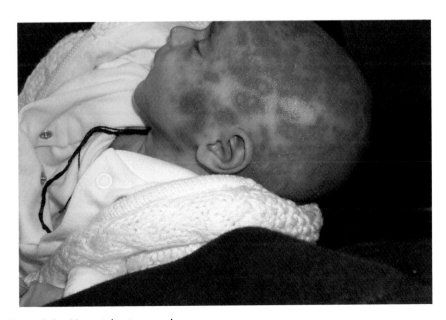

Figure 8.1 – Neonatal cutaneous lupus.

- The mechanism is not fully understood and no appropriate animal model exists. Reports of discordant twins suggest that fetal as well as maternal factors are involved.
- Although the fetal circulation is established by 12 weeks gestation, CHB is not usually detected until 18 to 30 weeks gestation. Once a fetal bradycardia is recognised, detailed scanning of the fetal heart, showing atrioventricular dissociation, confirms CHB.
- The pathogenesis is thought to involve inflammation and fibrosis of the conducting system. Maternal antibodies initiate transdifferentiation of cardiac fibroblasts to unchecked proliferating myofibroblasts, causing scarring of the atrioventricular node. Other cardiac tissues may be affected, and a pancarditis with myocarditis and pericardial effusion may accompany the CHB. This is supported by the demonstration of binding of IgG anti-Ro antibodies to fetal hearts.
- Maternal antibody profiling has revealed that the development of CHB is strongly dependent on a specific antibody profile to 52 kDa Ro (as opposed to 60 kDa Ro or La).
- It is likely that heart block progresses through first- and second-degree heart block before third-degree (complete) heart block develops. Fetuses and neonates of mothers with anti-Ro/La have been described with first- and second-degree block. Treatment with dexamethasone may reverse these lesser degrees of heart block, although progression to complete heart block is usual. For this reason it has been suggested that all neonates born to Ro/La positive mothers should have an ECG performed.
- There is no treatment that reverses CHB if the heart block is complete, although salbutamol given to the mother may be beneficial to the fetus if the bradycardia is causing fetal heart failure. This therapy may be limited by maternal side effects.
- If the fetal heart failure is thought to be because of myocarditis, dexamethasone and plasmapheresis may be successfully used, but these too have no effect on the conduction defect.
- The perinatal mortality rate is increased, with 19% of affected children dying in the early neonatal period. However, most infants who survive this period do well, although 50% to 60% require pacemakers in early infancy. All should be paced by their early teens to avoid the risk of sudden death.
- Prophylactic treatment with dexamethasone and/or intravenous immunoglobulin to prevent the development of CHB in fetuses of mothers, with previously affected fetuses, has not been studied in randomised controlled trials and is associated with a high incidence of serious maternal side effects.

Antiphospholipid syndrome

Anticardiolipin antibodies (aCL) and lupus anticoagulant (LA) are overlapping subsets of aPLs. The combination of either of these with one or more of the characteristic clinical features (Table 8.1) is known as the antiphospholipid syndrome (APS). Table 8.2 presents other features of APS.

Incidence

- APS was first described in patients with SLE, but it is now recognised both that most patients with APS do not fulfil the diagnostic criteria for SLE and that those with primary APS do not usually progress to SLE.
- The prevalence of aPL in the general obstetric population is low (<2%).
- Approximately 30% to 40% of women with SLE have aPL.

Table 8.1 –   Clinical criteria for the diagnosis of APS

Thrombosis	Venous—may be unusual sites
	Arterial
	Small vessel (e.g. thrombotic microangiopathy in kidney)
Pregnancy morbidity	≥3 consecutive miscarriages (<10 weeks gestation)
	≥1 fetal death (>10 weeks gestation with normal fetal morphology)
	≥1 premature birth (<34 weeks gestation with normal fetal morphology) because of pre-eclampsia or severe placental insufficiency

- Approximately 30% of those with aPL have thrombosis.
- Up to 30% of women with severe early onset pre-eclampsia may have aPL.

Clinical features

Although the clinical features of primary and SLE-associated APS are similar, and the antibody specificity is the same, the distinction is important, and patients with primary APS should not be labelled as having lupus.

Pathogenesis

- The binding of aCL to cardiolipin requires the presence of a co-factor, β_2-glycoprotein (β_2GPI). This co-factor, an endogenous coagulation inhibitor, plays a key role in APS-associated thrombosis.
- In APS-associated fetal loss, there is typically massive infarction and thrombosis of the placental and decidual vessels, probably secondary to spiral artery vasculopathy. Platelet deposition and prostanoid imbalance may be implicated in a similar way to pre-eclampsia.
- Many of the adverse outcomes described are the end result of defective or abnormal placentation and these findings support placental failure, being the mechanism by which aPLs are associated with late loss. But aPL-associated thrombosis within the placenta cannot explain all the recognised pregnancy complications in APS.

Table 8.2 – Other recognised features of APS

Thrombocytopenia	
Haemolytic anaemia	
Livedo reticularis	
Cerebral involvement	Epilepsy, cerebral infarction, chorea and migraine, transverse myelopathy/myelitis
Heart valve disease	Particularly mitral valve
Hypertension	
Pulmonary	
hypertension Leg ulcers	

- aPLs bind to human trophoblasts in vitro. Trophoblast cell membranes behave as targets for both β_2GPI-dependent and β_2GPI-independent aPL.
- aPLs reduce human chorionic gonadotrophin (hCG) release and inhibit trophoblast invasiveness.
- Lupus anticoagulant predicts venous thrombosis and fetal loss more strongly than do anticardiolipin antibodies.

Diagnosis

- Firm diagnosis of APS requires two or more positive readings for LA and/or aCL at least 12 weeks apart, plus at least one of the clinical criteria listed in Table 8.1.
- LA is a misnomer coined because it prolongs coagulation times in vitro. It is detected by the prolongation of the activated partial thromboplastin time (aPTT) or the dilute Russell's viper venom time (dRVVT). This prolongation fails to correct with the addition of platelet poor plasma, but corrects with excess phospholipid.
- aCLs are measured using commercially available enzyme-linked immunosorbent assay (ELISA) kits. Medium or high titres of IgG or IgM are required.

Pregnancy

Effect of pregnancy on APS

- The risk of thrombosis is exacerbated by the hypercoagulable pregnant state (see Chapter 3). If previous thromboses have been venous, the risk is of recurrent venous thrombosis. If there have been previous arterial events then the risk of recurrent arterial events such as stroke is increased.
- Pre-existing thrombocytopenia may worsen.

Effect of APS on pregnancy

- The risks of miscarriage, second and third trimester fetal death, pre-eclampsia, FGR and placental abruption are increased.
- Establishing causality for first trimester losses is difficult, since the risk of miscarriage is high (10–15%) in the normal population. aPLs are more common in women suffering three or more first trimester miscarriages, than in those with one or two miscarriages.
- Fetal death in APS is typically preceded by FGR and oligohydramnios.
- The risk of fetal loss is directly related to antibody titre, particularly the IgG aCL, although many women with a history of recurrent loss have only IgM antibodies. Women who are positive for lupus anticoagulant, anticardiolipin and β_2GPI have the highest risk for thrombosis and pregnancy morbidity.
- Quantifying the risk is difficult and the presence of aPL does not preclude successful pregnancy.
- Previous obstetric history is the best predictor of pregnancy outcome in women with APS.
- Reported outcomes vary depending on whether the study population is made up of those with predominantly recurrent miscarriage (in whom complications are less likely—10% risk of pre-eclampsia/preterm delivery) or those with SLE, thrombosis or previous late intrauterine death or severe early onset pre-eclampsia (in whom the risk of preterm delivery before 37 weeks gestation is 30–40% and the risk of FGR exceeds 30%).
- Pre-eclampsia is common and often severe, and of early onset in the latter group.

Management

Pre-pregnancy

- Women with a history of thrombosis, recurrent miscarriage, intrauterine fetal death, or severe early onset pre-eclampsia or FGR should be screened for the presence of LA or aCL.
- A detailed history of the circumstances of the fetal loss is essential to exclude other causes of late miscarriage, such as cervical incompetence or idiopathic preterm labour. The presence of aPL does not constitute a diagnosis of APS unless the clinical features are suggestive.

Antenatal

- Care of pregnant women with APS should be multidisciplinary and in centres with expertise in the management of this condition.
- Aspirin inhibits thromboxane and may reduce the risk of vascular thrombosis. There are many non-randomised studies suggesting that low-dose aspirin is effective and it can prevent pregnancy loss in experimental APS mice.
- Aspirin is a logical and safe treatment in those with aPLs but no clinical features of APS.
- Randomised, controlled trials of aspirin as a single agent in APS pregnancy do not support any benefit over placebo; however, such studies have been undertaken in low-risk women. Most centres now advocate treatment with low-dose aspirin for all women with APS, prior to conception, in the belief that the placental damage occurs early in gestation, and that aspirin may prevent failure of placentation.
- Women with APS and previous thromboembolism are at extremely high risk of further thromboembolism in pregnancy and the puerperium and should receive antenatal thromboprophylaxis with a high prophylactic dose or full anticoagulant doses of low-molecular-weight heparin (LMWH) (e.g. Enoxaparin 40 mg b.d.) (see Chapter 3). Many of these women are on life-long anticoagulation therapy with warfarin. The change from warfarin to LMWH should be achieved prior to six weeks gestation to avoid warfarin embryopathy.
- A few women with cerebral arterial thrombosis because of APS on long-term warfarin may experience transient ischaemic symptoms when LMWH is substituted for warfarin. If these do not improve on higher (full anticoagulant) doses of LMWH, the reintroduction of warfarin is justified to prevent maternal stroke.
- Opinion is divided about the best therapy for those with recurrent pregnancy loss, but without a history of thromboembolism.
- Treatment with high-dose steroids (in the absence of active lupus) to suppress LA and aCL, in combination with aspirin, is no longer recommended due to the maternal side effects from such prolonged high doses of steroids. This strategy has been abandoned in favour of anticoagulant treatment with aspirin and/or s.c. LMWH. Such regimens give equivalent fetal outcome with fewer maternal side effects than combinations of aspirin and steroids.
- Any additional benefit of heparin must be balanced against the risk of heparin-induced osteoporosis (0.04% with LMWHs), and the cost and inconvenience of daily injections.
- In women with recurrent miscarriage, but without a history of thrombosis, there is evidence to support the use of no therapy, aspirin alone, and aspirin and LMWH.

Table 8.3 – Therapeutic management of APS pregnancies

Clinical history	Anticoagulant therapy
No thrombosis, no miscarriage, no adverse pregnancy outcome	Aspirin 75 mg o.d. from pre-conception
Previous thrombosis	On maintenance warfarin: transfer to aspirin and LMWH (enoxaparin 40 mg b.d.) as soon as pregnancy confirmed Not on warfarin: aspirin 75 mg o.d. from pre-conception and commence LMWH (enoxaparin 40 mg o.d.) once pregnancy confirmed. Increase LMWH to b.d. at 16–20 wk
Recurrent miscarriage <10 weeks	No prior anticoagulant therapy: aspirin 75 mg o.d. from pre-conception Prior miscarriage with aspirin alone: aspirin 75 mg o.d. from pre-conception and LMWH (enoxaparin 40 mg o.d.) once pregnancy confirmed. Consider discontinuation of LWWH at 20 weeks gestation if uterine artery waveform is normal
Late fetal loss, neonatal death or adverse outcome because of pre-eclampsia, FGR or abruption	Aspirin 75 mg o.d. from pre-conception and LMWH (enoxaparin 40 mg o.d.) once pregnancy confirmed

Recent studies show that the live birth rate in women treated with aspirin alone is consistently 70% to 80%, and there is no demonstrable improvement when LMWH is added. A pragmatic approach is to offer aspirin alone, particularly if the history is of less than three miscarriages and then if miscarriage occurs despite aspirin therapy to offer LMWH in addition.

- Antithrombotic strategies vary in different centres around the world. A suggested protocol is given in Table 8.3.
- LMWH is given in prophylactic doses [enoxaparin (Clexane®) 40 mg o.d.; dalteparin (Fragmin®) 5000 units o.d.] when given for fetal indications, but in women with previous thrombosis higher doses [e.g. enoxaparin (Clexane®) 40 mg b.d.; dalteparin (Fragmin®) 5000 units b.d.] are indicated.
- Immunosuppression with azathioprine, i.v. immunoglobulin (IVIg) and plasmapheresis have all been tried. The numbers treated do not allow firm conclusions regarding efficacy. IVIg is extremely expensive, precluding its use outside a research setting.
- Close fetal monitoring is essential. Uterine artery Doppler waveform analysis at 20 to 24 weeks gestation helps predict the higher risk pregnancies. Monthly growth scans are performed from 28 weeks if the uterine artery Doppler waveform at 24 weeks shows pre-diastolic 'notching'.

- High-risk women require closer surveillance with regular blood pressure checks and urinalysis to detect early onset pre-eclampsia.
- Such intensive monitoring allows for timely delivery, which may improve fetal outcome.

Postpartum

- Women on long-term warfarin treatment may recommence this postpartum (starting after 5–7 days) and LMWH is discontinued when the international normalised ratio (INR) is >2.0.
- Women with previous thrombosis should receive postpartum LMWH or warfarin for six weeks.
- Women without previous thrombosis should receive postpartum LMWH for at least one week to six weeks depending on the presence of other risk factors.

Antiphospholipid syndrome—points to remember

- Not all women with APS have SLE.
- The important clinical features are recurrent miscarriage, intrauterine fetal death, uteroplacental insufficiency and arterial and venous thrombosis.
- Even in the absence of fetal loss, there is an increased risk of severe, early onset pre-eclampsia, FGR and placental abruption.
- Previous poor obstetric history is the most important predictor of fetal loss.
- Management should be multidisciplinary in centres with expertise in APS and with facilities for regular and close fetal surveillance.
- Treatment is with low-dose aspirin with or without LMWH.

Scleroderma

Incidence

Scleroderma is rare (2.3–12 cases per million per year) but more common in women (female to male ratio 3:1).

Clinical features

- Scleroderma may be divided into:
  - Localised cutaneous form (morphoea) with areas of waxy, thickened skin, usually on the forearms and hands
  - Systemic sclerosis associated with Raynaud's phenomenon and organ involvement
  - CREST syndrome (calcinosis, Raynaud's phenomenon, oesophageal involvement, sclerodactyly, telangiectasia).
- The skin in systemic sclerosis is typically bound down to produce sclerodactyly, beaking of the nose, a fixed facial expression and limitation of mouth opening. Skin ulceration and partial digit amputation are common.
- Systemic involvement usually takes the form of progressive fibrosis and includes the oesophagus most commonly (80%), lungs (45%), heart (40%) and kidneys (35%).

Pathogenesis and immunology

■ The aetiology is unknown.

■ Theories include a contribution from microchimerism. Male cells have been detected in affected tissues from skin and other organs. These persistent fetal cells may alternatively have a protective effect which could explain why nulliparous women have been found to have an increased risk of developing scleroderma when compared with parous women and why they have an earlier onset of the disease and have more pulmonary involvement and death than parous women.

■ There may be associated antinuclear, anticentromere (associated with limited cutaneous systemic sclerosis/CREST syndrome), antinucleolar or topoisomerase I (Scl-70) antibodies (associated with diffuse cutaneous scleroderma and lung involvement). RNA-polymerase I (U3RNP) antibodies are associated with pulmonary hypertension, but this may also develop secondary to lung disease.

Pregnancy

Effect of pregnancy on scleroderma

■ The prognosis for localised cutaneous scleroderma without organ involvement is good.

■ Those with early diffuse systemic sclerosis (<4 years) and/or renal involvement are at risk of rapid overall deterioration and renal crisis during pregnancy.

■ Raynaud's disease tends to improve as a result of vasodilation and increased blood flow.

■ Reflux oesophagitis may deteriorate due to lowered oesophageal tone.

■ Those with severe pulmonary fibrosis and pulmonary hypertension are at high risk of postpartum deterioration.

Effect of scleroderma on pregnancy

■ Overall success rates are 70% to 80%, but outcomes are improved in those without systemic disease.

■ There is an increased risk of preterm delivery. Late diffuse disease is associated with an increased risk of miscarriage.

■ Pre-eclampsia, FGR and perinatal mortality are risks for women with hypertension and renal disease.

■ Venepuncture, venous access and blood pressure measurement may be difficult because of skin or blood vessel involvement.

■ General anaesthesia may be complicated by difficult endotracheal intubation (partly related to limitation of mouth opening), and regional anaesthesia may also be difficult if there is skin involvement on the back.

Management

■ No treatment has been shown to influence the progress of scleroderma and management is therefore symptomatic. Some centres use regular prostacyclin infusions.

■ Women with early diffuse disease should be advised to delay pregnancy until the disease has stabilised.

■ Pre-pregnancy assessment with formal lung function tests and echocardiography is important.

- Women with multiple or severe organ involvement (pulmonary hypertension, severe pulmonary fibrosis, renal involvement) should be advised against pregnancy.
- Raynaud's phenomenon may be helped by heated gloves or nifedipine, which may be used safely in pregnancy.
- Regular multidisciplinary assessment for disease activity and fetal well-being, and blood pressure checks are essential.
- Although generally contraindicated in pregnancy, the benefits of angiotensin-inhibiting enzyme (ACE) inhibitors in scleroderma renal crisis outweigh the risks to the fetus, and their use is justified in this situation.
- Early assessment by an anaesthetist is advisable if problems with regional or general anaesthesia are anticipated.
- Steroid treatment (including for fetal lung maturity) should be avoided as this may precipitate a renal crisis.

Ehlers–Danlos syndrome (EDS)

- This group of disorders consists of inherited (predominantly autosomal dominant) defects of collagen metabolism, characterised by fragile skin and blood vessels, easy bruising, skin hyperelasticity and joint hypermobility.
- Types I (classic or gravis) and IV (ecchymotic or arterial) carry the highest risks in pregnancy, and maternal mortality with type IV may be as high as 20% to 25%.
- Types II (mitis) and X (fibronectin abnormality) have more favourable outcomes.
- Type III is the commonest form and causes joint hypermobility.

Pregnancy

Effect of EDS on pregnancy

Problems in pregnancy arise mostly at delivery and include the following:

- Spontaneous vaginal, perineal and other visceral tears
- Skin fragility and poor healing
- Great vessel rupture
- Uterine rupture
- Postpartum haemorrhage (common)
- Increased risk of preterm rupture of membranes
- Increased risk of malpresentation
- Increased risk of FGR.

Management

- Pre-conceptual categorisation of disorder and genetic counselling is essential.
- Avoidance or termination of pregnancy is advisable for those with type IV.
- Caesarean section may not result in fewer complications.

Vasculitis

Women with vasculitis will all, or should all, be under long-term follow-up with a rheumatologist.

Wegener's granulomatosus

- Wegener's granulomatosis is an anti-neutrophil cytoplasmic antibodies (ANCA)-related systemic vasculitis involving predominantly the upper respiratory system (causing haemoptysis because of alveolar haemorrhage), the cartilage of the nose, and the kidneys.
- Pregnancy is rare as Wegener is uncommon in women of child-bearing age.
- There is an increased risk of adverse pregnancy outcome particularly if the disease is active at conception or presents during pregnancy. This includes increased fetal and maternal mortality and morbidity.
- The major first-line therapeutic agent is cyclophosphamide. In pregnancy the mainstays of treatment are prednisolone and azathioprine. Septrin (co-trimoxazole = trimethoprim + sulphamethoxazole) or erythromycin may be used to reduce bacterial carriage in the nose and reduce flare. If co-trimoxazole is used in pregnancy it must be given with high dose (5 mg) folic acid. Rituximab may be used as a third-line treatment but is avoided if possible in pregnancy.

Takayasu's arteritis

- Takayasu's arteritis is a rare inflammatory arteritis, which predominantly affects large arteries, including the aorta and its major branches and the pulmonary arteries. Inflammation of the artery leads to fibrosis, stenosis and thrombosis. Aneurysms may also be a feature.
- It affects predominantly women of child-bearing age who present with hypertension (because of renal artery involvement), stroke and end organ or limb ischaemia. It is known as the 'pulseless' disease because often peripheral pulses will be absent in affected limbs. Vascular bruits are also common.
- Fever and raised ESR and/or CRP are important features but diagnosis is usually made with the finding of typical features on vascular imaging using angiography. Outwith pregnancy, positron emission tomography (PET) scanning is used to assess disease activity.
- Corticosteroids are first-line therapy and if there is evidence of disease activity with a rising CRP or ESR (beyond what would be expected in pregnancy), these should be increased or instituted in pregnancy. Azathioprine may also be used.
- Blood pressure control is important and often challenging in pregnancy.

Pregnancy-associated osteoporosis

Incidence

- Normal pregnancy is associated with a significant fall in bone density, and rarely idiopathic transient osteoporosis of pregnancy may develop.
- Osteoporosis is defined as bone density <2.5 (T score) standard deviations below the mean for young adults.

Clinical features

- Presentation is with hip joint or most frequently back pain, usually during the third trimester or puerperium of the first full-term pregnancy.

- Bone mineral density usually recovers within a year after delivery, although it may be delayed until the cessation of lactation, and recurrence in subsequent pregnancies is mild or absent.
- There is no correlation between bone mass and parity, suggesting full recovery between pregnancies.

Pathogenesis

- Reduction in bone density affects trabecular rather than cortical bone.
- Osteoporosis results from either excessive osteoclastic activity with accelerated bone resorption and remodelling or decreased osteoblastic activity.
- Osteoporosis may stem from a failure in the changes of calcitropic hormones [vitamin D, calcitonin and parathyroid hormone (PTH)] to cope with the increased demand for calcium in pregnancy.
- The condition may represent pre-existing osteopenia (bone density between 1 and 2.5 standard deviation below mean) and a low peak bone mass that is unmasked and becomes symptomatic during pregnancy. The latter may be a result of additional mechanical stresses or simply an exaggeration of the physiological changes that occur in bone during pregnancy and lactation.
- Continued lactation may exacerbate the problem, causing a further reduction in bone density, but it is unlikely to be the primary aetiological influence.
- Studies suggest an uncoupling of bone formation and bone resorption in the latter half of pregnancy. Although both increase in pregnancy, the rate of bone resorption exceeds the rate of bone formation.
- An aetiological role for PTH-related peptide, possibly placenta-associated, is also suggested.

Diagnosis

Radiological (if postpartum) or ultrasound or dual X-ray absorptiometry (DXA) investigations show signs of demineralisation of the femoral head or lumbar spine (80% trabecular bone), with non-traumatic compression vertebral fractures in severe cases.

Management

This usually requires avoidance of weight bearing to prevent pain and fractures. Bisphosphonates may be used in the post partum period.

Further reading

Bramham K, Hunt BJ, Germain S, et al. Pregnancy outcome in different clinical phenotypes of antiphospholipid syndrome. Lupus 2010; 19:58–64.

Branch DW, Khamashta MA. Antiphospholipid syndrome: Obstetric diagnosis, management, and controversies. Obstet Gynecol 2003; 101:1333–1344.

Buyon JP, Clancy RM. Neonatal lupus syndromes. Curr Opin Rheumatol 2003; 15:535–541.

Germain S, Nelson-Piercy C. Lupus nephritis and renal disease in pregnancy. Lupus 2006; 15:148–155.

Imbasciati E, Tincani A, Gregorini G, et al. Pregnancy in women with pre-existing lupus nephritis: Predictors of fetal and maternal outcome. Nephrol Dial Transplant 2009; 24:519–525.

Laskin CA, Spitzer KA, Clark CA, et al. Low molecular weight heparin and aspirin for recurrent pregnancy loss: Results from the randomized controlled HepASA trial. J Rheumatol 2009; 36:279–287.

McKillop L, Germain S, Nelson-Piercy C. SLE in pregnancy. BMJ 2007; 335:933–936.

Nelson JL, Ostensen M. Pregnancy and rheumatoid arthritis. Rheum Dis Clin North Am 1997; 23:195–212.

Ostenson M, Lockshin M, Doria A, et al. Update on safety during pregnancy of biological agents and some immunosuppressive anti-rheumatic drugs. Rheumatology (Oxford) 2008; 47(suppl 3):iii28–31.

Perez-Aytes A, Ledo A, Boso V, et al. In utero exposure to mycophenolate mofetil: A characteristic phenotype? Am J Med Genet A 2008; 146:1–7.

Sau A, Clarke SD, Bass J, et al. Azathioprine and breast feeding: Is it safe? BJOG 2007; 114:498–501.

Smith R, Athanasou NA, Ostlere SJ, et al. Pregnancy-associated osteoporosis. QJM 1995; 88:865–878.

Steen VD. Pregnancy in women with systemic sclerosis. Obstet Gynecol 1999; 94:15–20.

Vinet E, Pineau C, Gordon C, et al. Biologic therapy and pregnancy outcome in women with rheumatic diseases. Arthritis Rheum 2009; 61:587–592.

Youssef P, Kennedy D. Arthritis in pregnancy: The role and safety of biological agents. Obstet Med 2009; 2:134–137.

CHAPTER 9

Neurological problems

Epilepsy
Migraine and headache
Multiple sclerosis (MS)
Myasthenia gravis
Myotonic dystrophy
Idiopathic (benign)
 intracranial hypertension (IIH)
Stroke

Subarachnoid haemorrhage
 (SAH)
Cerebral vein thrombosis
Bell's palsy
Posterior reversible
 encephalopathy syndrome
 (PRES)
Entrapment neuropathies

Epilepsy

Incidence

Epilepsy affects approximately 0.5% of women of child-bearing age and is the commonest chronic neurological disorder to complicate pregnancy.

Clinical features

Epilepsy is classified according to the clinical type of seizure or specific electroencephalographic (EEG) features. Many types of epilepsy are characterised by more than one type of seizure. These may be broadly divided into:

- Primary generalised epilepsy (including tonic–clonic seizures, absences and myoclonic jerks)
- Partial (focal) seizures with or without loss of consciousness or secondary generalisation (complex partial seizures)
- Temporal lobe seizures, which are a form of partial seizures.

Temporal lobe seizures are often associated with an aura, a duration of one minute or more and confusion after the event. Absences (petit mal) in contrast are normally of short duration (a few seconds), have a rapid onset, rapid recovery and are precipitated by hyperventilation. Absences are associated with 3 Hz spike and wave discharge on the EEG.

The clinical features of tonic–clonic seizures due to primary generalised epilepsy and secondary generalised partial seizures may be similar as there may be no identifiable aura associated with the latter. Pointers to a diagnosis of primary generalised epilepsy are myoclonic jerks and photosensitivity.

Pathogenesis

Most cases of epilepsy are idiopathic and no underlying cause is found. Approximately 30% of these patients have a family history of epilepsy.

Secondary epilepsy may be encountered in pregnancy in patients who have the following:

- Previous surgery to the cerebral hemispheres
- Intracranial mass lesions (meningiomas and arteriovenous malformations enlarge during pregnancy. This should always be considered if the first seizure occurs in pregnancy)
- Antiphospholipid syndrome (see Chapter 8, p. 140).

Other causes of seizures in pregnancy (see also section B, Table 8) include the following:

- Eclampsia (see Chapter 1, p. 7)
- Cerebral vein thrombosis (CVT) (see Chapter 3, p. 55)
- Thrombotic thrombocytopenic purpura (TTP) (see Chapter 14, p. 255)
- Stroke (risk is increased in pregnancy and 4% have seizures, see p. 168)
- Subarachnoid haemorrhage (see p. 170)
- Drug and alcohol withdrawal
- Hypoglycaemia (diabetes, hypoadrenalism, hypopituitarism, liver failure)
- Hypocalcaemia (magnesium sulphate therapy, hypoparathyroidism)
- Hyponatraemia (hyperemesis, hypoadrenalism, pre-eclampsia)
- Infections (tuberculoma, toxoplasmosis)
- Postdural puncture. Seizures are rare and preceded by typical postdural puncture headache and other neurological symptoms. Seizures occur typically four to seven days after dural puncture
- Gestational epilepsy (seizures are confined to pregnancy)
- Pseudoepilepsy (also referred to as 'non-epileptic seizure disorder' or 'non epileptic attack disorder'; these patients may have true epilepsy as well). Useful distinguishing features to differentiate these 'pseudo fits' are:
  - Prolonged/repeated seizures without cyanosis
  - Resistance to passive eye-opening
  - Down-going plantar reflexes
  - Persistence of a positive conjunctival reflex.

Diagnosis

Most women with epilepsy in pregnancy have already been diagnosed, but when a first seizure occurs in pregnancy, the following investigations are appropriate:

- Blood pressure, urinalysis, uric acid, platelet count, clotting screen, blood film
- Blood glucose, serum calcium, serum sodium, liver function tests
- Computerised tomography (CT) or magnetic resonance imaging (MRI) of the brain. Although this is not necessarily recommended for the first seizure in the non-pregnant woman, there is no doubt of its value in pregnancy, bearing in mind the above differential diagnoses.
- EEG.

Pregnancy

Effect of pregnancy on epilepsy

- In most women pregnancy does not affect the frequency of seizures.
- In a recent prospective European study, compared with the first trimester, seizure control remained unchanged throughout pregnancy in 64%, 17% had an increase and 16% a decrease in seizures in pregnancy.
- A woman who has been seizure free for many years is unlikely to have seizures in pregnancy unless she discontinues her medication.
- Those with poorly controlled epilepsy, especially those whose seizure frequency exceeds once a month, are more likely to deteriorate in pregnancy.
- There is no relation to the seizure type or course of epilepsy during previous pregnancies.
- Women with multiple seizure types are also more likely to experience an increase in seizure frequency in pregnancy.
- The risk of seizures is highest peripartum (see later), and in the prospective EURAP study 3.5% of pregnancies were complicated by intrapartum seizures.
- Epilepsy is a common indirect cause of maternal death in the United Kingdom. The maternal death rate from epilepsy ranges from 5 to 10 per million maternities or approximately five cases per year in the United Kingdom. In many deaths the cause was aspiration, but epileptic seizures may be fatal in themselves. It is not known whether pregnancy increases the risk of sudden unexplained death in epilepsy (SUDEP), estimated at 1 in 500 woman-years outside pregnancy.
- Risk factors for SUDEP include high seizure frequency, increasing numbers of antiepileptic drugs, low IQ and early onset epilepsy. SUDEP is uncommon in those with good seizure control.

Possible reasons for deterioration in seizure control during pregnancy include the following:

- Pregnancy itself
- Poor compliance with anticonvulsant medication (because of fears regarding teratogenesis). One study using hair analysis confirmed that pregnant women commonly stop or reduce antiepileptic drugs (AEDs) in pregnancy.
- Decreased drug levels related to nausea and vomiting in early pregnancy.
- Decreased free drug levels.
- Lack of sleep towards term and during labour.
- Lack of absorption of AEDs from the gastrointestinal tract during labour.
- Hyperventilation during labour.

Effect of epilepsy on pregnancy

- The fetus is relatively resistant to short episodes of hypoxia and there is no evidence of adverse effects of single seizures on the fetus. Some have documented fetal bradycardia during and after maternal tonic–clonic convulsions, but cerebral damage in the long term is not a feature.
- Large prospective studies show no increased risk of miscarriage or obstetric complications in women with epilepsy unless a seizure results in abdominal trauma.
- Status epilepticus is dangerous for both mother and fetus and should be treated vigorously. Fortunately this complicates from <1% to 2.5% of pregnancies in women with epilepsy. In the EURAP study, status affected 1.8% of pregnancies.

- The main concern stems from the increased risk of congenital abnormalities (see later).
- The risk of the child developing epilepsy is also increased (4–5%) if either parent has epilepsy, and maternal epilepsy is associated with a higher risk.
- If there is a previously affected sibling, the risk is 10%.
- If both parents have epilepsy, the risk is 15% to 20%.
- The risk of a woman with idiopathic epilepsy having a child who develops epilepsy is increased if she herself had onset of epilepsy before the age of 10 years.

Teratogenic risks of antiepileptic drugs (AEDs)

- Phenytoin, primidone, phenobarbitone, carbamazepine, sodium valproate, lamotrigine, topiramate and levetiracetam all cross the placenta and are teratogenic.
- The major malformations caused by AEDs are:
  - Neural tube defects [particularly valproate (1–3.8%) and carbamazepine (0.5–1%)]
  - Orofacial clefts (particularly phenytoin, carbamezepine, phenobarbitone)
  - Congenital heart defects (particularly phenytoin, phenobarbitone and valproate).
- Minor malformations (fetal anticonvulsant syndrome) associated with AED use in pregnancy include the following:
  - Dysmorphic features (V-shaped eyebrows, low-set ears, broad nasal bridge, irregular teeth)
  - Hypertelorism
  - Hypoplastic nails and distal digits
  - Hypoplasia of the midface could be a marker for cognitive dysfunction.
- There is no association between different types of epilepsy and the risk of major congenital malformations.
- Data from many prospective registers demonstrate a particularly high risk associated with valproate.
- Metaanalysis of all studies show that the risk for any one drug is approximately 6% to 7% (i.e. two- to three-fold the background level of risk). The newer prospective registries suggest that for lamotrigine and topiramate there is an increased risk of oral clefts. They also show that valproate is associated with at least double the risk of the other AEDs.
- The risk increases with the number of drugs, so for those taking two or more AEDs, the risk is 10% to 15% in older studies and 6% in the newer prospective studies; polytherapy regimens containing valproate have higher rates of major malformations (8–9%) than those without valproate.
- For valproate and lamotrigine there is evidence of a dose-dependent teratogenic effect. Offspring of mothers using >1 g/day valproate are at a greater than two-fold increased risk of congenital malformations, particularly neural tube defects, compared with those exposed to 600 mg/day or less.
- In addition, studies have reported an association between maternal valproate use and impaired psychomotor development, and additional educational needs and reduced verbal IQ in the children. Furthermore, the relationship of valproate use in the mother and IQ in the infant at age 3 is also dose dependent. The effect on IQ is more marked with valproate polytherapy.

- Various theories exist to explain the mechanism for teratogenesis of AEDs, including:
  - A genetic deficiency of the detoxifying enzyme epoxide hydrolase leading to accumulation of toxic metabolites
  - Cytotoxic free radicals
  - Folic acid deficiency. Phenytoin and phenobarbitone particularly, but also carbamazepine and valproate, interfere with folate metabolism.
- These different mechanisms may explain why it has not been possible to show a reduction in the risk of neural tube, cardiovascular and urogenital defects and oral clefts with the use of pre-pregnancy and first trimester folic acid in women receiving AEDs. However, the recommendation to take folic acid supplements is still appropriate.
- The benzodiazepines (e.g. clobazam, clonazepam) used normally as add-on therapy are not teratogenic in monotherapy.

Management

Antenatal management in established epilepsy

- All women receiving AEDs should be advised to take folic acid 5 mg daily prior to conception. This should be continued throughout pregnancy, as there is also a small risk of folate-deficiency anaemia.
- There is no need to change the AED in pregnancy if epilepsy is well controlled with phenytoin, carbamazepine, valproate, lamotrigine, levetiracetam or phenobarbitone.
- Many women may stop their AED of their own volition because of fears about teratogenesis. In most cases, and certainly in women with regular seizures, it is appropriate to counsel restarting the AED. If the woman is seen after the first trimester she may be reassured that the risk of congenital abnormalities has passed.
- After careful counselling, women receiving valproate may wish to be weaned off or changed (under close supervision) to a different AED. If this is not deemed appropriate then the dose should if possible be reduced to 600 mg per day or less. To avoid the risk of congenital abnormalities this should be done pre-conception, but since it is not known at what gestation the effect on neurodevelopment occurs there may be some benefit to stopping valproate later in gestation. However, any risks of valproate must be balanced against the risk of seizures in pregnancy when considering reducing or stopping the drug.
- If continued, sodium valproate therapy should be changed to a three or four times daily regimen or a modified-release preparation (e.g. Epilim chrono®) to lower peak concentrations and reduce the risk of neural tube defects.
- Relatives, friends and/or partners should be advised on how to place the woman in the recovery position to prevent aspiration in the event of a seizure.
- Women should be advised to bathe in shallow water or to shower.
- Pre-natal screening for congenital abnormalities with nuchal translucency scanning and detailed ultrasound at 18 to 20 weeks should be offered. Scanning should include a fetal cardiology assessment.
- The altered pharmocokinetics in pregnancy mean that for most drugs concentration of the free drug falls. This is due to:
  - increased plasma volume
  - enhanced renal and hepatic drug clearance.

These effects are partially offset by changes in protein binding. Protein levels fall in pregnancy and protein binding of drugs decreases, resulting in increased free drug levels. For drugs that are largely protein bound, such as phenytoin, this effect partly counteracts the above factors leading to reduced free drug levels, so changes in dosage are rarely needed in pregnancy.

However, for drugs with very little protein binding, such as carbamezepine and lamotrigine, this effect of reduced protein binding is not significant and the predominant result of pharmacokinetic changes of pregnancy is marked reductions in free drug levels and thereby a need in many patients to increase the dosage during pregnancy.

- A baseline serum or salivary drug level is useful to establish compliance and inform future changes in drug doses.
- In women with regular seizures it is common to need to increase the dose of sodium valproate, carbamezepine and especially lamotrigine in pregnancy. Doses of lamotrigine may need to be increased two- to three-fold during pregnancy.
- If a woman is seizure free, there is no need to measure drug levels serially or adjust the dose unless she has a seizure. The exception to this is lamotrigine where profound reduction in drug levels mean that prophylactic increases in dose are appropriate in pregnancy.
- In women who have regular seizures and who are dependent on critical drug levels, it is worth monitoring drug levels since they are likely to fall, and increasing doses of AED should be guided by serum concentrations of the free drug.
- In general it is preferable to be guided by the patient and her seizure frequency rather than by drug levels.
- Although some authorities recommend an increased dose of corticosteroids [to compensate for increased metabolism in women receiving hepatic enzyme-inducing drugs (carbamezepine, phenytoin, phenobarbitone)] to induce fetal lung maturation, this recommendation has not been widely adopted.
- Vitamin K (10–20 mg orally) should be prescribed in the last four weeks of pregnancy for women with epilepsy taking hepatic enzyme-inducing drugs. This is because in babies of women receiving these drugs, vitamin K-dependent clotting factors may be reduced and the risk of haemorrhagic disease of the newborn is increased.

Intrapartum management

- The risk of seizures increases around the time of delivery. Women with major convulsive seizures should deliver in hospital.
- One to two percent of women with epilepsy will have a seizure during labour and 1–2% will have one in the first 24 hours postpartum. Women should not therefore be left unattended in labour or for the first 24 hours postpartum.
- Women should continue their regular AEDs in labour.
- To limit the risk of precipitating a seizure because of pain and anxiety, early epidural analgesia should be considered.
- If seizures that are not rapidly self-limiting occur in labour, oxygen and intravenous lorazepam (4 mg over two minutes) or diazepam [10–20 mg (rectal gel) or 10–20 mg intravenously at 2 mg/min] should be given.
- For women who have had seizures during previous deliveries, an option is to use rectal carbamezepine or intravenous sodium valproate or phenytoin to replace the usual oral therapy and ensure adequate absorption in labour. Alternatively oral clobazam may be used for short periods of time (e.g. starting the day before

planned delivery or at the onset of labour) to provide extra protection from seizures in labour.

■ Most women with epilepsy have normal vaginal deliveries and caesarean section is only required if there are recurrent generalised seizures in late pregnancy or labour.

Postnatal management

■ The neonate should also receive 1 mg vitamin K intramuscularly.

■ All women with epilepsy should be encouraged to breastfeed. Most AEDs are secreted into breast milk, but the dose received by the baby is only a fraction (3–5%) of the therapeutic level for neonates, and in any case is less than that received in utero.

■ Babies whose mothers received phenobarbitone in pregnancy may experience withdrawal symptoms if they are not breastfed, and although this is rare with the newer AEDs, it provides a logical reason to encourage breastfeeding in all mothers with epilepsy.

■ The only AEDs that cross in significant amounts (30–50%) to breast milk are lamotrigine and phenobarbitone.

■ In addition, phenobarbitone, primidone and lamotrigine can accumulate in a breastfed baby due to slow elimination. Lamotrigine is metabolised mainly by glucuronidation and the capacity to glucuronidate is not fully developed in newborns. Lamotrigine should not be initiated in breastfeeding mothers.

■ If the mother's dose of AED was increased during pregnancy, it may be gradually decreased again over a few weeks in the puerperium. Blood levels of phenytoin and lamotrigine increase rapidly following delivery, but carbamazepine and valproate take longer to return to pre-conception levels. Therefore, if doses of lamotrigine have been increased in pregnancy they should probably be decreased relatively rapidly postpartum.

■ If a baby of a mother taking AEDs is unusually sleepy or has to be woken for feeds, the mother should be encouraged to feed before rather than after taking her anticonvulsants. This should avoid peak serum and therefore breast-milk levels.

■ The mother should be advised of strategies to minimise the risk to her and her baby should she have a major convulsive seizure. This includes changing nappies with the baby on the floor and bathing the baby in very shallow water or with supervision.

Management of newly diagnosed idiopathic epilepsy in pregnancy

■ The annual incidence of new cases of epilepsy in women of child-bearing age is 20 to 30 per 100,000.

■ Having excluded all the secondary causes of seizures listed earlier, it is not obligatory to treat one isolated seizure.

■ If treatment is required, carbamazepine and lamotrigine are reasonable choices. However, it is the type of epilepsy that guides AED therapy; and generalised seizures with myoclonus and photosensitivity respond particularly well to sodium valproate.

Pre-pregnancy counselling

■ Ideally, this should form part of the routine management of epilepsy in pregnancy.

■ It should be assumed that all women of child-bearing age may become pregnant and therefore any opportunity to counsel such women should be taken.

- Control of epilepsy should be maximised prior to pregnancy with the lowest dose of the most effective treatment that gives best seizure control. Polytherapy should be avoided if possible.
- Review of AED medication should take into account the risk of teratogenesis and other adverse neurodevelopmental effects particularly of valproate. If there are any issues concerning fertility, it is important to remember the association between sodium valproate, weight gain and polycystic ovarian syndrome.
- Any changes to minimise the risk of neural tube defects (e.g. a decrease in the dose of sodium valproate) should ideally be made pre-conception since the neural tube closes at gestational day 26.
- Women who have been seizure-free for more than two years may wish to discontinue AEDs at least pre-conception and for the first trimester. This should be a fully informed decision after counselling concerning particularly the risk of losing a driving licence in the event of a seizure. It is not appropriate for women with juvenile myoclonic epilepsy to discontinue AEDs.
- The risk of recurrent seizures is approximately 25% by one year after drug withdrawal (80% of which will occur within four months after tapering of the dose begins).
- The risk of recurrence is approximately 40% by two years after drug withdrawal.
- Recurrence risk is increased to over 50% in women with
  - A known structural lesion
  - An abnormal EEG
  - Onset of seizures in adolescence
  - A history of frequent seizures requiring more than one AED.
- Factors associated with a low risk of recurrent seizures following discontinuation of AED are
  - A normal EEG
  - Onset in childhood
  - Seizures that have been easily controlled with one drug.
- If a decision is taken to stop treatment, AEDs should be withdrawn slowly in order to reduce the risk of withdrawal-associated seizures. This is particularly important for benzodiazepines and phenobarbitone.
- Patients with juvenile myoclonic epilepsy require lifelong treatment with AEDs.
- The current recommendations are to stop driving from the commencement of the period of drug withdrawal and for a period of six months after cessation of treatment, even if there is no recurrence of seizures.
- All women receiving AEDs should be advised to take pre-conception folic acid (5 mg/day).

Contraception

- Women taking hepatic enzyme-inducing drugs (phenytoin, primidone, carbamazepine, phenobarbitone) require higher doses of oestrogen to achieve adequate contraception. They should be given a combined oral contraceptive pill containing 50 μg ethinyloestradiol or be instructed to take two pills containing 30 μg. The combined oral contraceptive pill may still not be effective and an alternative method of contraception may be appropriate.
- The efficacy of the progesterone-only pill is also affected by enzyme-inducing antiepileptic medication. Women should be advised to take two rather than one daily pill of Micronor (norethisterone 350 μg) or Microval (levonorgestrel 30 μg).

■ Medroxyprogesterone injections (Depo-Provera®) are effective and larger doses are not needed since elimination is dependent on hepatic first-pass rather than enzyme activity.

■ The 'morning after pill' can be used if required, but again a double dose is advised.

■ Valproate, clonazepam, vigabatrin, lamotrigine, levetiracetam, gabapentin and tiagabine do not induce hepatic enzymes and all methods of contraception are suitable.

Epilepsy—points to remember

■ All women receiving antiepileptic drugs (AEDs) should receive pre-pregnancy counselling and be advised to take folic acid 5 mg daily pre-conception.

■ Most AEDs are teratogenic. The risk is lower with mono- rather than polytherapy and higher with sodium valproate.

■ Prenatal screening for congenital abnormalities should be offered.

■ In most women, the frequency of seizures is not altered by pregnancy provided there is compliance with AED regimens.

■ Free drug levels tend to fall in pregnancy and increased doses of AED may be required.

■ Vitamin K (10–20 mg orally daily) should be prescribed in the last four weeks of pregnancy for all women receiving enzyme-inducing AEDs.

■ Breastfeeding should be encouraged.

■ Hepatic enzyme-inducing drugs reduce the efficacy of most hormonal methods of contraception, particularly the combined oral contraceptive pill.

Migraine and headache

Incidence

■ Migraine is three times more common in women than men, and is common in the child-bearing years. Headaches including migraine are a common problem in pregnancy affecting up to 35% of women.

■ Differentiation between tension headache and migraine can be very difficult and not all migraine is 'classical'.

■ Migraine can occur and worsen in pregnancy in known migraine sufferers. It may also occur as a pregnancy-related phenomenon in women without any prior history of migrainous headaches.

■ Migraine and headache account for almost one-third of neurological problems encountered in pregnancy.

Clinical features

■ Features of a headache that make migraine a likely diagnosis are the following:
  – Throbbing, unilateral severe headache
  – Prodromal symptoms that are usually visual, including scotoma and teichopsia (fortification spectra; the sensation of a luminous appearance before the eyes, with a zigzag, wall-like outline)
  – Nausea and vomiting
  – Photophobia or noise sensitivity.

- During the prodromal phase of classical migraine, transient hemianopia, aphasia and sensory symptoms may occur. In hemiplegic migraine, the hemiparesis may last several hours and differentiation from a transient ischaemic attack is difficult, particularly if there is no headache.
- Hemiplegic migraine may rarely lead to cerebral infarction.
- Migraine associated with such focal signs may occur in up to 0.1% of pregnancies.
- Most cases occur in the third trimester and 40% occur in women with no previous history of migraine.

Pathogenesis

- Tension headaches are thought to be because of muscle contraction and are often related to periods of stress.
- Migraine is thought to be because of vasodilation of cerebral blood vessels, possibly related to platelet aggregation and serotonin [5-hydroxytryptamine (5-HT)] release with stimulation of nociceptors.
- Migraine may be precipitated by:
  - Certain dietary factors (e.g. chocolate, cheese)
  - Premenstruation
  - Oral contraceptive pill
  - Stress.

Diagnosis

- Diagnosis is made by taking a careful history and performing a neurological examination (in order to exclude focal signs, neck stiffness and papilloedema).
- The key issue is to distinguish the primary headache syndromes (tension, migraine, cluster) from secondary causes (see later)
- Any focal signs lasting longer than 24 hours warrant further investigation with cerebral imaging. There is no test to confirm the diagnosis of migraine. Aura is associated with a slow emergence of symptoms.
- The differential diagnosis (see also section B, Table 7) of headache in pregnancy and the puerperium include secondary causes:
  - Pre-eclampsia
  - Postdural puncture headache
  - Sub-arachnoid haemorrhage
  - Meningitis
  - CVT
  - Idiopathic (benign) intracranial hypertension
  - Intracranial mass lesions.

Pregnancy

Effect of pregnancy on migraine

- Fifty to ninety percent of women with pre-existing classical migraine improve during pregnancy, with reduction in frequency and severity of attacks.
- Improvement is most marked in the second and third trimesters.
- Improvement is more common in those with premenstrual migraine and migraine without aura.

- Migraine may present for the first time during pregnancy or women may develop aura for the first time. Pregnancy may also trigger attacks of aura without headache leading to diagnostic confusion.

Effect of migraine on pregnancy

- Pre-existing migraine is associated with an increased risk of pre-eclampsia.
- Outside pregnancy a case control study has also demonstrated an increased risk of stroke, ischaemic heart disease, thromboembolism, hypertension and diabetes.

Management

- For the acute attack, paracetamol-based analgesic with metoclopramide is the treatment of choice in pregnancy.
- Other antiemetics (e.g. buclizine, cyclizine) may be used.
- Codeine phosphate is also safe for use in pregnancy.
- Ergotamine is contraindicated.
- Sumatriptan (Imigran®) and other 5-HT$_1$ agonists are commonly used in non-pregnant women for control of acute attacks. There are limited data of their use in pregnancy and they are usually avoided, although there is no evidence of adverse effects. Birth registry data suggest no significant increase in the rate of birth defects. If these are the only agents that successfully treat an acute attack then it is reasonable to use them sporadically in pregnancy.
- Prophylaxis should be considered if attacks are frequent.
- Low-dose aspirin (75 mg daily) is safe and effective for prophylaxis of migraine complicating pregnancy, and should be considered as a first-line agent.
- β-Blockers (propranolol 10–40 mg t.d.s.) may be used in resistant cases without contraindications. These work in >80% of patients. The use of β-blockers, particularly atenolol, throughout pregnancy has been associated with growth restriction (see Chapter 1, p. 12).
- If both aspirin and β-blockers are ineffective in preventing headache and migraine in pregnancy, then tricyclic antidepressants such as amitriptyline (25–50 mg at night), calcium antagonists (e.g. Verapamil 40–80 mg nocte) or cyproheptadine (2–4 mg nocte) may prove useful and are safe for use in pregnancy.
- There are few data regarding pizotifen (Sanomigran®), a serotonin antagonist used for prevention of migraine outside pregnancy, but its use is justified after the first trimester if first- and second-line prophylactic agents are not effective.
- Valproate, gabapentin and topiramate, useful outside pregnancy, should be avoided.

Migraine—points to remember

- Migraine can occur as a pregnancy-related phenomenon in women without prior history of migraine.
- Those with pre-existing migraine often improve in pregnancy.
- Hemiplegic migraine, particularly aura without headache may mimic transient ischaemic attacks (TIAs).
- Ergotamine should be avoided in pregnancy.
- Low-dose aspirin, β-blockers, tricyclic antidepressants, and pizotifen may be used for prophylaxis.

Contraception

Women with classical migraine should not take oestrogen-containing oral contraceptives.

Multiple sclerosis (MS)

Incidence

This disease is relatively common (0.06–0.1% in the United Kingdom) and more commonly affects women, with the typical age of onset during the child-bearing years.

Clinical features

- MS typically runs a relapsing and remitting clinical course.
- Common presentations include optic neuritis, diplopia, sensory symptoms or weakness of the limbs.
- The course of MS is extremely variable; some are perfectly normal between relapses, others develop cumulative neurological disability.

Pathogenesis

- The cause is not known and prevalence is higher with increasing latitude, so the condition is uncommon in equatorial regions.
- There are multiple areas of demyelination within the brain and spinal cord.

Diagnosis

- There is no single diagnostic test. Most patients encountered in pregnancy are aware of their diagnosis.
- Cerebrospinal fluid examination, visually evoked responses and MRI are all used to help confirm the diagnosis.

Pregnancy

Effect of pregnancy on MS

- MS is less likely to present for the first time and less likely to relapse during pregnancy.
- The decrease in relapse rate during pregnancy is most marked in the third trimester, and accompanied by cessation of disease activity on MRI. This is possibly related to the decrease in cell-mediated immunity and the increase in humoral immunity characteristic of pregnancy.
- Those with neuropathic bladders may experience increased problems with urinary tract infection during pregnancy.
- The rate of relapse increases markedly in the first 3 months postpartum, but declines to pre-pregnant levels by 10 months after delivery.
- Exacerbation during the three to six months following delivery occurs in up to 40% of patients.
- Neither breastfeeding nor epidural analgesia have an adverse effect on the rate of relapse. Indeed there are some data to suggest that exclusive breast feeding may prevent relapse in the post partum period.

- The overall rate of progression of disability is not altered by pregnancy.
- There is no long-term effect of pregnancy or breastfeeding on the course of MS.

Effect of MS on pregnancy

There is little effect of MS on pregnancy outcome.

Management

- Severe acute relapses may be treated with high-dose steroids as in the non-pregnant.
- Agents used to reduce relapses such as β-interferons and glatiramer are usually discontinued during pregnancy because of a lack of safety data.

Multiple sclerosis—points to remember

- Pregnancy has no effect on the long-term prognosis of MS.
- Attacks are less likely during pregnancy but more likely in the postpartum period.
- Prophylactic treatments such as β-interferon and glatiramer are avoided in pregnancy.
- Those with disability may require extra help during pregnancy and while caring for the infant following delivery.
- There is no contraindication to epidural anaesthesia, except that careful documentation of pre-existing neurological deficit in the legs is necessary to avoid any postpartum exacerbation of MS being inappropriately attributed to the regional block.

Myasthenia gravis

Incidence

The prevalence is between 1 in 10,000 and 1 in 50,000, with a female to male preponderance of 2:1. Onset is usually in the second and third decades.

Clinical features

There may be exacerbations and remissions. The symptoms and signs include the following:

- Diplopia
- Ptosis
- Dysphagia
- Respiratory muscle weakness (in severe cases)
- Ten to fifty percent have a thymoma that is usually benign
- Ten percent have associated thyroid disease.

Pathogenesis

Myasthenia gravis is caused by IgG antibodies directed against the nicotinic acetylcholine receptor on the motor endplate. These blocks neuromuscular transmission at the postsynaptic level causing weakness and fatigue of skeletal, but not smooth muscle.

Diagnosis

- The diagnosis is made by administration of edrophonium chloride, a short-acting anticholinesterase. This produces prompt but transient improvement in muscle strength (the Tensilon test).
- Electromyography typically shows a reduction in evoked muscle potential following repetitive, supramaximal muscle motor-nerve stimulation.
- Acetylcholine receptor antibodies are found in up to 90% of patients and an associated thymoma in 10%.

Pregnancy

Effect of pregnancy on myasthenia gravis

- In approximately 40% of women, pregnancy is associated with exacerbation of the disease. In 30%, there is no change; in 30%, remissions occur.
- Exacerbation in pregnancy is less likely if the woman has undergone previous thymectomy.
- The course of myasthenia gravis is not necessarily the same in different pregnancies in the same woman.
- Postpartum exacerbations occur in 30% of women.
- The physiology of pregnancy may also indirectly influence the disease. For example, nausea and vomiting in early pregnancy, delayed gastric emptying and gastrointestinal absorption, and increased volume of distribution and renal clearance, may all lead to subtherapeutic levels of medication.

Effect of myasthenia gravis on pregnancy

- Transplacental passage of antibodies may rarely cause arthrogryposis multiplex congenital where the fetus develops contractures due to lack of movement.
- There is a high incidence of preterm delivery and growth restriction (40%).
- Since the uterus has smooth muscle, the first stage of labour is unaffected by myasthenia; however, maternal effort using voluntary striated muscle is required in the second stage, and this may be impaired.

Neonatal myasthenia gravis

- Up to 20% of neonates born to mothers with myasthenia may be affected by neonatal myasthenia due to transplacental passage of IgG antibodies. This usually becomes apparent in the first two days after birth, and is characterised by difficulty in feeding, crying, a floppy baby and respiratory embarrassment.
- It is transient, resolves within two months, corresponding to the disappearance of maternal antibodies in the neonate, and responds to anticholinesterase drugs.
- The delayed onset of neonatal myasthenia contrasts with congenital heart block (see Chapter 8, p. 140) caused by transplacental passage of anti-Ro antibodies, which usually affects the fetus in utero. The explanation may be:
  - Transfer of maternal drugs across the placenta

- Differences between fetal and adult acetylcholine receptors
- An inhibitory effect of the α-fetoprotein in amniotic fluid on the binding of antibody to the acetylcholine receptor.
■ There is no way to predict which neonates will be affected but it is related to the titre of acetylcholine receptor antibodies. The risk is lower in thymectomised women.

Management

■ Patients with myasthenia gravis are often treated with long-acting anti-cholinesterases, for example, pyridostigmine; this drug should be continued in pregnancy.
■ Increased doses may be required as pregnancy advances; this may be more appropriately achieved by decreasing the dosage interval rather than increasing each dose.
■ In large doses, these drugs may cause nausea, vomiting, diarrhoea and hypersalivation, and overdose can result in paradoxical weakness and respiratory failure.
■ A vaginal delivery should be the aim, although instrumental delivery may be required to prevent the woman from becoming exhausted. Caesarean section should only be performed for the usual obstetric indications.
■ Anticholinesterase drugs should be given parenterally in labour to avoid erratic absorption due to delayed gastric emptying.
■ Some patients receive immunosuppression with corticosteroids for disease control and these should be maintained in pregnancy.
■ Azathioprine and plasmapheresis (for crises) have also been used.
■ Thymectomy is also employed in the treatment of myasthenia gravis, but its use is not recommended in pregnancy.

Other drugs and women with myasthenia gravis

Certain drugs should be avoided or used with caution in women with myasthenia. These include the following:

■ Drugs that impair neuromuscular transmission and may increase weakness (aminoglycoside antibiotics such as gentamicin).
■ Drugs that may block neuromuscular transmission such as β-blockers (particularly propranolol).
■ Other drugs that may exacerbate or cause muscle fatigue such as β-adrenergics (ritodrine, salbutamol) and narcotics.
■ Although magnesium sulphate is the drug of choice for seizure prophylaxis in eclampsia and pre-eclampsia (see Chapter 1), it should be avoided in women with myasthenia gravis since it may precipitate a crisis.
■ Anaesthetic agents.
Women with myasthenia are more resistant to the depolarising neuromuscular blocking agents such as succinyl choline (suxamethonium) and therefore they will require a higher dose to achieve the same degree of muscle relaxation. By contrast women with myasthenia gravis are extremely sensitive to non-depolarising muscle relaxants (e.g. vecuronium), which may have an exaggerated or prolonged effect. Consultation with an experienced obstetric anaesthetist is advisable, preferably prior to delivery.

- Epidural analgesia and anaesthesia are safe to use but the ester type of local anaesthetics (e.g. chlorprocaine, tetracaine) depend on maternal plasma cholinesterase for their metabolism, and should be avoided if the mother is being treated with anticholinesterases.
- Lignocaine and the amide type of local anaesthetics are metabolised by a different pathway and are therefore safe for use in labour and delivery. Bupivicaine is safe to use.
- If an inhalational anaesthetic is required, ether and halothane should be avoided.

Myasthenia gravis—points to remember

- The course of myasthenia gravis in pregnancy is unpredictable.
- Postpartum exacerbations occur in 30% of women.
- Increased doses of long-acting anticholinesterases may be required as pregnancy advances.
- Many drugs should be avoided in myasthenia gravis and consultation with an experienced obstetric anaesthetist is recommended.
- Up to 20% of neonates born to myasthenic mothers may be affected by neonatal myasthenia due to transplacental passage of IgG antibodies.

Myotonic dystrophy

Incidence

- Myotonic dystrophy is a rare degenerative neuromuscular and neuroendocrine disease. Pregnancy in severely affected women is rare. In some milder cases, the disease may only be recognised in pregnancy.
- With increasing frequency women are presenting for pre-pregnancy counselling prior to in vitro fertilisation (IVF) and pre-implantation genetic diagnosis (PGD) to avoid bearing an affected child.

Pathogenesis

- Myotonic dystrophy type 1 is the commonest muscular dystrophy encountered in adulthood. This is an autosomal dominant inherited disorder. It is a tri-nucleotide repeat disorder, with the affected gene located on chromosome 19.
- The number of repeats affects the phenotype so that individuals with more repeats have an earlier onset and more severe form of the disease. Since the number of repeats increases with cell division and gametogenesis successive generations show anticipation.

Clinical features

The characteristic features include the following:

- Progressive muscular dystrophy
- Muscle weakness
- Myotonia (failure to relax after forceful contraction)

- Myopathic facies (because of weakness of facial muscles)
- Cataracts
- Frontal alopecia
- Cognitive problems
- Heart conduction defects
- Hypersomnia, dysphagia
- Pneumonia and hypoventilation.

Pregnancy

Effect of pregnancy on myotonic dystrophy

- Pregnancy may be associated with marked exacerbations of myotonia and muscle weakness, or symptoms may be unchanged.
- Deterioration may occur early in pregnancy, but is most severe in the third trimester.
- Improvement after delivery is rapid.

Effect of myotonic dystrophy on pregnancy

- There is an increased risk of:
  - First and second trimester miscarriage
  - Stillbirth
  - Polyhydramnios (indicative of an affected fetus)
  - Preterm delivery (also more common with an affected fetus)
  - Placenta praevia.
- The second trimester losses and preterm delivery may be related to abnormal myotonic involvement of the uterus.
- Abnormalities of all three stages of labour have been described. Both prolonged and rapid first and second stages are reported. Uterine inertia responds to oxytocin.
- Postpartum haemorrhage is common because of failure of uterine contractions in the third stage.
- The baby may be affected with congenital myotonic dystrophy, which is distinct from the adult form and probably arises from a combination of the autosomal dominant gene and an intrauterine environmental factor. The disease is rare with an affected father.
- The congenital syndrome includes the following:
  - Severe generalised hypotonia and weakness
  - Difficulties in breathing, sucking and swallowing
  - Talipes
  - Arthrogryposis
  - Mental retardation
  - Myotonia and cataracts are usually absent.

Management

- Prenatal diagnosis is possible by direct DNA analysis from PGD or chorion villus biopsy.
- General anaesthesia should be avoided and great care is needed with respiratory depressants such as opiates that may exacerbate pulmonary hypoventilation.
- Referral to an obstetric anaesthetist is recommended.

Idiopathic (benign) intracranial hypertension (IIH)

Incidence

This condition is rare but most common in obese, young women.

Clinical features

- Headache, often retro-orbital
- Obesity, rapid weight gain
- Diplopia (15%)
- Papilloedema
- Cerebrospinal fluid (CSF) pressure is increased.

Diagnosis

The combination of papilloedema and raised intracranial pressure without CT or MRI evidence of hydrocephalus or a space-occupying lesion.

Pregnancy

Effect of pregnancy on IIH

- IIH may present for the first time in pregnancy, commonly in the second trimester.
- Pre-existing IIH tends to worsen during pregnancy, possibly related to weight gain.

Management

- Limitation of weight gain.
- Monitor visual fields and visual acuity. In severe cases, infarction of the optic nerve may occur, leading to blindness. Any impairment of visual acuity or in the visual fields should prompt treatment with corticosteroids.
- The main problem in pregnancy is treatment of the headache, which may be persistent and severe.
- Thiazide diuretics and acetazolamide may reduce intracranial pressure and are often used to treat the condition. These may be used in pregnancy, although acetazolamide is usually avoided in the first trimester and thiazides may cause neonatal thrombocytopenia if used in the third trimester.
- Repeated CSF drainage or insertion of a shunt may provide relief from headache.
- In extreme cases where vision is threatened, surgery with optic nerve fenestration may be an option.

Stroke

The risks of arterial ischaemic stroke, cerebral venous thrombosis and intracranial haemorrhage are increased, particularly in the puerperium.

Ischaemic (non-haemorrhagic) stroke

Incidence

- Strokes are rare in women of child-bearing age (3.5 in 100,000).
- Pregnancy increases the risk of cerebral infarction (5–200 in 100,000), but this risk is largely due to a nine-fold increased risk during the puerperium.

- Epidemiological studies have shown that the excess risk of pregnancy is approximately 8 strokes per 100,000.
- Patients who have had stroke in the past may be reassured that they are very unlikely to have recurrence in pregnancy unless they have an obvious risk factor such as antiphospholipid syndrome (see Chapter 8, p. 140). In one study, the recurrence risk of stroke was 2% in pregnancy.

Clinical features

- Most strokes associated with pregnancy occur in the distribution of the carotid and middle cerebral arteries.
- Most cases occur in the first week after delivery.

Pathogenesis

- The risk factors of hypertension, smoking and diabetes for stroke in non-pregnant patients are found less commonly in pregnancy-associated strokes.
- Cerebral infarction may rarely occur following classical migraine.
- Unusual causes of strokes are more common in pregnancy, such as:
  - Cardiac causes of arterial emboli or arrhythmias
  - Mitral valve prolapse/disease
  - Peripartum cardiomyopathy (see Chapter 2, p. 30)
  - Infective endocarditis
  - Paradoxical embolus (in situations causing increased right compared with left atrial pressure) through an atrial septal defect (ASD) or patent foramen ovale (PFO)
  - Aortic dissection
  - Antiphospholipid syndrome (see Chapter 8, p. 140)
  - Vasculitis (systemic lupus erythematosus (SLE), Takayasu's disease)
  - Sickle-cell disease
  - TTP
  - Pre-eclampsia/eclampsia (see Chapter 1, p. 6).

Diagnosis

- MRI or CT is appropriate to confirm ischaemic stroke and differentiate haemorrhage from infarction.
- Investigations to establish a cause should include echocardiography and carotid Doppler scans.

Management

- This depends on the underlying cause.
- It is safe to continue or start low-dose aspirin in pregnancy.
- Anticoagulation may be appropriate.

Haemorrhagic stroke

Incidence

- This is very rare in women of child-bearing age (where there is a preponderance of cerebral infarction as a cause of stroke) outside pregnancy, but is almost as common as ischaemic stroke in pregnancy.

- The relative risk in pregnancy is 2.5 and during the puerperium is 28.
- There are approximately 2–4 maternal deaths annually in the United Kingdom due to intracerebral haemorrhage.

Pathogenesis

- *Pre-eclampsia/eclampsia.* Intraparenchymal haemorrhage is found in 40% of women dying from eclampsia. The haemorrhage is thought to be due to cerebral vasospasm, loss of autoregulatory control and breakthrough of the vessel wall (see Chapter 1, p. 7).
- *Ruptured vascular malformations.* Whether pregnancy increases the risk of rupture of arteriovenous malformations (AVMs) is controversial. The rate of first cerebral haemorrhage is not increased by pregnancy and the risk of a second haemorrhage is not known accurately.
- AVMs are oestrogen sensitive and therefore tend to dilate in pregnancy.
- Reported haemorrhages from AVMs occur fairly evenly throughout gestation and the postpartum period. Approximately 6% occur during labour and delivery.

Management

- If an AVM is diagnosed pre-pregnancy, pregnancy should be deferred until after treatment.
- AVMs may not be amenable to surgery. There are no data concerning embolisation of AVMs in pregnancy. Stereotactic radiotherapy is not used in pregnancy because it exposes the fetus to large amounts of gamma irradiation.
- In women with untreated AVMs, there is no advantage of caesarean over vaginal delivery and the former should be reserved for the usual obstetric indications.

Subarachnoid haemorrhage (SAH)

Incidence

- Twenty in 100,000 pregnancies.
- The risk of SAH is increased 2- to 3-fold during pregnancy and 20-fold in the puerperium.
- Bleeding from either an aneurysm or an AVM is associated with a high rate of maternal morbidity and mortality.
- There are four to five maternal deaths every year due to SAH in the United Kingdom and it remains one of the commonest indirect causes of maternal death.

Clinical features

- Headache (sudden and severe, often occipital)
- Vomiting
- Loss of or impaired consciousness
- Sudden collapse
- Neck stiffness
- Papilloedema
- Focal neurological signs are often, but not invariably present.

Pathogenesis

- SAH may be due to a ruptured arterial (berry) aneurysm or to AVM.
- Outside pregnancy, the ratio of aneurysm to AVM is 7:1.
- In pregnancy, relatively more cases are due to AVMs. The ratio is 1:1.
- The classic notion that rupture of an arterial aneurysm occurs more frequently during labour, related to Valsalva manoeuvres, has not been confirmed.
- In one study of ruptured aneurysms related to pregnancy, 90% occurred antenatally, 8% during the puerperium and only 2% during labour and delivery.
- The risk of bleeding from arterial aneurysms increases progressively with successive trimesters.
- This suggests haemodynamic, hormonal or other physiological changes of pregnancy may play a role in aneurysm rupture.

Diagnosis

- CT or MRI will confirm the diagnosis and determine the site of the bleed. CT is best to detect an acute bleed but if presentation is delayed MRI is more sensitive at detecting subarachnoid blood.
- If SAH is suspected but CT and MRI are negative then lumbar puncture to examine the CSF for blood, xanthochromia or bilirubin can diagnose SAH.
- Magnetic resonance or CT angiography is used to identify the cause of the bleeding.
- Angiography should not be withheld because of the pregnancy.

Management

- Neurosurgical or radiological management for SAH should not differ from that of the non-pregnant woman.
- There is neurosurgical consensus to treat asymptomatic aneurysms >7–10 mm.
- Clipping and endovascular treatment of aneurysms has been successful during all stages of pregnancy.
- Surgical management is associated with lower maternal and fetal mortality rates.
- The risk of re-bleeding from an AVM in the remainder of pregnancy may be as high as 50% with the greatest risk in the immediate period after haemorrhage.
- If the AVM or aneurysm is successfully operated upon, then vaginal delivery is preferable.
- If the lesion has not been operated on, elective caesarean section does not improve maternal or fetal outcome. It may be appropriate if there has been acute bleeding near term or for fetal salvage if the mother is moribund.
- Measures to decrease the risk of recurrent bleeding during vaginal delivery include epidural anaesthesia (which is also recommended to avoid the hypertensive response to intubation of the trachea, in the event of an emergency caesarean section), and a short second stage with possible low instrumental delivery.
- Regional anaesthesia is contraindicated in cases of recent SAH, when there is a risk of raised intracranial pressure.
- If general anaesthesia is used, β-adrenergic blockade will attenuate a hypertensive response to intubation.

Cerebral vein thrombosis

The reader should consult Chapter 3, p. 55.

Bell's palsy

Incidence

- This condition occurs much more commonly in pregnancy (10-fold increase).
- Incidence is approximately 45 in 100,000 pregnancies.

Clinical features

- There is a unilateral lower motor neurone lesion of the facial (VIIth cranial) nerve.
- This causes facial weakness, including loss of frontalis muscle (the patient cannot wrinkle her forehead) on the affected side.
- There may be associated pain around the ear or loss of taste on the anterior two-thirds of the tongue.
- Most cases in pregnancy occur around term, either in the two weeks before or after delivery.

Pathogenesis

- Outwith pregnancy most cases are due to latent herpes viruses (herpes simplex virus type 1 and herpes zoster virus), which are reactivated from cranial ganglia.
- Peripartum Bell's palsy may have a different aetiology, possibly related to swelling of the facial nerve within the petrous temporal bone. The reason for the increased incidence in late pregnancy and a possible increased incidence in pre-eclampsia may be related to oedema.
- Ramsay Hunt syndrome is herpes zoster (shingles) of the geniculate ganglion and causes a unilateral facial palsy (identical to Bell's) with herpetic vesicles in the external auditory meatus and occasionally the soft palate.
- Very rarely, Bell's palsy may be bilateral, in which case the differential diagnosis should include the following:
  - Guillain–Barré syndrome
  - Sarcoidosis
  - Lyme disease.

Diagnosis

The diagnosis is made on clinical grounds.

Management

- Bell's palsy usually (80–95%) improves spontaneously, but this may happen slowly over a period of months. Recovery is more likely with a partial (95%) rather than complete (85%) palsy.
- There is no evidence that pregnancy-associated Bell's palsy is associated with a worse outcome.
- A short (two-week) course of corticosteroids (prednisolone 40 mg/day, tapered after the first week) may speed or increase the chance of recovery, but this needs to be instituted as soon as possible (preferably within 24–72 hours after the onset of symptoms).
- Steroids should not be given in Ramsay Hunt syndrome and therefore it is imperative to examine the ear for vesicles prior to the prescription of corticosteroids.

Posterior reversible encephalopathy syndrome (PRES)

- This is transient neurological disturbance causing occipital lobe-related symptoms commonly headache, seizures and cortical blindness of acute or subacute onset.
- In pregnancy it is usually related to pre-eclampsia and eclampsia. Cortical blindness in pre-eclampsia typically is associated with:
  - Severe impairment of vision limited to distinguishing light and dark
  - Normal optic fundi
  - Normal pupillary reflex and is often preceded by blurred vision, photophobia, nausea and vomiting.
- The symptoms and signs normally recover relatively rapidly.
- MRI shows a characteristic bilateral involvement of white and grey matter in the posterior regions of the cerebral hemispheres.
- It is caused by vasogenic brain oedema.

Entrapment neuropathies

Carpal tunnel syndrome

Incidence

- This may affect 2% to 3% of women in pregnancy.

Clinical features

- Paraesthesiae and numbness in the thumb and lateral two and half fingers.
- Pain in the same distribution that may occasionally be experienced proximal to the wrist.
- More severe symptoms at night and in the dominant hand, relieved by shaking the wrist.
- Reproduction of symptoms on percussion over the carpal tunnel (Tinel's sign) or sustained flexion of the wrist (Phalen's sign).
- Severe cases may cause motor loss in the distribution of the median nerve and wasting of the thenar eminence.

Pathogenesis

This is caused by compression of the median nerve at the flexor retinaculum. It is more common in:

- Pregnancy
- Hypothyroidism
- Rheumatoid arthritis
- Acromegaly.

Diagnosis

This is usually obvious from the clinical features but may be confirmed by nerve conduction studies.

Management

- Reassurance that the condition is likely to improve or abate after delivery.

- Wrist splints to avoid flexion of the wrist.
- Severe cases may warrant local steroid injection or surgical division of the flexor retinaculum.

Meralgia paraesthetica

- This is numbness or pain in the distribution of the lateral cutaneous nerve of the thigh (anterolateral aspect of the thigh) caused by compression of this nerve at the lateral aspect of the inguinal ligament.
- It is more common in pregnancy and in obesity and tends to resolve following delivery.

Lumbosacral plexopathies

- Trauma to the lumbosacral plexus or specific nerves may occur usually as a result of pressure from the fetal head during a prolonged second stage, particularly if there is fetal macrosomia.
- The commonest of these is foot drop because of damage of the sciatic nerve (L4-S3), lumbosacral trunk (L4-5) or common peroneal nerve (L4-5). The latter occurs from pressure on the common peroneal nerve at the neck of the fibula, usually with the woman in the lithotomy or squatting position.
- It is important to distinguish these neuropraxias from a complication of regional anaesthesia, for example, epidural abscess or haematoma.

Further reading

Adab N, Kini U, Vinten J, et al. The longer term outcome of children born to mothers with epilepsy. J Neurol Neurosurg Psychiatry 2004; 75:1517–1518.

Briemberg HR. Neuromuscular diseases in pregnancy. Semin Neurol 2007; 27:460–466.

Ciafaloni E, Massey JM. Myasthenia gravis and pregnancy. Neurol Clin 2004; 22:771–782.

EURAP Study Group. Seizure control and treatment in pregnancy: Observations from the EURAP epilepsy pregnancy registry. Neurology 2006; 66:354–360.

Fairhall JM, Stoodley MA. Intracranial haemorrhage in pregnancy. Obstet Med 2009; 2:142–148.

Goadsby PJ, Goldberg J, Silberstein SD. Migraine in pregnancy. BMJ 2008; 336:1502–1504.

Grosset DG, Ebrahim S, Bone I, et al. Stroke in pregnancy and the puerperium: What magnitude of risk? J Neurol Neurosurg Psychiatry 1995; 58:129–131.

Kelly VM, Nelson LM, Chakravarty EF. Obstetric outcomes in women with multiple sclerosis and epilepsy. Neurology 2009; 73:1831–1836.

Kittner SJ, Stern BJ, Feeser BR, et al. Pregnancy and the risk of stroke. N Engl J Med 1996; 335:768–774.

Meador K, Reynolds MW, Crean S, et al. Pregnancy outcomes in women with epilepsy: A systematic review and meta-analysis of published pregnancy registries and cohorts. Epilepsy Res 2008; 81:1–13.

Meador KJ, Baker GA, Browning N, et al. Cognitive function at 3 years of age after fetal exposure to antiepileptic drugs. N Engl J Med 2009; 360:1597–1605.

Mas J-L, Lamy C. Stroke in pregnancy and the puerperium. J Neurol 1998; 245:305–313.

Morrow J, Russel A, Guthrie E, et al. Malformation risks of antiepileptic drugs in pregnancy: A prospective study from the UK Epilepsy and Pregnancy Register. J Neurol Neurosurg Psychiatry 2006; 77:193–198.

Rudnik-Schoneborn S, Zerres K. Outcome in pregnancies complicated by myotonic dystrophy: A study of 31 patients and review of the literature. Eur J Obstet Gynecol Reprod Biol 2004; 114:44–53.

Sibai BM, Coppage KH. Diagnosis and management of women with stroke during pregnancy/postpartum. Clin Perinatol 2004; 31:853–868.

Scottish Intercollegiate Guideline Network (SIGN). Diagnosis and management of epilepsy in adults. http://www.sign.ac.uk/guidelines/fulltext/70/section4.html. Accessed March 2010.

Sullivan FM, Swan IR, Donnan PT, et al. A randomised controlled trial of the use of aciclovir and/or prednisolone for the early treatment of Bell's palsy: The BELLS study. Health Technol Assess 2009; 13:iii–iv, ix–xi 1–130.

Turan TN, Stern BJ. Stroke in pregnancy. Neurol Clin 2004; 22:821–840.

CHAPTER 10

Renal disease

Physiological adaptation	**Pregnancy in dialysis patients**
Urinary tract infection	**Renal transplant recipients**
Chronic kidney disease	**Acute kidney injury**
Specific types of renal disease	

Physiological adaptation

- There is a dramatic dilatation of the urinary collecting system during pregnancy. This may be the result of ureteral smooth-muscle relaxation induced by progesterone, or compression of the ureters by the enlarging uterus or iliac vessels. Caliceal and ureteral dilatation is more pronounced on the right.
- The 'physiological hydronephrosis' of pregnancy can be dismissed as normal up to a pelvicalceal diameter of approximately 2 cm.
- Renal plasma flow (RPF) rises very early in pregnancy and it increases up to 60% to 80% by the second trimester of pregnancy. See Table 10.1.
- RPF falls throughout the third trimester but is maintained at 50% greater than pre-pregnancy values at term.
- Glomerular filtration rate (GFR) also increases significantly and creatinine clearance rises by approximately 50%. This results in a fall in the serum urea and creatinine levels.
- The use of eGFR (estimated GFR) from the Modification of Diet in Renal Disease (MDRD) formula is not recommended for use in pregnancy.
- Protein excretion is increased and the upper limit of normal in pregnancy is taken as 300 mg/24 hours or a protein creatinine ratio of 30 mg/mmol.
- Microscopic haematuria, in the absence of proteinuria, renal impairment or infection, is not uncommon in pregnancy and may relate to bleeding from small venules in dilated collecting systems. If renal ultrasound (US) is normal no further investigation is required unless the haematuria persists postpartum.
- There is physiological sodium (and water) retention during pregnancy; 80% of pregnant women develop some oedema, especially towards term, so it is usually not a pathological sign. The pregnant woman has a decreased ability to excrete a sodium and water load and this is most marked near term.
- Renal secretion of vitamin D, renin and erythropoietin are all increased in pregnancy.

Table 10.1 – Physiological renal changes in pregnancy

Physiological variable	Direction of change	Percentage increase or normal range for pregnancy
RPF	↑	60–80%
GFR	↑	55%
Creatinine clearance	↑	120–160 mL/min
Protein excretion	↑	<300 mg/24 hr
Urea	↓	2.0–4.5 mmol/L
Creatinine	↓	25–75 mmol/L
Bicarbonate	↓	18–22 mmol/L
Uric acid	↑	With gestation (see appendix 2)

Abbreviations: GFR, glomerular filtration rate; RPF, renal plasma flow.

Urinary tract infection

This may be divided into the following:

- Asymptomatic bacteriuria
- Acute cystitis
- Acute pyelonephritis.

Although urinary tract infection (UTI) is a common and important problem in pregnancy, it should never be assumed to be the cause of abdominal pain and/or proteinuria before further investigation (see section B) to confirm or refute the diagnosis is undertaken.

Asymptomatic bacteriuria

Incidence

- This affects 4% to 7% of pregnant women of whom up to 40% will develop symptomatic UTI and 30% acute pyelonephritis if untreated in pregnancy.
- Women who have a history of previous UTI and are found to have bacteriuria have a 10-fold increased risk of developing cystitis or acute pyelonephritis in pregnancy.

Pathogenesis

- Seventy-five to ninety percent of bacteriuria in pregnancy is because of *Escherichia coli*, probably derived from the large bowel.
- Colonisation of the urinary tract results from ascending infection from the perineum and may be related to sexual intercourse.

Diagnosis

- Most women with asymptomatic bacteriuria are infected during early pregnancy. Very few subsequently acquire asymptomatic bacteriuria.
- Bacteriuria is only considered significant if the colony count exceeds 100,000/mL on a mid-stream urine (MSU) specimen.
- Urine culture resulting in a non-significant or mixed growth should be repeated on a fresh MSU specimen.
- Dipsticks for nitrites and leucocyte esterase may be used to help exclude UTI.

Management

- Because dilation of the upper renal tract during pregnancy increases the risk of pyelonephritis (see later), asymptomatic bacteriuria should be treated.
- Treating asymptomatic bacteriuria reduces the risk of preterm delivery and low birthweight babies.
- The choice of antibiotic depends on the sensitivities of the causative organism.
- Ampicillin, amoxycillin and the cephalosporins are safe and appropriate antibiotics for use in pregnancy. Treatment with cefadroxil or cefalexin 500 mg b.d. is effective against the majority of urinary pathogens.
- Nitrofurantoin 100 mg t.d.s. and trimethoprim 200 mg b.d. are safe alternatives. Nitrofurantoin used in the third trimester may precipitate neonatal haemolytic anaemia. Trimethoprim should be avoided in the first trimester due to its antifolate action.
- Long-acting sulphonamides should be avoided in the last few weeks of pregnancy because they increase the risk of neonatal kernicterus. Septrin (co-trimoxazole = trimethoprim + sulphamethoxazole) is no longer recommended for treatment of UTI.
- Treatment for three days is sufficient for asymptomatic bacteriuria. Regular urine cultures should be taken following treatment to ensure eradication of the organism. Approximately 15% of women will have recurrent bacteriuria during their pregnancy and require a second course of antibiotics.

Acute cystitis

Incidence

Cystitis complicates approximately 1% of pregnancies.

Clinical features

- These include urinary frequency, urgency, dysuria, haematuria, proteinuria and suprapubic pain.
- UTI in pregnancy is more common in women with diabetes (both pre-existing and gestational), in those receiving systemic corticosteroids or other immunosuppressant drugs and in those with a history of previous recurrent UTIs (with or without structural renal abnormalities).

Pathogenesis

See 'Asymptomatic Bacteriuria' (earlier). Most infections are due to *E. coli.*

Diagnosis

- This is confirmed by the finding of significant bacteriuria (see earlier) following culture of an MSU specimen.
- Microscopy of the urine may reveal organisms, white cells and occasionally red cells, but the false–positive rate is very high and it is no longer recommended for diagnosis of UTI.
- The presence of nitrites and leukocytes is suggestive but not diagnostic of UTI.

Management

- This is the same as for asymptomatic bacteriuria (see earlier).
- Antibiotic therapy is guided by sensitivities of the organism. If the organism is resistant to penicillins, cephalosporins, nitrofurantoin and trimethoprim then ciprofloxacin may be appropriate, but this is not used as first-line therapy in pregnancy as it has caused arthropathy in animal studies.
- Antibiotics should be continued for five to seven days.
- Several non-pharmacological manoeuvres may help prevent recurrent infection in those women troubled by UTIs in pregnancy. These include the following:
  - Increasing fluid intake. This ensures frequent voiding and a high-volume dilute urine, all of which reduce the risk of symptomatic infection.
  - Emptying the bladder following sexual intercourse. This 'washes away' organisms massaged up the urethra from the perineum into the bladder during coitus, before they have a chance to replicate in urine within the bladder.
  - Double voiding (to ensure no residual urine is left in the bladder following micturition).
  - The perineum should be cleaned from 'front to back' following defaecation to minimise the risk of bowel organisms colonising the urethra.

Acute pyelonephritis

Incidence

- This complicates 1% to 2% of pregnancies.
- It is more common in pregnancy due to the physiological dilatation of the upper renal tract.

Clinical features

- These include fever, loin and/or abdominal pain, vomiting, rigors, as well as proteinuria, haematuria and concomitant features of cystitis (see earlier).
- Like cystitis, it is more common in women with diabetes, those on steroid and other immunosuppressant therapy and those with previous recurrent UTIs.

Other risk factors include the following:

- Polycystic kidneys
- Congenital abnormalities of the renal tract (e.g. duplex kidney or ureter, reflux nephropathy)
- Neuropathic bladder (e.g. in those with spina bifida or multiple sclerosis) and,
- Urinary tract calculi.

Pathogenesis

See 'Asymptomatic Bacteriuria' (earlier). Most infections are due to *E. coli*. Cultures yielding significant growths of mixed organisms should prompt a search for underlying renal calculi.

Diagnosis

- This is confirmed by the finding of significant bacteriuria (see earlier) following culture of an MSU specimen.
- Differential diagnosis includes pneumonia (especially right lower lobe), viral infections, cholecystitis and biliary colic, pre-eclampsia, acute appendicitis, gastroenteritis, placental abruption and a degenerating uterine fibroid (see also section B, Tables 12 and 17).
- Investigation in women with fever should include blood cultures and a full blood count.

Pregnancy

- Acute pyelonephritis increases the risk of preterm labour at least in part because of associated pyrexia.
- There is also evidence for an increased risk of low birthweight babies, but this is partly related to an increase in preterm delivery.

Management

- This should be undertaken in hospital.
- Once the diagnosis is suspected and a urine sample obtained, antibiotic treatment with appropriate i.v. antibiotics should begin immediately, before awaiting the results of urine culture or sensitivities.
- I.v. penicillins or cephalosporins (e.g. cefuroxime) are usually the first choice, although in the case of septicaemia or resistant organisms or women who are allergic to both penicillins and cephalosporins, an aminoglycoside such as gentamicin may be used. There is a theoretical risk of fetal ototoxicity with the use of gentamicin in pregnancy, but provided drug levels are measured and kept within the therapeutic range, this should not be a problem encountered in clinical practice.
- Antibiotics should be given intravenously for at least 24 hours, when they may be changed to an appropriate oral formulation. Antibiotics should be continued for a period of at least two weeks.
- Renal function should be checked regularly since renal impairment may complicate acute pyelonephritis in pregnancy, especially if there is associated sepsis.
- I.v. fluids may also be required if the woman is volume depleted as a result of inadequate intake, vomiting or sweating.
- An US examination of the kidneys should be undertaken to exclude hydronephrosis, congenital abnormalities and renal calculi.

Prophylaxis

- Women who usually take antibiotic prophylaxis against UTIs should continue this in pregnancy.
- Suitable regimes in pregnancy include low-dose amoxycillin or low-dose oral cephalosporins (cephalexin 250 mg), or nitrofurantoin 50 mg o.d., but depend on the sensitivities of the usual infecting organisms. The prophylactic agent may

need to be changed in pregnancy if there is intervening infection with a resistant organism.
- Once a woman has had two or more confirmed and documented UTIs in pregnancy, renal US should be performed and antibiotic prophylaxis considered.

Urinary tract infection—points to remember

- UTI is more common in pregnancy.
- Asymptomatic bacteriuria should be treated because there is a significant risk of acute pyelonephritis.
- Acute pyelonephritis increases the risk of preterm labour.
- Acute pyelonephritis should be managed in hospital with i.v. antibiotics.
- Once antibiotic treatment has rendered the urine sterile, regular MSU specimens are necessary to exclude reinfection.
- Amoxycillin and cephalosporins are appropriate antibiotics for the treatment and prevention of UTI in pregnancy.
- Gentamicin may be required for severe or resistant infections.
- Investigations in cases of pyrexia and suspected acute pyelonephritis should include blood cultures, a full blood count, renal function and a renal US.

Chronic kidney disease

Pregnancy

Effect of pregnancy on chronic kidney disease

The risks include the following:

- Possible accelerated decline in renal function
- Escalating hypertension during pregnancy
- Worsening proteinuria during pregnancy
- A flare/relapse of glomerulonephritis (particularly with lupus).

Increased proteinuria is a physiological response to pregnancy and may not necessarily indicate superimposed pre-eclampsia or deteriorating renal disease.

Effect of chronic kidney disease on pregnancy

The risks include the following:

- Miscarriage
- Pre-eclampsia
- Fetal growth restriction (FGR)
- Preterm delivery
- Fetal death.

Factors influencing outcome

The outcome of pregnancy and any adverse effect on underlying renal disease are both influenced by:

- Presence and degree of renal impairment (see later)
- Presence and severity of hypertension

- Presence and degree of proteinuria
- Underlying type and class of chronic kidney disease (CKD) (see later).

In general, women without hypertension or renal impairment prior to conception have successful pregnancies and pregnancy does not adversely influence the progression of the kidney disease.

Degree of renal impairment

- Degree of renal impairment was traditionally divided into mild (plasma creatinine <125 μmol/L), moderate (plasma creatinine 125–250 μmol/L) and severe (plasma creatinine >250 μmol/L).
- Absolute creatinine levels may be misleading if allowance is not made for the size of the woman. For example, a plasma creatinine level of 200 μmol/L in a woman weighing 50 kg represents a greater reduction in renal function than the same level in a woman weighing 80 kg. The GFR may be calculated using the Cockcroft Gault equation that takes account of the age, weight and sex of the patient.
- It is now conventional to classify renal disease by stages of CKD according to GFR in mL/min as follows:

CKD stage	GFR in mls/min/1.73 metre squared
CKD 1	>90
CKD 2	60–89
CKD 3	30–59
CKD 4	15–29
CKD 5	<15

- Women with severe renal impairment (CKD 5, serum creatinine >250 μmol/L) should be advised against pregnancy.

Effect of pregnancy on renal impairment

- Women with more severe renal impairment are more likely to have an accelerated decline and/or a permanent worsening of renal function as a result of the pregnancy (Table 10.2).
- Initially in all but those with very severe renal impairment, the usual increase in GFR occurs, leading to a fall in the serum creatinine level early in pregnancy. However, in those with moderate and severe renal impairment, the serum creatinine level usually begins to rise to and beyond pre-pregnancy levels during the second trimester.

Effect of degree of renal impairment on pregnancy outcome

- Women with more severe renal impairment are at increased risk of adverse pregnancy outcome and complications—especially pre-eclampsia, FGR and preterm delivery (Table 10.3).
- Polyhydramnios (and the accompanying risks of preterm rupture of the membranes and cord prolapse) may complicate pregnancies where the maternal urea level is

Table 10.2 – Effect of pregnancy on renal impairment

Degree of renal impairment	Mild Cr <125 μmol/L	Moderate Cr 125–180 μmol/L	Severe Cr >180 μmol/L	On dialysis
Loss of function (%)	2	40	70	n/a
Reduced function persisting postpartum (%)	0	20	50	n/a
End-stage renal failure (%)		2	35	n/a

Abbreviation: Cr, creatinine.

greater than 10 mmol/L. This results from fetal polyuria due to the osmotic load from the high maternal urea level.
■ Once the maternal urea level is greater than 20–25 mmol/L, there is a risk of fetal death.

Specific types of renal disease

Glomerulonephritis

■ The type of glomerulonephritis has less impact on pregnancy outcome than the level of renal impairment. Most pregnancies are successful. Those with hypertension are at increased risk of superimposed pre-eclampsia.
■ Fetal loss and preterm delivery rates are approximately 20%.
■ Less than 10% have a reversible and 3% have a progressive decrease in renal function related to pregnancy.

Table 10.3 – Effect of degree of renal impairment on pregnancy outcome

Degree of renal impairment	Mild Cr <125 μmol/L	Moderate Cr 125–180 μmol/L	Severe Cr >180 μmol/L	On dialysis
Pre-eclampsia (%)	22	40	60	75
FGR (%)	25	40	65	>90
Preterm delivery (%)	30	60	>90	>90
Perinatal mortality (%)	1	5	10	50

Abbreviation: Cr, creatinine.

- Over 25% have a reversible and <10% have a permanent increase in blood pressure.
- In those with normal renal function at conception, pregnancy does not affect the course of renal disease or the occurrence of end-stage renal failure. Hypertension and proteinuria accelerate the rate of decline in renal function, whether or not a woman has been pregnant.

Reflux nephropathy

- This is one of the most common renal diseases in women of child-bearing age.
- Women with reflux nephropathy should be screened regularly for UTI and treated promptly if it occurs.
- Overall approximately 25% of women develop pre-eclampsia and this risk is increased in cases of bilateral renal scarring, hypertension and serum creatinine >110 μmol/L.
- Even those with normal renal function and without hypertension pre-pregnancy are at increased risk of hypertension (33%) and pre-eclampsia (15%).
- Those with renal impairment may experience rapid worsening of renal function.
- There is a particular association between reflux nephropathy in the mother and severe FGR.
- Reflux nephropathy may be inherited as an autosomal dominant condition, and therefore offspring of affected mothers should be screened with a micturating cystogram, as US may miss the diagnosis. It is common to start prophylactic antibiotics if there is suspicion that the child may have reflux nephropathy.

Diabetic nephropathy (see also Chapter 5)

- Adverse pregnancy outcome and maternal complications are doubled compared with pregnant women with diabetes without nephropathy.
- The specific risks are UTI, pre-eclampsia, proteinuria and oedema that may be severe but usually revert after delivery to pre-pregnancy levels.
- Nephrotic syndrome can be severe with marked hypoalbuminaemia and the associated risks of pulmonary oedema and thrombosis.
- Anaemia is often out of proportion to the degree of renal impairment, and may become severe in pregnancy. This is due to a combination of deficient erythropoeitin secretion in the presence of renal impairment and haemodilution.
- Over 30% of affected women have preterm deliveries and over 50% have an increase in blood pressure.
- Most women with diabetic nephropathy show the normal increase in GFR and pregnancy does not increase the rate of deterioration in renal function.

SLE nephritis

See Chapter 8, p. 135.

Polycystic kidney disease

- This is an autosomal dominant disorder usually presenting in the fourth decade with hypertension, recurrent UTIs, haematuria or renal impairment. Some asymptomatic

women are aware of their diagnosis because of affected family members and positive screening. Women may remain undiagnosed throughout pregnancy.
- The risks in pregnancy are of pre-eclampsia, which is more common in those with pre-existing hypertension or renal impairment, and UTIs.
- Loin pain and haematuria may occur without UTI, related to bleeding into a renal cyst, or may occur in the absence of these complications.
- Pregnancy has no adverse long-term effect on renal function.
- Polycystic kidney disease (PKD) may be associated with polycystic liver disease and subarachnoid haemorrhage from intracranial aneurysms. Liver cysts may enlarge during pregnancy and those with a family history of intracranial aneurysms should be screened for aneurysms prior to pregnancy.
- Since PKD is an autosomal dominant disorder, there is a 50% chance of transmission to the affected woman's offspring.

Management of pregnancies complicated by chronic kidney disease

- Management should begin with pre-pregnancy counselling. Assessment of renal function, proteinuria and blood pressure enables accurate counselling and provides a baseline with which to compare trends in pregnancy.
- Obstetricians and physicians who have expertise in the care of renal disease in pregnancy should jointly manage women with CKD.
- In view of the increased risk of pre-eclampsia, treatment with low-dose aspirin from the first trimester should be advised, especially in those with hypertension and renal impairment or a previous poor obstetric history.
- Careful monitoring and control of blood pressure both pre-pregnancy and antenatally is important. Treatment for hypertension is no different from the management of pregnant women without renal disease (see Chapter 1, p. 10); however, the threshold for treatment may be lower, since good control of hypertension is important to preserve renal function. Blood pressure should be kept <140/90 mm/Hg.
- Regular assessment of renal function by serum creatinine and proteinuria by 24-hour protein excretion or protein creatinine ratio is essential. It may be useful to give the woman urine testing strips so that she can monitor the presence and severity of any proteinuria or haematuria.
- It is also important to monitor serum albumin, bicarbonate, calcium, haemoglobin and platelet levels.
- The fetus should be monitored with regular US assessment of growth and liquor volume. Doppler assessment of uterine artery blood flow at 20 to 24 weeks is useful to predict pre-eclampsia and FGR and assessment of the umbilical flow is useful in the presence of FGR.
- Admission should be considered if the woman develops worsening hypertension, deteriorating renal function or proteinuria, superimposed pre-eclampsia, or polyhydramnios.
- As discussed in Chapter 8, the differentiation between pre-eclampsia and deterioration of pre-existing renal disease may be extremely difficult. However, the indications for renal biopsy during pregnancy are mostly limited to early gestations where the result of the biopsy is likely to influence or change the management (i.e. before 28 weeks gestation where a diagnosis of a steroid- or immunosuppressant-responsive lesion is suspected).

CKD—points to remember

- Women with CKD are at increased risk of pre-eclampsia, FGR, preterm delivery and caesarean section; the perinatal mortality rate is increased.
- These obstetric complications and the risk of permanent deterioration in renal function are increased by the presence and severity of any renal impairment or hypertension.
- For women with moderate or severe renal impairment (plasma creatinine >125 μmol/L), 60% to 90% of infants are born preterm and the risk of acceleration of decline in renal function is 20% to 50%.
- An increase in the degree of proteinuria is very common in pregnancy and does not necessarily imply pre-eclampsia or worsening renal disease.
- Management should include regular monitoring of blood pressure, renal function and fetal well-being.
- In view of the increased risk of pre-eclampsia, treatment with low-dose aspirin should be advised, especially in those with hypertension and renal impairment or a previous poor obstetric history.

Pregnancy in dialysis patients

- Fertility is reduced in women on haemodialysis or chronic ambulatory peritoneal dialysis (CAPD). The pregnancy rate is approximately 1 in 200 women per year.
- The chance of successful pregnancy outcome is low (50%) with both haemodialysis and CAPD.
- Poor prognostic features for pregnancy in dialysis patients include the following:
  - Age >35 years
  - More than five years on dialysis
  - Delayed diagnosis of pregnancy (leading to late increase in dialysis times).

Effect of pregnancy on renal replacement therapy

- Anaemia is exacerbated by pregnancy, and transfusion requirements increase. Erythropoietin and i.v. iron can be used safely and doses increased in pregnancy.
- Pregnancy is associated with markedly increased requirements for dialysis.
- Doses of heparin may need to be increased to prevent clotting of dialysis lines.
- Pregnancy causes fluctuations in fluid balance and blood pressure.
- Doses of vitamin D and calcium may need to be reduced.

Effect of dialysis on pregnancy

- The risks include the following:
  - Miscarriage
  - Intrauterine death
  - Hypertension and pre-eclampsia
  - Preterm labour
  - Preterm rupture of membranes
  - Polyhydramnios related to uraemia
  - Placental abruption.
- Full heparinisation requirements during haemodialysis increase the risk of bleeding.

- The specific problems with CAPD include peritonitis and limitation in the volume of exchanges in later pregnancy.

Management

- In women on haemodialysis, the duration and/or the frequency of dialysis must be increased, to more than 20 hr/wk, and often dialysis is required on five to six days per week.
- The aim should be to maintain the pre-dialysis urea at less than 15 to 20 mmol/L.
- Dietary restrictions can usually be lifted, although continued adherence to fluid restriction is important to avoid large fluid shifts during dialysis.

Renal transplant recipients

- Women receiving renal transplants should be warned that as renal function returns to normal (usually rapidly after successful transplantation), ovulation, menstruation and fertility also resume.
- Women desiring pregnancy are usually advised to wait approximately one to two years after transplantation, by which time graft function has stabilised and maintenance levels of immunosuppressive drugs would have been reached, thus minimising any risk to the fetus.
- Graft survival is improved for recipients of living, related donors compared with cadaveric donors.
- Successful pregnancy outcome for those transplant recipients who become pregnant and do not miscarry before 12 weeks is now >95%.
- As with CKD, pregnancy outcome and effects on the renal allograft are both dependent on the baseline serum creatinine level and the presence of hypertension; the poorer the graft function at conception, the higher the risk of complications and deterioration in graft function.

Pregnancy

Effect of pregnancy on renal transplants

- Pregnancy has no adverse long-term effect on renal allograft function or survival in women with baseline creatinine levels of <100 μmol/L.
- For women who enter pregnancy with a serum creatinine level >130 μmol/L, renal graft survival is only 65% at three years.
- Renal allografts adapt to pregnancy in the same way as native kidneys, and exhibit an increase in GFR and collecting-system dilatation. As with native kidneys, the GFR may decrease again in the third trimester.
- As with other causes of renal impairment, the risk of deterioration in renal function is increased in those with higher baseline serum creatinine and hypertension.
- More than 10% of women are likely to develop new long-term problems following pregnancy, although whether this is as a direct result of pregnancy is difficult to ascertain. The risk of long-term problems is higher in women developing pregnancy complications prior to 28 weeks gestation.

Effect of renal transplants on pregnancy

- Outcome is optimal in those without hypertension, proteinuria or recent episodes of graft rejection as well as in those with normal or near-normal renal function (serum creatinine level <125 μmol/L).

- The chance of successful outcome beyond 12 weeks is 97% with a baseline creatinine level <125 μmol/L, but this is reduced to 75% if the baseline creatinine level is >125 μmol/L.
- The complication rate is higher for women with diabetes and those with poor graft function.
- The risks of pre-eclampsia, FGR and preterm delivery are increased in the presence of renal impairment and hypertension. The incidence of a complicated pregnancy overall is approximately 50% and includes the following:
  - Hypertension/pre-eclampsia (20–30%)
  - Graft rejection (10%)
  - FGR (20–40%)
  - Preterm delivery (45–60%)
  - Infection, especially UTI.

Antenatal management

- Women should be jointly managed by nephrologists and obstetricians with expertise in the care of pregnant renal transplant recipients.
- Careful monitoring and control of blood pressure is important.
- Regular assessment of renal function and proteinuria is essential.
- A full blood count and liver function tests should also be checked regularly. Anaemia is common and haematinics should be prescribed. Maternal hypocalcaemia and hypercalcaemia are both potential problems, and calcium status should be carefully monitored. Doses of calcium and vitamin D may need to be altered in pregnancy.
- An MSU specimen should be taken and sent at each visit and any infection treated promptly. Some women require prophylactic antibiotics.
- Cytomegalovirus (CMV) titres should be checked in each trimester if the woman is CMV negative at the onset of pregnancy.
- The fetus should be monitored with regular US assessment of growth and Doppler assessment of uterine and umbilical circulation.
- Provided proteinuria is not accompanied by deteriorating renal function or hypertension, this is not an indication for delivery.
- The differential diagnosis of deteriorating renal function includes the following:
  - Reversible causes, for example, infection (e.g. UTI), dehydration, obstruction
  - Pre-eclampsia
  - Ciclosporin/Tacrolimus nephrotoxicity
  - Acute and/or chronic rejection.
- The features of acute rejection include the following:
  - Deteriorating renal function
  - Fever
  - Oliguria
  - Graft swelling and tenderness
  - Altered echogenicity of renal parenchyma and blurring of corticomedullary junction on US.
- Definitive diagnosis of rejection is only possible with renal biopsy.

Immunosuppressive therapy

- The levels of immunosuppressive drugs are maintained at pre-pregnancy levels. Regimes vary but include treatment with:

- Prednisolone
- Azathioprine
- Ciclosporin
- Tacrolimus
- Mycophenolate mofetil (MMF)
- Sirolimus (rapamycin).

- Women require reassurance regarding the relative safety of their drugs, as reduction or cessation of immunosuppressive therapy may provoke rejection.
- Side effects of prednisolone and azathioprine are discussed in Chapters 4 (p. 61) and 8 (p. 132), respectively.
- Azathioprine dose may be monitored via maternal white cell count.
- Both the calcineurin inhibitors (CNIs), ciclosporin and tacrolimus, appear to be safe for use in pregnancy. Plasma levels should be measured regularly. The risk of diabetes is increased with tacrolimus.
- Pregnancy success rates are similar in women taking azathioprine and ciclosporin, but the incidence of FGR is higher (30–40% vs. 20%) in women taking ciclosporin.
- Sirolimus should also be avoided if possible because of known toxicity in animals. Few data are available in human pregnancy and a potent adverse effect on wound healing is reported; however, successful pregnancies have been reported.
- MMF is generally contraindicated in pregnancy, as there is an increased risk of malformations (see Chapter 8, p. 133). In women where MMF is used because of an episode of rejection and it is deemed to be the only drug to adequately control disease or rejection, changing to a safer alternative such as azathioprine in preparation for pregnancy may not be appropriate and, after counselling, women may opt to go ahead with pregnancy despite the unknown risk of teratogenesis. However, often it may be a reasonable compromise to change immunosuppression from MMF to azathioprine, particularly if MMF has been used as a first-line agent and it is likely that adequate immunosuppression will be achieved with a switch over to azathioprine prior to conception. Women should be counselled regarding possible detrimental effects on graft function from such a change in therapy, and pregnancy should be delayed for at least 3 months to ensure function remains stable following any change in immunosuppressant therapy.

Delivery

- Caesarean section is only required for obstetric indications, although the overall section rate is increased compared with background rates, largely because of increased rates of preterm delivery. The renal allograft does not obstruct vaginal delivery.
- Prophylactic antibiotics should be given to cover any surgical procedure, including episiotomy.
- Parenteral steroids are necessary to cover labour, as with any woman on maintenance steroids (see Chapter 4, p. 64).

Neonatal problems

These are largely related to preterm delivery but also include the following:

- The response of neonates to routine childhood immunisations may be altered after exposure to ciclosporin in utero and may be better delayed.

■ Transient reduced levels of T and B lymphocytes in neonates exposed to CNIs that normalise in a few months.

Simultaneous pancreas kidney transplants

■ Increasing numbers of women with type 1 diabetes and nephropathy are receiving simultaneous pancreas kidney (SPK) transplants.
■ The principles of management in pregnancy are the same as for women with renal allografts. However those with SPK transplants experience increased complications related to
  – infection (when the pancreas drains into the bladder this may result in a chemical cystitis which can predispose to infection.
  – obstruction (related to the renal allograft being intraperitoneal)
  – increased rates of renal (but not pancreatic) allograft rejection
  – acidosis (related to bicarbonate loss when the pancreas drains in to the bladder)
■ Most SPK performed now have the pancreas draining into the bowel which reduces complication rates.

Renal transplants—points to remember

■ If graft function is normal, pregnancy outcome is excellent and there is no adverse long-term effect on renal allograft function or survival.
■ The chance of successful pregnancy outcome is reduced and the risk of long-term deterioration in graft function increased with poor baseline graft function.
■ Pregnancy outcome is optimal in those without hypertension, proteinuria or recent episodes of graft rejection.
■ The doses of immunosuppressive drugs are maintained at pre-pregnancy levels.
■ Prednisolone, azathioprine, ciclosporin and tacrolimus are safe for use in pregnancy without any reported increase in the risk of congenital malformations. MMF and sirolimus are usually contraindicated.
■ The risks of pre-eclampsia, graft rejection, FGR, preterm delivery and infection are increased.
■ Caesarean section is only required for obstetric indications, but the rate is increased.
■ Prophylactic antibiotics should be given to cover any surgical procedure.

Acute kidney injury

Incidence

■ Acute renal failure is rare in pregnancy (<0.005%), but mild-to-moderate transient renal impairment is more common.
■ In the developing world, acute kidney injury (AKI) remains a common cause of maternal mortality.
■ In the developed world, renal impairment is much less dangerous than iatrogenic fluid overload, particularly in the context of pre-eclampsia.

Clinical features

- AKI most commonly presents in the postpartum period.
- Anuria is unusual and should prompt a search for urinary retention, a blocked urinary catheter or damage to the ureters.
- Oliguria, especially intra- and postpartum, is common and does not indicate AKI unless there is a concomitant increase in urea and creatinine.
- Urea may rise in isolation following corticosteroid administration; this does not indicate AKI.
- The serum sodium level is low; there may be hyperkalaemia and a metabolic acidosis.
- Oliguria may be followed by a period of polyuria. This may occur physiologically after delivery, or in the recovery phase of acute tubular necrosis.
- There may be evidence of pre-existing renal impairment.

Pathogenesis (see also section B, table 13)

The causes of AKI in pregnancy include the following:

- *Infection*: septic abortion, puerperal sepsis, rarely acute pyelonephritis.
- *Blood loss*: postpartum haemorrhage, abruption.
- *Volume contraction*: pre-eclampsia, eclampsia, hyperemesis gravidarum.
- *Post-renal failure*: ureteric damage or obstruction.
- *Drugs*: non-steroidal anti-inflammatory drugs (NSAIDs), antibiotics.

In many of these situations, there is an associated coagulopathy. The constellation of acute renal failure, microangiopathic haemolytic anaemia and thrombocytopenia may be due to the following:

- Pre-eclampsia (see Chapter 1).
- Haemolysis, Elevated Liver enzymes, and Low Platelets (HELLP) syndrome (7% have acute renal failure) (see Chapter 11, p. 206).
- Thrombotic thrombocytopenic purpura (TTP)/haemolytic uraemic syndrome (HUS) (see Chapter 14, p. 255).
- Acute fatty liver of pregnancy (AFLP) (see Chapter 11, p. 203).

The commonest cause of AKI in the context of pre-eclampsia is HELLP syndrome (approximately 50%).

Diagnosis

- The underlying cause of AKI may be obvious, for example, in the case of abruption and postpartum haemorrhage, although abruption occurs in 16% of women with HELLP syndrome and this may be the true underlying cause.
- Blood loss may not be recognised or may be underestimated, and the diagnosis only made upon the finding of a low central venous pressure (CVP). Hypotension may be absent or masked by co-existent pre-eclampsia.
- The differentiation between pre-renal (volume depletion or blood loss) and renal (acute tubular or cortical necrosis) causes is important, since the treatment of each is different.

- Often AKI is seen postpartum, where there are features of pre-eclampsia with thrombocytopenia, and differentiation of HELLP syndrome from HUS may be difficult. Indeed the conditions are closely related and HUS may evolve from HELLP.
- Pointers to HELLP syndrome, which is far more common, are abnormal liver function, a coaguloapthy (not seen in HUS) and a lower grade haemolysis.
- Pointers to HUS are profound thrombocytopenia and florid microangiopathic haemolytic anaemia.

Management

- This depends on the underlying cause, but in all cases accurate assessment of fluid balance, usually with a urinary catheter and CVP line, is essential. Measurements of fluid input and output should be made hourly.
- The treatment of pre-renal failure is adequate replacement of blood and fluid losses. Diuretics should be avoided until volume depletion has been corrected.
- Any associated coagulopathy must be treated (see Chapter 14, p. 252).
- Once volume depletion has been excluded or treated, fluids are infused at a rate of 20 mL/hr (to allow for insensible losses) plus the volume of the previous hour's urine output. This can be averaged out over 24 hours to allow for i.v. drug administration and equates to approximately 500 mL plus the total output of the previous day.
- Fluid overload must be prevented, especially in pre-eclampsia, because of the susceptibility of these women to pulmonary oedema (see Chapter 1, p. 15).
- There is no place for 'fluid challenges' in the context of a high or normal CVP.
- Acute tubular necrosis is reversible and supportive management is continued until recovery is apparent.
- Plasmapheresis is not needed for HELLP syndrome, which usually improves with conservative therapy.
- Dialysis may become necessary in AKI to prevent or treat uraemia, acidosis, hyperkalaemia or fluid overload, but a requirement for long-term renal replacement therapy is very unusual.

Further reading

Armenti VT, Constantinescu S, Moritz MJ, et al. Pregnancy after transplantation. Transplant Rev (Orlando) 2008; 22:223–240.

Davison J, Nelson-Piercy C, Kehoe S, et al., eds. Renal Disease in pregnancy. Report of RCOG Study Group. London: RCOG, 2008.

Hou SH. Pregnancy in women with chronic renal insufficiency and end stage renal disease. Am J Kidney Dis 1999; 33:235–252.

Jones DC, Hayslett JP. Outcome of pregnancy in women with moderate or severe renal insufficiency. N Engl J Med 1996; 335:226–232.

Jungers P, Chauveau D. Pregnancy in renal disease. Kidney Int 1997; 52:871–885.

Jungers P, Houllier P, Forget D, et al. Influence of pregnancy on the course of primary chronic glomerulonephritis. Lancet 1995; 346:1122–1124.

Schnarr J, Smaill F. Asymptomatic bacteriuria and symptomatic urinary tract infections in pregnancy. Eur J Clin Invest 2008; 38(suppl 2):50–57.

Williams DJ, Davison J. Chronic kidney disease in pregnancy. BMJ 2008; 336:211–215.

CHAPTER 11

Liver disease

Physiological changes	Acute fatty liver of pregnancy
Hyperemesis gravidarum	HELLP syndrome
Viral hepatitis	Pre-existing liver disease
Obstetric cholestasis	Gall bladder disease

Physiological changes

- Pregnancy is associated with increased liver metabolism.
- The total serum protein concentration decreases, largely due to the 20% to 40% fall in serum albumin concentration. Some of this decrease may be explained by dilution due to the increase in total blood volume.
- Concentrations of fibrinogen are dramatically increased, and there are rises in the concentrations of caeruloplasmin, transferrin and many of the specific binding proteins such as thyroid-binding globulin (TBG) and corticosteroid-binding globulin (CBG).
- There is no significant change in bilirubin concentration during normal pregnancy, but the alkaline phosphatase concentration increases dramatically two- to four-fold. This is largely due to placental production, which increases with successive trimesters. The upper limit of normal for alkaline phosphatase increases from approximately 130 U/L in the first trimester to more than 400 U/L in the third trimester.
- Occasionally pregnant women are encountered with isolated, markedly raised alkaline phosphatase (>1000 /L). This is invariably of placental origin, but if reassurance is required isoenzymes may be requested to exclude a liver or bone origin.
- There is a fall in the upper limit of the normal ranges of alanine transaminase (ALT), serum glutamic pyruvic transaminase (SGPT), aspartamine transaminase (AST), and serum glutamic-oxaloacetic transaminase (SGOT) throughout pregnancy from approximately 40 U/L in the first trimester to below 30 U/L in the third. The concentrations of other liver enzymes are not substantially altered. (See table of normal ranges, appendix 2.)

Hyperemesis gravidarum (see also Chapter 12)

Hyperemesis with severe or protracted vomiting in early pregnancy, sufficient to cause fluid, electrolyte and nutritional disturbance, may be associated with abnormal liver function tests in up to 50% of cases. The most usual abnormalities are:

- A moderate rise in transaminases (50–200 U/L)
- Slightly raised bilirubin (jaundice is uncommon).

Hyperemesis is a diagnosis of exclusion (see 'Differential Diagnosis of Abnormal Liver Function Tests' in section B, Table 15).

- Associated epigastric pain should raise the possibility of peptic ulcer, pancreatitis, cholecystitis or ischaemic heart disease.
- Significant elevation of transaminases, especially in the presence of jaundice, should prompt a search for viral hepatitis.

As the hyperemesis improves spontaneously or is treated (see Chapter 12), the abnormalities in liver function resolve.

Viral hepatitis

Worldwide, viral hepatitis is the commonest cause of hepatic dysfunction in pregnancy. Causes include the following:

- Hepatitis viruses A, B, C, D or E (Table 11.1)
- Cytomegalovirus (CMV)
- Epstein–Barr virus (EBV)
- Herpes simplex virus (HSV).

With the important exception of hepatitis E and herpes simplex infection, the clinical features of viral hepatitis in the pregnant woman do not differ from those in the non-pregnant woman.

Table 11.1 – Viral hepatitis in pregnancy

Virus	Transmission	Vertical transmission	Timing of maternal infection giving maximum risk to fetus/neonate	Treatment to protect neonate
Hepatitis A	Faecal–oral	Rare	Near delivery	Immune globulin at birth
Hepatitis B	Blood	Common (especially if HbeAg positive)	Puerperium (i.e. infectious at delivery)	Hepatitis B Ig Hepatitis B vaccine
Hepatitis C	Blood	Uncommon	Third trimester	None
Hepatitis D	Blood	Uncommon		Hepatitis B Ig Hepatitis B vaccine
Hepatitis E	Faecal–oral	? Common	? Near delivery	

Hepatitis A

This is caused by a virus transmitted via the faecal–oral route, and is an acute, self-limited illness that does not result in chronic infection. Maternal–fetal transmission is rare, but may result if the mother develops hepatitis A at or around the time of delivery. In such cases, the neonate should be given immune globulin at birth.

Hepatitis B (HBV)

- Hepatitis B is a blood-borne virus and transmission is sexual, vertical or via blood.
- More than 250 million people are chronically infected with hepatitis B world-wide. The prevalence in developed countries is 0.5% to 5%. Carriage among pregnant women in the United Kingdom is 0.5%, but up to 1% in inner city areas.
- The risk of perinatal infection from asymptomatic mothers is high, and greatest for mothers who are both hepatitis B surface antigen (HBsAg) positive and hepatitis B e-antigen (HbeAg) positive (vertical transmission 95%).
- Chronic carriers of hepatitis B have a 25% chance of dying of liver cirrhosis or liver cancer.
- Women who are HBsAg positive, but HbeAg negative, have a 2% to 15% vertical transmission risk. Measurement of HB virus DNA has replaced e-antigen as the most sensitive test of viral activity. Vertical transmission is higher with a higher viral load.
- Outside pregnancy patients with elevated aminotransferase (>twice the upper limit of normal) and serum HBV DNA above 20,000 IU/mL are offered treatment with antivirals (lamivudine or tenofovir) or pegylated interferon-α. Liver biopsy may help inform therapeutic decisions.
- One-year courses with pegylated interferon-α induce sustained remission in approximately 30% of patients with HBeAg-positive chronic hepatitis B and approximately 15% in patients with HBeAg-negative chronic hepatitis B. However interferon is associated with side effects. Oral antivirals achieve initial responses in the majority of patients, but are intended as long-term therapies. Lamivudine has been shown to prevent progression to liver cirrhosis and liver cancer.
- In pregnancy antiviral therapy during the third trimester of pregnancy in high-risk women with chronic HBV infection reduces viral load in the mother and may decrease the risk of perinatal transmission. Safety data in pregnancy are most robust with lamivudine and tenofovir compared with other therapies.
- Tenofovir is now the preferred agent as monotherapy with lamivudine can cause resistance. Therapy is considered when the viral load is 10^6 to 10^8 U/mL. If therapy is continued postpartum, women are advised not to breastfeed.
- Maternal–neonatal transmission usually occurs at delivery, but may also be transplacental (5%).
- Neonates infected at birth have a >90% chance of becoming chronic carriers of HBV with the associated risks of subsequent cirrhosis and hepatocellular carcinoma.
- All neonates born to women with acute or chronic HBV should be given hepatitis B immune globulin and HBV vaccine within 24 hours of birth. Immunisation is 85% to 95% effective at preventing both HBV infection and the chronic carrier state.
- Provided babies are immunised, there is no need to prevent HBsAg-positive mothers from breastfeeding.

Hepatitis C (HCV)

- Up to 300 million people worldwide have chronic hepatitis C infection. Prevalence in the United Kingdom is approximately 0.3% to 0.7%.
- Hepatitis C is the primary cause of non-A, non-B hepatitis and the commonest cause of posttransfusion hepatitis [approximately 85% of patients contracting posttransfusion non-A, non-B hepatitis prior to 1991 are hepatitis C virus (HCV)-antibody positive].
- However, only 15% of those infected in the United Kingdom have a history of transfusion of blood or blood products.
- The commonest (75%) risk factor for hepatitis C infection in the United Kingdom is past or current i.v. drug use.
- Of i.v. drug users in the United Kingdom, 50% to 90% are HCV infected.
- Sexual transmission is unusual and <5% of long-term sexual partners become infected.
- There is a significant risk (80%) of chronic infection. Approximately 20% of those with chronic infection develop slowly progressive cirrhosis over a period of 10 to 30 years. Detection of HCV antibody implies persistent infection rather than immunity.
- The risk of progressive liver disease is lower in women, those aged <40 years, and those who do not abuse alcohol.
- Interferon-α combined with ribavirin (tribavirin) is more effective than interferon-α alone. Approximately 30% of those with viral genotypes 0, 1 or 2 will have a sustained response following one year of combination therapy. Of those with viral genotypes 3, 4 or 5 treated for six months, 54% will demonstrate a sustained response.
- Side effects of interferon therapy include a fever or flu-like illness in 80%, fatigue in 50%, depression in 25% and haematological abnormalities in 10%. Only 15% of patients receiving interferon therapy experience no side effects.

Pregnancy

- Pregnancy does not induce deterioration in liver disease.
- There is no evidence of increased risk of adverse pregnancy outcome; however, women with hepatitis C antibodies have an increased risk of obstetric cholestasis (OC) that may present earlier than usual (see later).
- Vertical transmission occurs in approximately 3% to 5% of cases.
- Viral load is an important risk factor for vertical transmission that occurs predominantly in women positive for HCV RNA as well as anti-HCV antibody (Table 11.2). In women with chronic HCV, maternal ALT levels do not affect rates of transmission.
- Co-infection with human immunodeficiency virus (HIV) and active i.v. drug use are major risk factors for vertical transmission of HCV.
- In the neonate, HCV infection can only be reliably detected using the polymerase chain reaction to detect HCV RNA, as all infants of HCV antibody-positive mothers will have detectable levels of maternal HCV antibody for the first few months of life.
- There are no vaccines to prevent HCV infection. Immune globulin is not recommended for infants of HCV-positive mothers.
- Interferon and ribavirin treatment are not recommended in pregnancy.
- Transmission by breast milk is uncommon.

Table 11.2 – Vertical transmission rate for HBV and HCV related to the serostatus of the mother

Infection	Serostatus of mother		Vertical transmission rate (%)
HBV	HBsAg+	HbeAg⁻ and HBV DNA⁻	2–15
	HBsAg+	HBeAg⁺ and HBV DNA⁺	80–95
HCV	HCV Ab+	HCV RNA⁻	<1
	HCV Ab+	HCV RNA⁺	11
	HCV Ab+	HCV RNA⁺ and HIV Ab⁺	16

Abbreviations: HbsAg, Hepatitis B surface antigen; HBV DNA, hepatitis B virus DNA; HBeAg, hepatitis B e-antigen; HCV Ab, hepatitis C virus antibodies; HCV RNA, hepatitis C virus RNA; ⁻, negative; ⁺, positive.

Hepatitis delta virus

This virus is only found in HBsAg-positive people, most of whom are HbeAg negative. Prevention of HBV infection or transmission will also prevent hepatitis delta virus (HDV) infection.

Hepatitis E (HEV)

- This is transmitted via the faecal–oral route.
- It has caused several epidemics in association with contaminated water in developing countries. Outbreaks have been reported in India, Ethiopia, Mexico and the Middle East.
- It causes a mild, self-limiting disease, similar to hepatitis A virus infection, in the non-pregnant woman.
- There is a dramatically increased mortality rate in pregnant women, particularly if the virus is acquired in the third trimester. There is an increased incidence of hepatic encephalopathy and fulminant hepatic failure.
- The risk of fulminant hepatic failure with acute hepatitis E infection in pregnancy is 15% to 20%, with a mortality rate of 5%. Maternal death is more likely with infection in late pregnancy.
- The virus has a predilection for pregnant women; the reason for this is not known.
- If this diagnosis is suspected or confirmed, expeditious transfer to a liver unit is advised.

Herpes simplex virus

- This is rare but may cause fulminant hepatitis in the pregnant woman, with an associated high mortality rate.
- Most cases are due to primary HSV type 2 infections, although oral or vulval vesicles may only appear after presentation with liver failure.
- Clinical features include fever and abdominal pain. Jaundice is unusual, but there is usually marked elevation in the transaminases, and there may be prolongation of the prothrombin time.

- Since the infection is usually disseminated, patients may have associated pneumonitis or encephalitis. Immunosuppression is an important risk factor.
- Diagnosis is made on liver biopsy, which shows extensive focal haemorrhagic necrosis and intranuclear inclusion bodies adjacent to the necrotic areas. Electron microscopy may reveal viral particles and the biopsy can also be stained with HSV antibodies. Viral culture of the liver biopsy and serology detecting IgG and IgM HSV antibodies may be helpful.
- Disseminated HSV should be treated with i.v. antiviral therapy. Aciclovir therapy for the infant can also be used to prevent transmission.

Obstetric cholestasis

Incidence

- OC is a disease unique to pregnancy. The exact incidence is not known, but it is more prevalent in certain populations, particularly those of Scandinavia (incidence 1.5%), Chile (incidence up to 12%), Bolivia and China.
- The prevalence in European countries is approximately 0.5% to 1%, although women of Indian and Pakistani descent seem to have a higher risk.

Clinical features

- Severe pruritus affecting the limbs and trunk, particularly the palms and soles, developing in the second half of pregnancy (usually during the third trimester).
- Associated insomnia and malaise are common.
- There may be excoriations, but no rash.
- Liver function tests are abnormal.
- There may be associated dark urine, anorexia and malabsorption of fat with steatorrhoea.
- If OC develops in HCV antibody-positive women, onset of symptoms is earlier in gestation (mean 29 weeks) than HCV antibody-negative women (mean 34 weeks).
- Complete recovery is usually rapid following delivery, although rarely the condition may worsen postpartum. In some women, abnormal liver function tests may return to normal only slowly, taking four to six weeks to reach normal values.

Pathogenesis

The pathogenesis involves a predisposition to the cholestatic effect of increased circulating oestrogens, and progestogens may also play a role. Environmental factors may also contribute and there are seasonal variations in the incidence.

Genetic factors

- Positive family history may be found in approximately 35% of patients and 12% of parous sisters are affected.
- Family studies suggest autosomal dominant sex-limited inheritance.

Oestrogen

- Exogenous oestrogens (combined oral contraceptive pill) may precipitate a similar syndrome.

- Elevated oestrogens are associated with significant impairment in sulphation capacity (sulphation of bile acids is important in attenuating their cholestatic potential).
- Reproductive hormones also affect the function of bile acid transports within the hepatocytes.
- A decrease in hepatocyte membrane fluidity is also implicated, possibly correlated with a defect in the methylation of membrane phospholipids and a modification in the cholesterol:phospholipid ratio.

Diagnosis

OC is a diagnosis of exclusion. The diagnosis is therefore made in three steps:

- A typical history of pruritus without rash
- Abnormal liver function tests (see appendix 2)
- Exclusion of other causes of itching and abnormal liver function.

The usual pattern of abnormal liver function tests is as follows:

- Moderate (less than three-fold) elevation in transaminases (ALT is the most sensitive)
- Raised alkaline phosphatase (beyond normal pregnancy values)
- Raised gamma-glutamyl transpeptidase (γGT) (approximately 20% of cases)
- Mild elevation in bilirubin (less common)
- Increased serum total bile acid concentration
- Primary bile acids (cholic acid and chenodeoxycholic acid) may increase 10- to 100-fold
- In some instances, an increased concentration of bile acids may be the only biochemical abnormality or raised bile acids may precede other liver function abnormality
- Pruritus may precede the derangement of liver function tests and serial measurements are advised in women with persistent typical itching.

To exclude other common causes of pruritus and abnormal liver function, the following investigations are recommended:

- Liver ultrasound (the presence of gallstones without evidence of extrahepatic obstruction does not exclude a diagnosis of OC). Gallstones are also found more commonly in women with OC
- Viral serology (for hepatitis A, B, C and E, EBV, CMV)
- Liver autoantibodies (for pre-existing liver disease; anti–smooth muscle antibodies suggest chronic active hepatitis; antimitochondrial antibodies suggest primary biliary cirrhosis).

The differential diagnoses of pruritus and jaundice in pregnancy are discussed in section B, Tables 14 and 15.

Pregnancy

Maternal risks

- Vitamin K deficiency (malabsorption of fat-soluble vitamins)
- Increased risk of postpartum haemorrhage.

Fetal considerations

- Intrapartum fetal distress (abnormal intrapartum fetal heart rate, e.g. fetal brady-cardia, tachycardia or decelerations, delivery for fetal distress) (12–22%)
- Amniotic fluid meconium (25–45%)
- Spontaneous preterm delivery (12–44%)
- Intrauterine fetal death

The exact magnitude of these risks is difficult to determine, especially as management protocols have included early delivery before the perceived maximum time of risk for the fetus. Thus, reported perinatal mortality rates have fallen from 11% in earlier studies to 0% to 2% in more recent series in which women were delivered before 38 weeks gestation. Further considerations include the following:

- The mechanisms whereby OC may adversely affect the fetus are not known.
- The risk of stillbirth increases towards term, but does not correlate with maternal symptoms or transaminase levels.
- The fetal risk may be related to the serum concentration of maternal bile acids:
  - In a prospective Swedish study, no increase in fetal risk was detected in women with bile acid levels <40 μmol/L, and the risk of fetal complications (spontaneous preterm deliveries, asphyxial events and meconium staining) increased by 1% to 2% per additional μmol/L of serum bile acids.
  - High concentrations of bile acids have been found in amniotic fluid and fetal circulation.
  - Bile acids, especially cholic acid, cause a dose-dependent vasoconstrictive effect on isolated human placental chorionic veins. An abrupt reduction of oxygenated blood flow at the placental chorionic surface leading to fetal asphyxia may be an explanation for fetal distress and demise.
  - Bile acids are toxic to rat cardiac myocytes.

Prediction of fetal compromise
- This remains the most difficult aspect in the management of OC.
- No effect has been demonstrated on the Doppler blood-flow analysis in the uterine, umbilical or fetal cerebral arteries, even in severe cases of OC with high levels of bile acids.
- The risk of a given complication of OC is higher if a woman has suffered that complication in a previous pregnancy.
- Amniocentesis to detect meconium may offer the best predictor of fetal compromise.

Management

- Once a diagnosis of OC is made, the affected woman should be counselled concerning the possible risks to the fetus and the need for close surveillance.
- Liver function tests including, bile acids, should be checked weekly.
- Prothrombin time should be measured prior to delivery or if there is severe derangement of liver function.
- There is no evidence that monitoring fetal well-being with cardiotocography (CTG), ultrasound scans for fetal growth, liquor volume and umbilical artery Doppler blood-flow analyses predict fetal compromise or improve outcome.

- Randomised controlled trials are in progress to determine whether active management with early delivery at 37 to 38 weeks improves outcome.

Drug therapy

Vitamin K
- Vitamin K (10 mg orally, daily) given to the mother may reduce the risk of maternal and fetal bleeding.
- Vitamin K is mandatory for women with a prolonged prothrombin time.
- It is preferable to use a water-soluble formulation (menadiol sodium phosphate) in view of the often co-existent fat malabsorption.
- Vitamin K therapy is commenced at 32 weeks or from diagnosis (if after 32 weeks). This is earlier than institution of vitamin K for women receiving antiepileptic drugs (AEDs) (36 weeks) due to the increased incidence of preterm labour in OC.

Antihistamines
Chlorpheniramine (Piriton®) 4 mg t.d.s. or promethazine (Phenergan®) 25 mg at night may help relieve pruritus.

Ursodeoxycholic acid (UDCA)
- Ursodeoxycholic acid (UDCA) is an endogenous hydrophilic bile acid that acts by altering the bile acid pool, and reducing the proportion of hydrophobic, and therefore hepatotoxic, bile acids.
- It is a choleretic agent that reduces serum bile acids. UDCA stimulates the expression of transporters for canalicular and basolateral bile acid export as well as the canalicular phospholipid flippase.
- It has been used extensively outwith pregnancy in other conditions associated with bile salt retention, such as primary biliary cirrhosis.
- Doses of 1000 to 1500 mg daily in two to three divided doses lead to impressive relief or improvement of pruritus and reduction of total bile acid and liver enzyme levels in most (80–90%) patients.
- UDCA is not licensed for use in pregnancy, but there are no reports of adverse fetal or maternal effects.
- There is currently no evidence to support or refute a beneficial effect of UDCA on the risk of fetal compromise and death, although theoretically as they lower bile acids one may expect a beneficial effect. This is currently being explored in a randomised placebo controlled trial.

Dexamethasone
- Dexamethasone suppresses fetoplacental oestrogen production. Given in one study at doses of 12 mg orally, daily, it relieved pruritus and lowered bile acids and transaminases.
- When used as a second-line therapy in women who have not responded to UDCA, dexamethasone led to a partial clinical and/or biochemical response in 70% of women.
- It is important to consider the potential adverse fetal and maternal side effects from such high doses of corticosteroids.

Rifampicin
- Rifampicin improves symptoms and biochemical markers of liver injury in cholestatic liver disease outwith pregnancy. It enhances bile acid detoxification as well as bilirubin conjugation and export systems.
- The complementary effects of rifampicin and UDCA may justify a combination of both these agents for the treatment of cholestatic liver diseases including OC. There are anecdotal reports of a beneficial effect of 150 mg rifampicin daily used in this context.

Cholestyramine
Cholestyramine, given at a dose of 4 g two to three times daily, is a bile acid chelating agent that may relieve itching in some women, but is poorly tolerated because it is so unpalatable and may cause gastrointestinal upset. It increases the risk of vitamin K deficiency.

S-Adenosylmethionine
S-Adenosylmethionine (sAME) therapy given intravenously may restore normal hepatocyte membrane fluidity. It has improved pruritus and liver biochemistry in some but not all studies.

Activated charcoal
This lowers total bile acid concentrations but has no effect on pruritus.

Epomediol
Epomediol is a synthetic terpenoid compound that has been reported to reduce ethinyloestradiol-induced cholestasis. It may reduce pruritus in OC.

Intrapartum management

- Where there is concern about the risk of intrauterine death in women who do not deliver preterm and have persistently raised bile acid levels (>40 μmol/L), labour may be induced at 37 to 38 weeks gestation.
- Equally if bile acids are <40 micromol/L then it is probably reasonable to await the onset of spontaneous labour. The result of a multicentre randomized controlled trial should address this controversial area.
- Due to the high risk of fetal distress, close monitoring is required throughout induction and labour.
- The neonate should receive i.m. vitamin K.

Recurrence risk/pre-pregnancy counselling

- Risk of developing OC in future pregnancies is approximately 90%.
- Women who have had OC should avoid oestrogen-containing oral contraceptives. If they are used, liver function should be monitored. The risk of cholestasis with the progesterone-only pill seems to be less, but it is prudent to monitor the liver function tests (LFTs) if this is initiated.
- Hormone replacement therapy need not be avoided, as this provides only physiological levels of oestrogen.

Obstetric cholestasis—points to remember

- Pruritus in the third trimester should prompt a request for LFTs.
- The most usual abnormality is elevated transaminases, which may only be mild and raised bile acids.
- Frank jaundice is rare.
- There is a risk to the fetus, which is difficult to predict and not mirrored by maternal symptoms. This risk relates to bile acid levels.
- Management should focus on relief of maternal symptoms, and monitoring of bile acids levels.
- There is no evidence that fetal surveillance improves outcome.
- It is as yet unknown whether elective early delivery before 38 weeks gestation improves outcome.
- Vitamin K should be given to the mother and neonate.
- The risk of recurrence in future pregnancies is approximately 90%.
- Women who have had OC should be advised to avoid oral contraceptives containing oestrogen.

Acute fatty liver of pregnancy

- Acute fatty liver of pregnancy (AFLP) is rare (1 in 7000 to 1 in 20,000 pregnancies), but potentially lethal for both the mother and fetus, especially if diagnosis is delayed.
- AFLP is commoner in primigravidae (although this predilection is not as marked as in pre-eclampsia).
- There is an association with male fetuses (ratio 3:1) and multiple pregnancy (20% of cases).
- The high maternal and fetal mortality rate may be lower than originally believed, as milder cases are recognised and appropriately treated. Previous studies suggest figures around 10% to 20% for maternal mortality and 20% to 30% for perinatal mortality.
- The more recent UKOSS (UK Obstetric Surveillance System) study of AFLP found a maternal mortality rate of 2% and a perinatal mortality rate of 11%.

Clinical features

- Usually presents after 30 weeks gestation, and often near term (35–36 weeks), with gradual onset of nausea, anorexia and malaise.
- Severe vomiting (60%) and abdominal pain (60%) should alert the clinician to the diagnosis.
- There are often co-existing features of mild pre-eclampsia, but hypertension and proteinuria are usually mild.
- Jaundice usually appears within two weeks of the onset of symptoms and there may be ascites.
- Liver function is abnormal and there is a variable (3- to 10-fold) elevation in transaminase levels and raised alkaline phosphatase.
- Coagulopathy due to disseminated intravascular coagulation (DIC) (90%) is often the presenting feature postpartum and may be severe.

- There is usually associated renal impairment.
- The woman may develop fulminant liver failure with hepatic encephalopathy.
- Hypoglycaemia may be severe and affects approximately 70% of women.
- There may be polyuria and features of diabetes insipidus (DI), and the association of transient DI and AFLP is well described (see Chapter 7, p. 115).

Pathogenesis

- AFLP may be a variant of pre-eclampsia.
- A subgroup of women with AFLP and Haemolysis, Elevated Liver enzymes and Low Platelets (HELLP) syndrome is heterozygous for long-chain 3-hydroxy-acyl-coenzyme A dehydrogenase (LCHAD) deficiency, a disorder of mitochondrial fatty acid oxidation. These women may succumb to AFLP or HELLP syndrome when the fetus is homozygous for β-fatty acid oxidation disorders.
- The mechanism of hepatocellular damage may involve the affected fetus producing abnormal fatty acid metabolites.

Diagnosis

Differential diagnosis from HELLP syndrome is shown in Table 11.3.

Distinctive features of AFLP that may help in its distinction from HELLP syndrome are as follows:

- Profound hypoglycaemia (70%)
- Marked hyperuricaemia (which is out of proportion to the other features of pre-eclampsia—90%)
- Coagulopathy (90%) in the absence of thrombocytopenia.

Radiological evaluation with magnetic resonance imaging (MRI), computerised tomography (CT) or ultrasound may sometimes show hepatic steatosis, but the liver may appear normal (as the fat is microvesicular). CT may show decreased attenuation suggestive of fatty infiltration.

Liver biopsy with special stains for fatty change or electron microscopy has been considered the gold standard for diagnosis. The characteristic histopathological lesion is microvesicular fatty infiltration (steatosis) of hepatocytes, most prominent in the central zone, with periportal sparing but little or no inflammation or hepatocellular necrosis. Liver biopsy is not always necessary or practical in the presence of coagulopathy.

Management

- The optimal management of AFLP involves expeditious delivery and this practice has led to improved prognosis for mother and baby.
- Severely ill patients require a multidisciplinary team in an intensive care setting. Early liaison with a regional liver unit is advisable.
- Coagulopathy and hypoglycaemia should be treated aggressively before delivery. Large amounts of 50% glucose may be needed to correct the hypoglycaemia, and fresh frozen plasma and albumin should be given as necessary.
- The best markers of severity in AFLP are as follows:
  - Prothrombin time
  - Glucose

Table 11.3 – Differential diagnosis of HELLP syndrome and AFLP

Symptom	HELLP	AFLP
Epigastric pain	++	+
Vomiting	±	++
Hypertension	++	+
Proteinuria	++	+
Elevated liver enzymes	+	++
Hypoglycaemia	±	++
Hyperuricaemia	+	++
DIC	+	++
Thrombocytopenia (without DIC)	++	±
White blood count	+	++
Ultrasound/CT	Normal/hepatic haematoma	See text
Multiple pregnancy		+
Primiparous	++	+
Male fetus	50%	70% (M:F = 3:1)

Abbreviations: CT, computerised tomography; DIC, Disseminated intravascular coagulation.

- – Acidosis and raised lactate
- – Encephalopathy.
- ■ Plasmapheresis has been used in some cases.
- ■ *N*-acetylcysteine (NAC), an antioxidant and glutathione precursor, promotes selective inactivation of free radicals and is a logical treatment in hepatic failure and often given or advised by liver units in AFLP.
- ■ Multiple system failure may necessitate ventilation and dialysis.
- ■ Patients with fulminant hepatic failure and encephalopathy should be referred urgently to a specialist liver unit.
- ■ Orthotopic liver transplantation should be considered in patients with fulminant hepatic failure and those who manifest signs of irreversible liver failure despite delivery of the fetus and aggressive supportive care.

Prompt reversal of the clinical and laboratory findings usually follows delivery and may be very dramatic; however, significant morbidity is common (33%) and often related to severe coagulopathy and the need for repeated operations to control postpartum haemorrhage. If the woman survives the initial episode, a complete recovery without long-term liver damage is the norm.

Recurrence

There are limited data but recurrence has been described and liver function should be closely monitored in subsequent pregnancies. Recurrence is particularly likely in women who are heterozygous for disorders of β-fatty acid oxidation, so screening for LCHAD deficiency may be indicated. The simplest way to do this is to send a neonatal blood spot for acylcarnitine analysis using tandem mass spectrometry.

Acute fatty liver of pregnancy—points to remember

- This condition is rare, but potentially fatal.
- The diagnosis should be considered, and liver function measured, especially if there is vomiting and abdominal pain.
- Differential diagnosis includes HELLP syndrome.
- Liver dysfunction is usually marked with hypoglycaemia, hyperuricaemia, renal impairment and coagulopathy.
- The woman is at risk of fulminant hepatic failure and encephalopathy and may require transfer to a regional liver unit.
- Delivery of the fetus is the correct treatment once hypoglycaemia, coagulopathy and hypertension have been controlled.

HELLP syndrome

- HELLP syndrome is one of several possible crises that may develop as a variant of severe pre-eclampsia (see Chapter 1, p. 6).
- The incidence in pre-eclamptic pregnancies is approximately 5% to 20%, although many more women with pre-eclampsia, perhaps 20% to 50%, have mild abnormalities of hepatic enzymes without full-blown HELLP syndrome.
- There is increased maternal (1%) and perinatal mortality (reported rates vary from approximately 10% to 60%).

Clinical features

- Epigastric or right upper quadrant pain (65%)
- Nausea and vomiting (35%)
- Tenderness in the right upper quadrant
- Hypertension with or without proteinuria
- Other features of pre-eclampsia
- Acute kidney injury (AKI) (7%)
- Placental abruption (16%). This may be the presenting feature and should always prompt investigation for HELLP syndrome or pre-eclampsia as underlying causes
- Metabolic acidosis.

Pathogenesis

■ See under 'Pre-eclampsia' (Chapter 1, p. 7).
■ The pathogenesis of HELLP syndrome involves endothelial cell injury, microangiopathic platelet activation and consumption.
■ Differential diagnosis includes AFLP (see earlier and Table 11.3) and haemolytic uraemic syndrome (HUS)/thrombotic thrombocytopenic purpura (TTP) (see p. 255). These conditions (AFLP, HELLP, HUS, TTP, pre-eclampsia) may all form part of a spectrum of endothelial disease.

Diagnosis

■ Low-grade haemolysis evident on peripheral blood smear, rarely enough to cause severe anaemia
■ Low (usually $<100 \times 10^9/L$) or falling platelets
■ Elevated transaminases
■ Elevated lactate dehydrogenase (LDH) (indicative of haemolysis)
■ Raised bilirubin (unconjugated, reflecting the extent of haemolysis).

The platelet count may fall below $30 \times 10^9/L$ in severe cases and some women develop DIC (20%).

■ Ultrasound may be useful to exclude hepatic haematoma or other causes of acute upper abdominal pain, for example cholecystitis.
■ Liver biopsy is rarely performed in this syndrome, and therefore reports of the histological changes are sparse. Most reports describe changes similar to patients with pre-eclampsia and liver involvement but without HELLP. There is fibrin deposition in the periportal regions and along the hepatic sinusoids, and periportal haemorrhage. Unlike AFLP, there may be hepatic cell necrosis and subcapsular haemorrhages.
■ Differential diagnosis from TTP and HUS is important since delivery rather than plasmapheresis is the optimal management for HELLP syndrome. Remember the following:
  – TTP and HUS are both rare compared with HELLP syndrome.
  – Abnormal liver function and coagulopathy suggest HELLP rather than TTP, even in the presence of frank haemolysis.
  – Co-existence of AKI is well recognised in HELLP syndrome and does not necessarily imply a diagnosis of HUS.
  – Profound thrombocytopenia ($<10 \times 10^9/L$) is unusual in pre-eclampsia and HELLP syndrome.
  – As the conditions are closely related HUS may evolve from HELLP.

Effect of HELLP syndrome on pregnancy

Factors contributing to maternal morbidity and mortality include the following:

■ Abruption
■ Subcapsular liver haematoma
■ AKI

- Massive hepatic necrosis
- Liver rupture.

Management

- Prompt delivery, especially if there is severe right upper quadrant pain and tenderness, since this is usually the result of liver capsule distension.
- As with all cases of pre-eclampsia, it is important to ensure adequate control of blood pressure prior to delivery.
- Platelet transfusion should be reserved for active bleeding or prior to surgery or regional anaesthesia/analgesia if the platelet count is below 50×10^9/L.
- Fresh frozen plasma (FFP) should be given to correct any coagulopathy.
- Corticosteroids given to induce fetal lung maturity have been shown to significantly improve both haematological and hepatic abnormalities in HELLP syndrome. It has also been demonstrated that if delayed delivery is achievable following steroid administration, then platelet counts are higher and in turn general anaesthesia rates are lowered and regional anaesthesia rates increased. However corticosteroids (other than those given for fetal lung maturation) are not recommended to treat maternal HELLP syndrome.

Postpartum Course

- Since delivery is usually expedited in diagnosed cases, a woman may deteriorate before she improves after delivery, developing a very low platelet count, severe hypertension and proteinuria.
- Up to 30% of cases arise postpartum, in women thought to have no or uncomplicated pre-eclampsia. These women are at particularly high risk of pulmonary oedema and renal failure. Management in such cases should be supportive, with strict adherence to fluid management protocols to avoid iatrogenic pulmonary oedema, and control of the blood pressure.
- Recovery from HELLP syndrome is usually rapid and complete with no hepatic sequelae. The liver enzymes often recover before the thrombocytopenia, although as in other cases of pre-eclampsia, antihypertensives may be required temporarily postpartum.
- Whether to give corticosteroids to women with HELLP syndrome who have not received antenatal steroids for fetal indications is controversial and they probably do not improve outcome or hasten recovery.

Recurrence

- In future pregnancies, women who have had HELLP syndrome are at a substantially increased risk of developing pre-eclampsia, preterm delivery and fetal growth restriction.
- The risk of recurrent pre-eclampsia is about 25% in women who had HELLP necessitating delivery before 34 weeks.
- The risk of recurrent HELLP syndrome, on the other hand, is low (3–5%). For women with pre-existing hypertension that predates the pregnancy complicated by HELLP syndrome, the risk of pre-eclampsia in subsequent pregnancies may be as high as 75%.

HELLP syndrome—points to remember

- This is one of the potential 'crises' that may develop in pre-eclampsia.
- Other features of pre-eclampsia including hypertension and proteinuria may be only mild.
- The typical features are right upper quadrant pain, abnormal liver function, low platelets and mild haemolysis.
- There is a risk of DIC, abruption, liver haematoma and liver rupture.
- Delivery of the fetus is the correct treatment once any hypertension has been controlled. Platelet transfusion is usually not required.
- Women may present or deteriorate postpartum and renal impairment is not uncommon.
- Women are at a greatly increased risk of developing pre-eclampsia in future pregnancies.
- The risk of recurrent HELLP syndrome is low.

Pre-existing liver disease

Autoimmune chronic active hepatitis

- Mild treated disease is unlikely to cause problems in pregnancy. The issues relate to immunosuppressive drug regimens (usually predinisolone ± azathioprine) (see Chapter 8, p. 132), which should be continued in pregnancy to prevent relapse.
- Withdrawal of immunosuppression is associated with a high risk of relapse during pregnancy or postpartum.

Primary biliary cirrhosis (PBC)

- This condition usually presents with pruritus and is associated with a raised alkaline phosphatase and γGT. Diagnosis is confirmed by the finding of antimitochondrial antibodies.
- Reported pregnancy outcomes are variable although stable, non-advanced disease is unlikely to cause problems. Pruritus may worsen in pregnancy and women may develop OC.

Sclerosing cholangitis

- This is a rare chronic, fibrosing, inflammatory disorder of unknown aetiology affecting the biliary tree. It is associated with inflammatory bowel disease, although the severities of the two conditions are not related.
- Clinical features include obstructive jaundice and diagnosis is supported by characteristic findings at endoscopic retrograde cholangiopancreatography (ERCP) and MRI.
- There is a significant risk of cholangiocarcinoma, which has a very poor prognosis.
- In the only reported series of pregnancies in women with sclerosing cholangitis (SC), pregnancy outcome was good. The only serious complication was severe pruritus.

Cirrhosis

- Severe hepatic impairment is associated with infertility.
- Liver disease may decompensate during pregnancy, and pregnancy should be discouraged in women with severe impairment of hepatic function.
- Progressive hepatic fibrosis with the development of cirrhosis is a feature of almost all chronic liver diseases. The degree of fibrosis can be measured non-invasively using transient elastography (FibroScan) that measures liver stiffness.
- Bleeding from oesophageal varices is a risk in women with portal hypertension, especially in the second and third trimesters.
- Those with portal hypertension stabilised on β-blockers should be advised to continue this in pregnancy since the risks to mother and fetus from variceal bleeding far outweigh any risk of β-blocker therapy in pregnancy.
- Similarly those with documented portal hypertension should commence β-blocker therapy in the second trimester.
- Splenomegaly is often associated with thrombocytopenia.

Liver transplants

- Fertility may return to normal after transplantation.
- Pregnancy should be postponed for 18 months to a year after transplantation to allow stabilisation of function and reduction to maintenance levels of immunosuppressive drugs.
- Immunosuppression must be continued and carefully monitored in specialist units throughout pregnancy. Tacrolimus, prednisolone and azathioprine are not associated with teratogenesis (see 'Renal Transplants', Chapter 10, p. 188).
- Pregnancy in liver transplant recipients is associated with an increased risk of preterm delivery, and maternal and fetal complications but pregnancy outcome is usually good.

Gall bladder disease

Incidence

- Gallstones are found in 6.5% to 8.5% of nulliparous women, and in 18% to 19% of women with two to three or more pregnancies.
- In women followed throughout pregnancy, neoformation of gallstones was documented in 3% (equivalent to the incidence outside pregnancy) to 8% depending on the population. Some 20% to 30% of these gallstones redissolve postpartum.
- Echogenic bile, or biliary sludge, may be present in over one-third of pregnant women.
- The prevalence of acute cholecystitis in pregnancy is approximately 0.1%.

Clinical features

- These are similar to those in the non-pregnant woman.
- Pain is present in the right upper quadrant or epigastrium, and it may radiate through to the back and tip of the scapula.
- Nausea, vomiting and indigestion are common.

- Acute cholecystitis may occur at any time in pregnancy and causes more severe pain than biliary colic. There is associated tenderness and guarding in the right hypochondrium. There may be fever and shock depending on the severity of the gall bladder sepsis.
- Complications include the following:
  - Jaundice secondary to oedema or stones in the common bile duct
  - Pancreatitis.

Pathogenesis

- Formation of cholesterol gallstones is increased by increasing concentrations of bile cholesterol or decreasing concentrations of bile acids.
- Pregnancy and the oral contraceptive pill increase cholesterol saturation of bile and the rate of secretion of cholesterol. They also increase the ratio of cholic acid to chenoxycholic acid. The net result is increased bile lithogenicity.
- Pregnancy also impairs gall bladder contractility, leading to gall bladder stasis.
- The combination of gall bladder stasis and the secretion of lithogenic bile increases the formation of both sludge and stones during pregnancy, but both may disappear either during or after pregnancy.

Diagnosis

- Ultrasound provides a safe and accurate method of detecting gallstones.
- Endoscopic ultrasound may also be safely performed in pregnancy
- Acute cholecystitis is suggested if there is, in addition, a raised white blood cell count, abnormal LFTs, pericholecystic fluid, distension and thickening of the gall bladder wall and ultrasound transducer-induced pain over the gall bladder.
- A mildly (two-fold) raised amylase is also consistent with a diagnosis of acute cholecystitis, although greater rises suggest pancreatitis or common bile duct stones.
- The differential diagnosis of acute cholecystitis in pregnancy (see also section B, Table 17) includes the following:
  - Appendicitis (see Chapter 12)
  - Pancreatitis (see Chapter 12)
  - Peptic ulcer (see Chapter 12)
  - Pneumonia, particularly of the right lower lobe (see Chapter 4, p. 65)
  - Acute fatty liver of pregnancy (see earlier)
  - HELLP syndrome (see earlier, p. 206)
  - Viral hepatitis (see earlier)
  - OC (see earlier).

Management

- This is the same as in the non-pregnant patient.
- Conservative management, with withdrawal of oral food and fluids, nasogastric aspiration, i.v. fluids, antibiotics and analgesia, leads to resolution of symptoms in over three-quarters of women.
- If surgery is required, this is best done during the second trimester, when the risk of miscarriage is low and the uterus is not yet large enough to obscure or distort the surgical field.
- Laparoscopic cholecystectomy has been safely performed in pregnancy.

- Endoscopic removal of common bile duct stones using ERCP and stent drainage in experienced hands may be performed with minimal radiation, but there is an associated risk of pancreatitis.
- Sphincterotomy may also be performed in pregnancy but is associated with a risk of bleeding.

Further reading

Ch'ng CL, Morgan M, Hainsworth I, et al. Prospective study of liver dysfunction in pregnancy in Southwest Wales. Gut 2002; 51:876–880. Erratum in: Gut 2003; 52:315.

Coffin CS, Shaheen AA, Burak KW, et al. Pregnancy outcomes among liver transplant recipients in the United States: A nationwide case-control analysis. Liver Transpl 2010; 16:56–63.

Geenes V, Williamson C. Intrahepatic cholestasis of pregnancy. World J Gastroenterol 2009; 15:2049–2066.

Gilat T, Konikoff F. Pregnancy and the biliary tract. Can J Gastroenterol 2000; 14(suppl D):55D–59D.

Giraudon I, Forde J, Maguire H, et al. Antenatal screening and prevalence of infection: Surveillance in London, 2000–2007. Euro Surveill 2009; 14:8–12.

Girling JC, Dow E, Smith JH. Liver function tests in pre-eclampsia: Importance of comparison with a reference range derived for normal pregnancy. Br J Obstet Gynaecol 1997; 104:246–250.

Glantz A, Marschall HU, Mattsson LA. Intrahepatic cholestasis of pregnancy: Relationships between bile acid levels and fetal complication rates. Hepatology 2004; 40:467–474.

Gurung V, Williamson C, Chappell L, et al. Pilot study for a trial of ursodeoxycholic acid and/or early delivery for obstetric cholestasis. BMC Pregnancy Childbirth 2009; 9:19.

Haram K, Svendsen E, Abildgaard U. The HELLP syndrome: Clinical issues and management. A Review. BMC Pregnancy Childbirth 2009; 9:8.

Janczewska I, Olsson R, Hultcrantz R, et al. Pregnancy in patients with primary sclerosing cholangitis. Liver 1996; 16:326–330.

Knight M, Nelson-Piercy C, Kurinczuk JJ, et al. UK Obstetric Surveillance System. A prospective national study of acute fatty liver of pregnancy in the UK. Gut 2008; 57:951–956.

Locatelli A, Roncaglia N, Arreghini A, et al. Hepatitis C virus infection is associated with a higher incidence of cholestasis of pregnancy. Br J Obstet Gynaecol 1999; 106:498–500.

Marschall HU, Wagner M, Zollner G, et al. Complementary stimulation of hepatobiliary transport and detoxification systems by rifampicin and ursodeoxycholic acid in humans. Gastroenterology 2005; 129:476–485.

Nesbitt TH, Kay HH, McCoy MC, et al. Endoscopic management of biliary disease during pregnancy. Obstet Gynecol 1996; 87:806–809.

Rahman TM, Wendon J. Severe hepatic dysfunction in pregnancy. QJM 2002; 95:343–357.

Stone S, Girling JC. Deranged liver function tests in pregnancy: The importance of postnatal follow-up. Obstet Med 2009; 2:32–33.

CHAPTER 12

Gastrointestinal disease

Physiological changes	Irritable bowel syndrome
Hyperemesis gravidarum	Coeliac disease
Constipation	Abdominal pain
Gastro-oesophageal reflux	Appendicitis
disorder (GORD)	Pancreatitis
Peptic ulcer disease	
Inflammatory bowel disease	
(IBD)	

Physiological changes

- Changes in gastrointestinal motility during pregnancy include decreased lower oesophageal pressure, decreased gastric peristalsis and delayed gastric emptying.
- Gastrointestinal motility is inhibited generally during pregnancy, with increased small- and large-bowel transit times.
- These changes may in part be responsible for the common symptoms of constipation and nausea and vomiting in early pregnancy.

Hyperemesis gravidarum

Incidence

- Nausea and vomiting are both common in pregnancy, affecting at least 50% of pregnant women.
- Hyperemesis gravidarum occurs in 0.1% to 1% of pregnancies.

Clinical features

- Onset is always in the first trimester, usually weeks 6 to 8.
- Persistent vomiting and severe nausea progress to hyperemesis when the woman is unable to maintain adequate hydration, and fluid and electrolyte as well as nutritional status are jeopardised.
- There is weight loss and ketosis and there may be muscle wasting.
- In addition to nausea and vomiting, there may be ptyalism (inability to swallow saliva) and associated spitting.
- There are usually signs of dehydration with postural hypotension and tachycardia.

Investigations

These usually reveal the following:

- Hyponatraemia
- Hypokalaemia
- Low serum urea
- Metabolic hypochloraemic alkalosis
- Ketonuria
- Raised haematocrit level and increased specific gravity of the urine
- Abnormal liver function tests (found in up to 50% of cases—see Chapter 11, p. 193)
- Abnormal thyroid function tests (found in up to 66% of cases).

The picture is that of a biochemical hyperthyroidism with a raised free thyroxine and/or a suppressed thyroid-stimulating hormone (TSH).

Patients with these abnormalities are clinically euthyroid without thyroid antibodies, except in the very rare case of thyrotoxicosis presenting in early pregnancy.

The abnormal thyroid function tests do not require treatment with antithyroid drugs and resolve as the hyperemesis improves.

There is an increased incidence of gestational thyrotoxicosis demonstrated in Asians compared with Europeans.

Pathogenesis

- The pathophysiology of hyperemesis is poorly understood. Various hormonal, mechanical and psychological factors have been implicated.
- There is a direct relationship between the severity of hyperemesis and the degree of biochemical hyperthyroidism, and it has been suggested that the raised thyroxine levels or suppressed TSH may be causative.
- The level of human chorionic gonadotropin (hCG), which shares a common α-subunit with TSH, is directly correlated with the severity of vomiting and free thyroxine concentrations, and inversely correlated with TSH levels. hCG probably acts as a thyroid stimulator in patients with hyperemesis. There is structural homology not only in the hCG and TSH molecules but also in their receptors, and this suggests the basis for the reactivity of hCG with the TSH receptor.
- The positive correlation between severity of hyperemesis and hCG levels explains the increased incidence of this condition in multiple pregnancy and hydatidiform mole. The theory is also supported by the fact that the peak in hCG levels (in weeks 6–12) coincides with the presentation of hyperemesis.
- Other hormonal deficiencies or excesses, involving follicle-stimulating hormone (FSH), progesterone, cortisol and adrenocorticotrophic hormone (ACTH), have been proposed as aetiological factors, but never proven.
- The physiological changes in oesophageal pressure, gastric peristalsis and gastric emptying may well exacerbate the symptoms of hyperemesis, but are unlikely to be causative in isolation.
- Many psychological and behavioural theories have been suggested to explain hyperemesis, usually involving hyperemesis as an expression of rejection of the pregnancy. Although there is often a psychological component to the condition, it is very difficult to prove causation since hyperemesis itself may cause extreme psychological morbidity. This relates to separation from family, inability to work, anger at being

214

unwell and guilt when this anger is turned inwards towards the fetus and resentment of the pregnancy results.

■ Certainly psychological factors do play a role in a proportion of cases and this may be evident by the rapid improvement on admission to hospital and consequent removal from a stressful home environment.

■ It is, however, extremely dangerous to assume psychological or psychiatric factors are solely responsible for the clinical picture in cases of severe hyperemesis. Maternal deaths are reported following inappropriate transfer to a psychiatric ward.

Diagnosis

■ Hyperemesis is a diagnosis of exclusion.

■ There is no single confirmatory test.

■ Vomiting beginning after week 12 of amenorrhoea should not be attributed to hyperemesis.

■ Other causes of nausea and vomiting must be considered, most commonly urinary tract infection and, more rarely, Addison's disease (insidious onset with some features predating the pregnancy), peptic ulceration or pancreatitis (abdominal pain is not a prominent symptom in hyperemesis).

■ Differentiation from true thyrotoxicosis in the presence of abnormal thyroid function tests relies on a history of symptoms, particularly weight loss, preceding the pregnancy and the presence of thyroid-stimulating antibodies.

■ The finding of thyroid eye disease (particularly lid lag) would make true thyrotoxicosis a more likely diagnosis.

■ Hyperemesis tends to recur in subsequent pregnancies, so a previous history makes the diagnosis more likely.

Effect of hyperemesis on pregnancy

Maternal complications

■ There were three deaths in the Confidential Enquiry into Maternal Deaths in the United Kingdom between 1991 and 1993, but none have been reported since. Two deaths were probably the result of Wernicke's encephalopathy (see later) and one the result of aspiration of vomitus.

■ Serious morbidity and mortality may result if hyperemesis is inadequately or inappropriately treated.

Wernicke's encephalopathy

Wernicke's encephalopathy because of vitamin B_1 (thiamine) deficiency is characterised by ophthalmoplegia, diplopia, ataxia and confusion. The typical ocular signs are a sixth nerve palsy, gaze palsy or nystagmus.

■ Wernicke's encephalopathy may be precipitated by i.v. fluids containing dextrose.

■ There is an increased incidence of abnormal liver function tests in women with hyperemesis complicated by Wernicke's encephalopathy compared with the incidence in hyperemesis in general. As in alcoholics, the abnormal functioning liver may participate in the development of Wernicke's encephalopathy by decreased conversion of thiamine to its active metabolite thiamine pyrophosphate and by a decreased capacity to store thiamine.

- Diagnosis of Wernicke's encephalopathy may be confirmed by the finding of a low red cell transketolase (thiamine-dependent enzyme).
- Enhanced magnetic resonance imaging (MRI) in acute Wernicke's encephalopathy may reveal symmetrical lesions around the aqueduct and fourth ventricle, which resolve after treatment with thiamine.
- Although institution of thiamine replacement may improve the symptoms of Wernicke's encephalopathy, if retrograde amnesia, impaired ability to learn and confabulation (Korsakoff psychosis) have supervened, the recovery rate is only approximately 50%.

Hyponatraemia

Hyponatraemia (plasma sodium <120 mmol/L) causes lethargy, seizures and respiratory arrest.

- Both severe hyponatraemia and, particularly, its rapid reversal may precipitate central pontine myelinolysis (osmotic demyelination syndrome). This is associated with symmetrical destruction of myelin at the centre of the basal pons and causes pyramidal tract signs, spastic quadraparesis, pseudobulbar palsy and impaired consciousness.
- Central pontine myelinolysis and Wernicke's encephalopathy may co-exist during pregnancy and thiamine deficiency may render the myelin sheaths of the central pons more sensitive to changes in serum sodium.

Other vitamin deficiencies

Other vitamin deficiencies occur in hyperemesis, including cyanocobalamin (vitamin B_{12}) and pyridoxine (vitamin B_6) causing anaemia and peripheral neuropathy.

Mallory–Weiss tears

Prolonged vomiting may lead to Mallory–Weiss tears of the oesophagus and episodes of haematemesis.

Malnutrition

Protein and calorie malnutrition results in weight loss, which may be profound (10–20%), and muscle wasting with consequent weakness.

Psychology

The psychological problems (see earlier) resulting from severe hyperemesis are often underestimated. Certain problems may pre-date the onset of hyperemesis, but others result from the condition itself. Requests for termination of pregnancy should not be assumed to indicate or confirm that the pregnancy was not wanted, but rather this should be an indication of the degree of desperation felt by the patient.

Total parenteral nutrition

If total parenteral nutrition (TPN) is required, this is usually given via a central venous catheter, and this has its own problems (e.g. infection, pneumothorax).

Thrombosis
Since hyperemesis results in dehydration and is usually associated with bed rest, it constitutes a risk factor for thromboembolism (see Chapter 3, p. 41).

Fetal complications

■ Wernicke's encephalopathy is associated with a 40% incidence of fetal death.
■ Initially it was thought that hyperemesis was not associated with any adverse fetal outcome and there is indeed no increase in the risk of congenital malformations for affected individuals. However, it has been shown that infants of mothers with severe hyperemesis (associated with abnormal biochemistry and weight loss >5%) have significantly lower birthweights and birthweight percentiles compared with infants of mothers with mild hyperemesis and those of the general antenatal population.
■ Women admitted repeatedly for hyperemesis have a more severe nutritional disturbance, associated with a significantly reduced maternal weight gain. Infants of women admitted on multiple occasions for hyperemesis have significantly lower birthweights than infants of mothers requiring only a single admission.

Management

■ The potential maternal and fetal complications of hyperemesis argue for early and aggressive treatment.
■ Any woman who is ketotic and unable to maintain adequate hydration should be admitted to hospital. With the advent of emergency gynaecology/early pregnancy units, it should be possible to manage women with less severe degrees of hyperemesis as day cases by administration of intravenous fluid therapy and antiemetics as required.
■ An ultrasound scan of the uterus should be performed to confirm gestational age, and to diagnose multiple pregnancy and exclude hydatidiform mole, both of which are associated with an increased incidence of hyperemesis.

I.V. fluid therapy

■ Adequate and appropriate fluid and electrolyte replacement is the most important component of management.
■ Infusion of dextrose-containing fluids (dextrose saline, 5% dextrose, 10% dextrose) is mistakenly thought by some to be desirable to provide the patient with at least some calories, but this assumption is erroneous and dangerous. Firstly, as discussed earlier, Wernicke's encephalopathy may be precipitated by carbohydrate-rich foods or dextrose administered intravenously. Secondly, the hyponatraemia demands the infusion of sodium-containing fluids (dextrose saline contains only 30 mmol/L of Na^+ and 5% dextrose contains none).
■ Normal saline (sodium chloride 0.9%; 150 mmol/L Na^+) or Hartmann's solution (sodium chloride 0.6%; 131 mmol/L Na^+) are appropriate solutions. To correct the hypokalaemia, it is usually necessary to use infusion bags containing 40 mmol/L of potassium chloride. There is no place for the use of double-strength saline (2N saline), even in cases of severe hyponatraemia, as this results in too rapid a correction of serum sodium with the risk of central pontine myelinolysis.
■ Fluid and electrolyte regimes must be adapted daily and titrated against daily measurements of serum sodium and potassium and fluid-balance charts.

- Due to the practical difficulties of maintaining fluid-balance charts over many days in busy wards, the patient should be weighed at least twice weekly to obtain an objective assessment of improvement or deterioration.

Thromboprophylaxis

Hyperemesis is a risk factor for venous thrombosis probably because of dehydration. Therefore, all women admitted with hyperemesis should receive appropriate doses of low-molecular-weight heparin (LMWH) (see Chapter 3, p. 47).

Thiamine therapy

- Thiamine supplementation should be given to anyone suffering from prolonged vomiting. Requirements for thiamine increase during pregnancy to 1.5 mg/day, and women admitted with a diagnosis of hyperemesis have usually been vomiting for at least one to two weeks prior to admission. If women can tolerate tablets, thiamine can be given as thiamine hydrochloride tablets 25 to 50 mg t.d.s. If i.v. treatment is required for those unable to tolerate tablets, this is given as thiamine 100 mg diluted in 100 mL of normal saline and infused over 30 to 60 minutes. Alternatively this may be given as Pabrinex® which contains 250 mg of thiamine hydrochloride per pair of ampules. The i.v. preparation is only required weekly. Treatment (as opposed to prevention) of Wernicke's encephalopathy requires much higher doses of thiamine.
- Drugs that may cause nausea and vomiting should be temporarily discontinued. The commonest example is iron supplements.
- All patients with hyperemesis require emotional support with frequent reassurance and encouragement from nursing and medical staff. Psychiatric referral may be appropriate in certain cases, but only after electrolyte and vitamin deficiencies have been corrected.
- The natural history of hyperemesis is gradual improvement with increasing gestation, although in a minority of women symptoms may persist beyond 20 weeks gestation.
- The only definitive cure is termination of the pregnancy.

Pharmacological treatment

Antiemetics

Antiemetics should be offered to women failing to respond to i.v. fluids and electrolytes alone.

- Extensive data exist to show a lack of teratogenesis with:
  - Antihistamines (H_1-receptor antagonists, e.g. promethazine, cyclizine)
  - Phenothiazines (chlorpromazine, prochlorperazine)
  - Dopamine antagonists (metoclopramide, domperidone).

Post-thalidomide anxiety has resulted in an understandable reluctance to prescribe antiemetics for hyperemesis.

- Possible regimens include the following:
  - Cyclizine 50 mg p.o./i.m./i.v. t.d.s.

- Promethazine 25 mg p.o. nocte
- Prochlorperazine (Stemetil®) 5 mg p.o. t.d.s.; 12.5 mg i.m./i.v. t.d.s; 25 mg p.r.
- Metoclopramide 10 mg p.o./i.m./i.v. t.d.s.
- Domperidone 10 mg p.o. q.d.s.; 30 to 60 mg p.r. t.d.s.
- Chlorpromazine 10 to 25 mg p.o.; 25 mg i.m. t.d.s.

■ If symptoms do not improve, the antiemetic should be *prescribed and given regularly* rather than on an 'as required'/p.r.n. basis.

■ Side effects include drowsiness, particularly with the phenothiazines, and extrapyramidal effects and oculogyric crises, particularly with metoclopramide and the phenothiazines. Extrapyramidal effects usually abate after discontinuation of the drug and oculogyric crises may be treated with antimuscarinic drugs such as benzatropine 1 to 2 mg i.m. or i.v.

Ondansetron

■ This highly selective 5-HT$_3$ (serotonin) antagonist is used with dramatic effect for postoperative and chemotherapy-induced nausea and vomiting.

■ It has been used with success in intractable hyperemesis, but in a comparative study i.v. ondansetron 10 mg was no better than i.v. promethazine 50 mg. However, in this study the hyperemesis was not very severe, which may explain the lack of difference in efficacy.

■ There is no evidence to support a teratogenic effect of ondansetron.

Histamine$_2$-receptor blockers and proton pump inhibitors (PPIs)

Histamine$_2$ (H$_2$)-receptor blockers (e.g. ranitidine) and the proton pump inhibitors (e.g. omeprazole) are used in cases where dyspeptic symptoms accompany the nausea and vomiting of hyperemesis. They appear to be safe for use in pregnancy.

Corticosteroids

■ Corticosteroids have resulted in dramatic and rapid improvement in case series of women with severe refractory hyperemesis. Randomised studies also support a beneficial effect.

■ They should not be used until conventional treatment with i.v. fluid replacement and regular antiemetics has failed.

■ Suggested doses are prednisolone 40 to 50 mg p.o. daily or hydrocortisone 100 mg i.v. b.d.

■ In cases that do respond to steroid therapy, the dose must be reduced slowly and prednisolone cannot usually be discontinued until the gestation at which the hyperemesis would have resolved spontaneously (in some extreme cases this occurs at delivery).

■ In cases that do not respond to steroid therapy, it should be discontinued.

Enteral feeding

■ When the gastrointestinal tract is intact and usable, it is preferable to use enteral rather than parenteral hyperalimentation to treat malnutrition.

■ Enteral hyperalimentation may be poorly tolerated because of nausea and vomiting and may even be contraindicated due to the risk of aspiration.

- Frequent tube displacement may also be a problem. Poor tolerance of a nasogastric tube can be bypassed by use of a gastrostomy feeding tube.
- To minimise the risk of aspiration, a nasojejunal feeding tube may be placed beyond the pylorus, but this necessitates radiation exposure for correct positioning of the tube or insertion under endoscopic guidance.
- The cost of enteral feeding is considerably less than that of TPN (see below).
- The successful use of enteral feeding via a nasogastric tube in hyperemesis unresponsive to antiemetics has been reported in women with meal-related nausea and vomiting only.

Total parenteral nutrition

- TPN may become necessary supportive therapy in very severe cases of hyperemesis.
- TPN has also been shown to have a rapid therapeutic effect in some cases.
- Metabolic and infectious complications are a risk, and strict protocols and careful monitoring are obligatory. The central line site must be inspected regularly for signs of infection.
- Phlebitis and thrombosis are other recognised complications of TPN. Line-related endothelial disruption may provoke thrombosis, but in addition the direct endothelial injury secondary to a hyperosmolar infusate is likely to contribute.
- Because TPN involves the use of high concentrations of glucose, thiamine supplementation is mandatory.
- In addition, parenteral hyperalimentation is expensive and is usually reserved for extremely severe life-threatening cases.
- The author would not recommend TPN for hyperemesis until optimal rehydration, antiemetic therapy and a trial of corticosteroids and/or ondansetron have failed to result in improvement.

Pre-pregnancy counselling/recurrence

- Hyperemesis almost invariably recurs in subsequent pregnancies.
- In very severe cases, especially those necessitating TPN or termination of the pregnancy, women may be advised that studies suggest a beneficial effect of steroids, which may provide a therapeutic option in subsequent pregnancies.

Hyperemesis gravidarum—points to remember

- Hyperemesis is a diagnosis of exclusion.
- Hyperemesis may be associated with both abnormal liver and thyroid function tests.
- The main risk in hyperemesis is from Wernicke's encephalopathy, resulting from thiamine deficiency.
- Adequate and appropriate (normal saline and potassium chloride) fluid and electrolyte replacement is the most important component of management.
- Thiamine supplementation and thromboprophylaxis should be given to all women admitted with hyperemesis.
- The common antiemetics are not teratogenic.
- Corticosteroids or ondansetron may have a role to play in severe resistant cases.

Constipation

Incidence

This is very common, experienced by up to 40% of women, especially in early pregnancy.

Clinical features

- Decreased frequency of defaecation
- Increased consistency of the stool, which may be fragmented and lumpy
- Increased difficulty in passing a stool
- Some women may complain of bloating, lower abdominal discomfort and increased flatus
- Constipation may well be associated with, and exacerbate, both haemorrhoids and anal fissures. Bleeding, itching and pain on defaecation are not uncommon.

Pathogenesis

- Decreased colonic motility because of vasodilatory prostaglandins and vascular endothelial substances.
- Oral iron supplements may cause gastrointestinal upset with either constipation or diarrhoea.
- Poor fluid and food intake related to nausea and vomiting in the first trimester will exacerbate constipation.
- Pressure on the rectosigmoid colon by the gravid uterus may explain constipation in the third trimester.

Management

- Women often require reassurance that constipation is a normal feature of pregnancy.
- Advice to increase fluid intake and dietary modification with particular attention to increasing the fibre content may suffice.
- Temporary cessation of oral iron supplements may help alleviate symptoms.
- Laxatives should only be used in severe cases and if the earlier mentioned measures fail.

Laxatives

Bulk-forming drugs
Unprocessed bran, methyl cellulose, ispaghula husk or sterculia may be used in pregnancy. These should all be taken with adequate fluids to prevent intestinal obstruction.

Stimulant laxatives
Glycerol suppositories and senna (Senokot®) tablets are safe for use in pregnancy. Danthron should be avoided.

Faecal softeners
Liquid paraffin, castor oil and soap enemas should be avoided in pregnancy. Docusate sodium (dioctyl sodium sulphosuccinate), which acts as a stimulant as well as a softening agent, is safe for use in pregnancy.

Osmotic laxatives
Lactulose and magnesium hydrochloride are also both safe for use in pregnancy.

Gastro-oesophageal reflux disorder (GORD)

Incidence

Oesophageal reflux is almost universal during pregnancy. Approximately 60% of women experience heartburn at some time in the third trimester.

Clinical features

- Reflux may be asymptomatic or may present with heartburn, 'water brash', nausea and vomiting, cough or wheezing or aspiration pneumonia.
- Recurrent or forceful vomiting may cause haematemesis from a Mallory–Weiss (oesophageal mucosal) tear or abrasion.

Pathogenesis

- Decreased lower oesophageal pressure, decreased gastric peristalsis and delayed gastric emptying all make reflux more likely.
- Later in pregnancy, the enlarging uterus exacerbates oesophageal reflux.
- Reflux of acid or alkaline gastric contents into the oesophagus causes inflammation of the oesophageal mucosa.

Management

- Antacids are safe to use in pregnancy and should be used liberally.
- Many formulations in liquid and tablet or capsule form are available. The liquid forms are more effective; they are best given to prevent symptoms before meals or at bedtime, but may be taken to relieve symptoms at any time.
- Aluminium-containing antacids tend to cause constipation and magnesium-containing antacids have a laxative effect. Both are safe for use in pregnancy.
- Reflux in late pregnancy may be relieved with postural changes, and some women find that sleeping in a sitting or semi-recumbent position will prevent symptoms at night.
- Avoiding food or fluid intake immediately before retiring at night may also help.
- Metoclopramide increases lower oesophageal pressure, speeds gastric emptying and may help relieve reflux.
- Sucralfate is also safe to use in pregnancy.
- H_2-receptor blockers, such as ranitidine, have been used throughout pregnancy without adverse effects.
- Omeprazole, a PPI, is more effective than ranitidine at suppressing gastric acid secretion, and may be used in conjunction with antiemetics in hyperemesis. It should only be used for GORD when H_2-receptor blockers have failed.

Peptic ulcer disease

Incidence

- Peptic ulceration is less common in pregnant than non-pregnant women, but data may be inaccurate due to the reluctance to fully investigate symptoms of dyspepsia with endoscopy during pregnancy.
- Complications of peptic ulcer disease, such as gastrointestinal haemorrhage and perforation, are very rare in pregnancy.

Clinical features

- Epigastric pain, which may be relieved by food in the case of duodenal ulcer, may be aggravated by food with a gastric ulcer.
- Heartburn and nausea make differentiation from reflux oesophagitis difficult.
- Ulcers that remain quiescent during pregnancy may cause resurgence of symptoms in the puerperium.

Pathogenesis

- Increased acid secretion and decreased mucosal resistance contribute to the aetiology.
- *Helicobacter pylori* is found in the stomach of almost 100% of patients with duodenal ulceration and is felt to have a causal role, since eradication with antibiotic therapy increases ulcer healing and decreases relapse.
- Smoking reduces mucosal resistance.
- The increase in prostaglandins induced by pregnancy has a protective effect on the gastric mucosa.

Diagnosis

- A high index of suspicion is needed, but this is an uncommon diagnosis in pregnancy.
- Although nausea, vomiting and heartburn are common in pregnancy, epigastric pain is not, and should lead the clinician to suspect a diagnosis of peptic ulcer disease. (See 'Differential Diagnosis of Abdominal Pain', Section B, Table 17.)
- In experienced hands, upper gastrointestinal endoscopy can be used safely in pregnancy and should not be withheld. Sedation with benzodiazepines can be given in the usual way.
- Haematemesis is most often due to a Mallory–Weiss tear and is not associated with a fall in haemoglobin. But repeated or severe episodes should be investigated with endoscopy as in the non-pregnant woman.

Management

- Regular antacids, sucralfate, H_2-receptor blockers and PPIs can all be used safely in pregnancy. Ranitidine is the most suitable H_2-receptor blocker.
- *H. pylori* eradication therapy can usually be deferred until after delivery.
- The prostaglandin analogue, misoprostol, protects the gastric mucosa, but is contraindicated during pregnancy due to the risk of inducing uterine contraction and abortion.

Inflammatory bowel disease (IBD)

This is divided into Crohn's disease and ulcerative colitis (UC).

Incidence

- Incidence of UC is approximately 5 to 10 in 100,000 and prevalence is approximately 0.8 to 1 in 1000.

- Incidence of Crohn's disease is approximately 5 in 100,000 and prevalence is approximately 0.5 in 1000.
- UC affects more women than men, but in Crohn's disease both sexes are affected equally.
- IBD usually presents in young adulthood and 25% of female patients will conceive after the diagnosis.

Clinical features

Ulcerative colitis

This is always confined to the colon and causes:

- Liquid diarrhoea
- Lower abdominal pain
- Urgency of defaecation
- Passage of blood and mucus per rectum.

Crohn's disease

Crohn's disease affects the terminal ileum alone in 30%, the ileum and colon in 50% and the colon alone in 20% of cases. Crohn's disease may affect any part of the gastrointestinal tract from the mouth to the anus.

Cases with involvement of the colon may present with any of the earlier mentioned features, although bleeding is more common in UC than in Crohn's disease. Cases with ileitis present with:

- Cramping mid-abdominal pain
- Diarrhoea
- Weight loss.

Complications

Crohn's disease

- Perforation
- Stricture formation
- Perianal problems
- Fistulae
- Abscess formation.

Ulcerative colitis

- Colonic dilation/toxic megacolon
- Malignancy.

Extraintestinal manifestations

These include the following:

- Arthritis (sacroileitis, ankylosing spondylitis)
- Aphthous ulcers (Crohn's disease)
- Gallstones

- Ascending cholangitis
- Sclerosing cholangitis
- Conjunctivitis/irodocyclitis/episcleritis.

Pathogenesis

- The cause of IBD is not known.
- Infection, autoimmunity, genetic factors and environmental toxins may all be involved.
- Patchy or segmental inflammation (skip lesions) is typical of Crohn's disease.

Diagnosis

Flexible sigmoidoscopy or colonoscopy and mucosal biopsy are safe in pregnancy and may confirm mucosal inflammation and allow histological examination to differentiate UC and Crohn's disease.

Pregnancy

Effect of pregnancy on IBD

- Pregnancy has little effect on the course of IBD.
- Risk of exacerbation of UC during pregnancy is approximately 50% (i.e. similar to the annual risk in non-pregnant patients).
- This risk is reduced to approximately 30% if colitis is quiescent at the time of conception.
- Exacerbations of UC are usually mild and occur during the first two trimesters.
- Crohn's disease remains quiescent in approximately three-quarters of pregnant patients, and improves in approximately one-third of those whose disease is active at the time of conception.
- Most exacerbations of inactive Crohn's disease occur during the first trimester.
- The highest risk relates to those women with active disease at the time of conception, and those who develop IBD for the first time in pregnancy. In these instances, it usually occurs during the first or second trimesters.
- Postpartum flare of UC is no more common than in the non-pregnant patient, but may occur in Crohn's disease.

Effect of IBD on pregnancy

- Fertility may be decreased in active Crohn's disease.
- In women with quiescent disease at the time of conception, the rates of miscarriage, stillbirth, fetal abnormality and livebirth are not increased.
- The majority (80–90%) of women have full-term normal pregnancies.
- Active disease at the time of conception is associated with an increased miscarriage rate.
- Active disease may adversely affect pregnancy outcome, with an increased rate of preterm delivery.
- Women with prior surgery, including ileostomy and proctocolectomy, and pouch surgery tolerate pregnancy well. Most women with stomas and quiescent disease have full-term normal deliveries, but those with previous surgery and active disease do less well. Ileostomy dysfunction may occur in the second trimester. The most serious

complication is intermittent intestinal obstruction, but peristomal cracking and bleeding may result from stretching of the abdominal wall. Successful pregnancies and vaginal deliveries have also been reported following ileoanal anastomosis and ileal pouches.

Management

- Women should be encouraged to conceive during periods of disease remission and to avoid/postpone pregnancy if their disease is active.
- The management of acute attacks and chronic disease is not substantially affected by pregnancy.
- Deterioration of symptoms may be investigated with a full blood count, stool culture, serum albumin (allowing for the normal fall in pregnancy) C reactive protein (CRP) and flexible sigmoidoscopy or rigid proctoscopy to assess the activity of colitis.
- The aminosalicylate sulfasalazine (Salazopyrin®) may be safely used throughout pregnancy and breastfeeding, and is particularly used for maintaining and inducing remission in women with UC and colonic Crohn's disease. The drug is split in the colon into sulfapyridine and the active moiety 5-aminosalicylic acid. The theoretical risk of kernicterus because of displacement of bilirubin from fetal albumin has been discounted by studies. Sulfasalazine may also be used rectally.
- Sulfasalazine is a dihydrofolate reductase inhibitor that blocks the conversion of folate to its more active metabolites. The use of supplemental folic acid 5 mg/ day pre-conceptually and in pregnancy is therefore important to reduce the increased risk of neural tube defects, cardiovascular defects, oral clefts and folate deficiency.
- The closely related aminosalicylate, mesalazine (Asacol®), is also safe.
- Oral and rectal preparations of corticosteroids are safe for use in pregnancy. For acute colonic disease, initial treatment is with topical corticosteroid enemas and oral sulfasalazine or mesalazine. Oral steroids (20–40 mg) may be required.
- There are extensive data regarding the safety of azathioprine in renal transplants and systemic lupus erythematosus (SLE) in pregnancy, and its active metabolite, 6-mercaptopurine (6MP), sometimes used in IBD, seems also to be safe in pregnancy [see also Chapter 4, p. 62 (steroids) and Chapter 8, p. 132 (azathioprine)]. Those who require azathioprine or 6MP to remain in remission should continue use of this drug in pregnancy.
- Metronidazole has been used extensively for other conditions in pregnancy and is safe to use.
- Data are accumulating for the safety of anti-TNFalpha agents and other biologics in pregnancy (see Chapter 8, p. 134). Etanercept, infliximab and adalimumab have all been used for IBD in pregnancy. Ideally they should be discontinued by 30 to 32 weeks gestation to allow time for the fetus to clear the drug prior to delivery. Evidence suggests that these drugs are not transferred to breast milk.
- Rarely, surgery for obstruction, haemorrhage, perforation, toxic megacolon, or failed medical treatment may be required during pregnancy, and should not be delayed due to the pregnancy.
- Caesarean section is only required for obstetric indications. In cases of severe peri-anal Crohn's disease resulting in a deformed or scarred rectum and perineum, vaginal delivery should be avoided due to perineal inelasticity. Similarly, active peri-anal Crohn's disease may prevent healing of an episiotomy.

- In women with pouches, there may be concern regarding maintenance of an intact external anal sphincter and the individual colorectal surgeon should be consulted regarding mode of delivery.

Inflammatory bowel disease—points to remember

- Pregnancy does not usually affect the course of IBD and symptoms generally remain stable if present at conception.
- Most changes in disease activity occur early in pregnancy.
- Pregnancy outcome is not affected by quiescent IBD, but active disease at conception or during pregnancy may adversely affect the pregnancy.
- Both aminosalicylates (sulfasalazine, mesalazine) and corticosteroids are safe to use in pregnancy and whilst breastfeeding.
- Azathioprine and 6mercaptopurine are safe in pregnancy and azathioprine is safe in breast feeding.
- Etanercept, infliximab and adalimumab are probably safe in the second and third trimesters and while breastfeeding.
- Elective caesarean section is not usually necessary, even in women with ileostomies, except for obstetric indications or in women with perianal Crohn's disease or some women with pouches.

Irritable bowel syndrome

Incidence

Irritable bowel syndrome (IBS) is common, and most sufferers encountered in pregnancy will already be aware of their diagnosis. Since it is a diagnosis of exclusion, new onset of symptoms in pregnancy is more likely to be attributed to the pregnancy than to IBS.

Clinical features

- Recurrent episodes of abdominal pain, typically in the left iliac fossa, but may occur anywhere in the abdomen.
- Altered bowel habit with, most commonly, constipation, but also diarrhoea.
- The history is usually long and there may be long symptom-free periods.
- The woman with IBS looks well despite frequent episodes of abdominal pain.
- There are no abnormal findings on examination.

Pathogenesis

- The cause of IBS is not known.
- Abnormal gut motility may be a contributory factor, and symptoms are usually exacerbated or brought on by stress.

Diagnosis

- IBS is a diagnosis of exclusion, and the extent of investigation depends on the age of the patient and the length of the history, plus the presence of any 'red flag' symptoms or signs.

- Most young women with a long history of intermittent abdominal pain require little in the way of invasive investigations.
- Rectal examination and sigmoidoscopy should be performed (pre-pregnancy), and although the colonic and rectal mucosa are normal, air insufflation may reproduce the pain.
- If diarrhoea is a feature, a rectal biopsy should be taken (pre-pregnancy) to exclude IBD.

Management

- Women should be reassured of the benign nature of IBS, and this in itself may help alleviate symptoms.
- Symptoms of IBS may be exacerbated by pregnancy, especially if constipation is a prominent feature.
- A high-fibre diet may help some women.
- Stool-bulking agents (see earlier) are preferred to unprocessed bran, which may worsen symptoms, in particular bloating.
- Antispasmodic agents act to relax intestinal smooth muscle and are used widely in the management of IBS in the non-pregnant woman. There is no evidence for teratogenesis with anticholinergic agents such as hyoscine (Buscopan®) and dicyclomine (Merbentyl®). Smooth muscle relaxants such as mebeverine (Colofac®) are not recommended in pregnancy.

Coeliac Disease

- This autoimmune disease affects 0.1–1% of people and is due to an inflammatory reaction in the small bowel as a result of ingesting gluten found in wheat, barley and rye.
- It is diagnosed by the presence of IgA antiendomysial antibodies or antitransglutamidase antibodies.
- Coeliac disease may cause diarrhoea, abdominal pain or steatorrhea. The diagnosis should be considered in those with weight loss, fat soluble vitamin deficiency and anaemia (B12, folate or iron deficiency).
- Management in pregnancy is the same as outwith pregnancy; that is strict adherence to a gluten free diet.

Abdominal pain

A full differential diagnosis is given in Section B, Table 17.

The commonest causes of abdominal pain in pregnancy are constipation, urinary tract infection and uterine contractions. The common non-obstetric surgical conditions are appendicitis, gall bladder disease (see Chapter 11) and pancreatitis.

Appendicitis

Incidence

- This is the commonest non-obstetric indication for laparoscopic surgery/ laparotomy in pregnancy.
- It usually presents in the first two trimesters with an incidence of approximately 1 in 3500.

Clinical features

■ The symptoms and signs are similar to those in the non-pregnant woman, with abdominal pain, rebound tenderness, nausea and vomiting. However, the abdominal pain may not be in the classical right iliac fossa position.
■ An aggressive course with complications such as perforation, wall abscess and paralytic ileus is not uncommon, perhaps because of delay in diagnosis due to pregnancy.
■ Preterm labour and perinatal mortality complicate 20% of cases with perforation.

Diagnosis

■ Ultrasound has improved diagnostic accuracy and reduced the negative laparotomy rate in cases of suspected appendicitis.
■ The normal appendix is not visualised in most cases.
■ The inflamed appendix is characterised by an outer diameter of >6 mm, non-compressibility, lack of peristalsis or presence of a periappendiceal fluid collection.
■ A posterolateral approach allows evaluation of the retrocaecal appendix, and transvaginal scanning that of a pelvic appendix.
■ Sometimes further imagining with CT or MRI is appropriate.

Management

If the diagnosis is confirmed (or the index of suspicion remains high even without radiological confirmation), a Lanz incision (transverse gridiron) or a laparoscopic approach for appendectomy is recommended.

Pancreatitis

Incidence

This rarely complicates pregnancy and the incidence is approximately 0.1 in 1000.

Clinical features

■ These are similar to those in the non-pregnant woman.
■ Most attacks occur in the third trimester and are mild.
■ Epigastric pain radiating to the back associated with nausea and vomiting.
■ Severe pancreatitis causes pulmonary, cardiac, renal and gastrointestinal complications with shock.

Pathogenesis

■ The commonest cause of pancreatitis is gallstones and this is also the case for attacks occurring in pregnancy. The next commonest cause is alcohol.
■ Pancreatitis is not more common in pregnancy.
■ Very rarely pancreatitis in pregnancy may be precipitated by hypertriglyceridaemia, although the physiological rise in triglycerides occurring in normal pregnancy is unlikely to be sufficient to cause pancreatitis without an underlying lipid disorder.
■ Primary hyperparathyroidism (see Chapter 6, p. 108) is another rare cause of pancreatitis during pregnancy.

Diagnosis

■ The serum amylase is invariably raised and levels >1000 U/L suggest pancreatitis or common bile duct stones.

■ Pregnancy itself does not cause changes in amylase, but a raised amylase level is not specific for pancreatitis; mild elevations in amylase level occur in cholecystitis, peptic ulcer perforation and bowel obstruction.

■ The absence of a diagnostic rise in serum amylase may be due to associated hyperlipidaemia that masks the rise in amylase.

Management

■ There is no specific cure for pancreatitis; management should be supportive and usually involves a period of fasting with nasogastric suction if there is evidence of paralytic ileus.

■ I.v. fluids and analgesia are given as required, and most cases resolve spontaneously.

■ Approximately 10% of patients may develop serious complications and an important feature of management is to identify this subgroup and ensure their rapid transfer to an intensive care unit.

■ Regular monitoring of cardiovascular status, haemoglobin, white cell count, amylase, renal function, oxygen saturation, liver function, prothrombin time, glucose and calcium is essential.

Further reading

Alstead EA, Nelson-Piercy C. Inflammatory bowel disease in pregnancy. Gut 2003; 52:159–161.

Bergin PS, Harvey P. Wernicke's encephalopathy and central pontine myelinolysis associated with hyperemesis gravidarum. Br Med J 1992; 305:517–518.

Diavcitrin O, Park YH, Veerasuntharam G. The safety of mesalazine in human pregnancy: A prospective cohort study. Gastroenterology 1998; 114:23–28.

Festin M. Nausea and vomiting in early pregnancy. Clin Evid (Online) 2007; pii:1405.

Jewell D, Young G. Interventions for nausea and vomiting in early pregnancy. Cochrane Database Syst Rev 4:CD000145.

Mahadevan U, Kane S, Sandborn WJ, et al. Intentional infliximab use during pregnancy for induction or maintenance of remission in Crohn's disease. Aliment Pharmacol Ther 2005; 21(6):733–738.

Mazzotta P, Magee LA. A risk–benefit assessment of pharmacological and non-pharmacological treatments for nausea and vomiting of pregnancy. Drugs 2000; 59:781–800.

Moran P, Taylor R. Management of hyperemesis gravidarum: The importance of weight loss as a criterion for steroid therapy. QJM 2002; 95:153–158.

Nelson-Piercy C, Fayers P, de Swiet M. Randomized, placebo-controlled trial of corticosteroids for hyperemesis gravidarum. Br J Obstet Gynaecol 2001; 108:1–7.

CHAPTER 13
Skin disease

Physiological changes	Dermatoses specific to
Pre-existing conditions	pregnancy
Eczema	Polymorphic eruption
Psoriasis	Pemphigoid gestationis
	Atopic eruption of pregnancy

Co-incident conditions

Acne

Erythema nodosum

Erythema multiforme

Pityriasis rosea

Physiological changes

- Increased pigmentation. This begins in the first trimester and fades after delivery. Existing pigmented areas (e.g. areolae and axillae) become darker. Specific areas (e.g. linea nigrum) appear.
- Melasma is the name given to the patches of light-brown facial pigmentation that develops in approximately 70% of women in the second half of pregnancy. The usual distribution involves the forehead, cheeks, upper lip and chin.
- Spider naevi. These occur on the face, upper trunk and arms. They can be numerous and in some cases almost confluent. Most appear in early pregnancy and regress following delivery, although 25% may persist.
- Palmar erythema. Present in up to 70% of women by the third trimester. Fades within one week of delivery.
- Hair loss. This is a normal feature of the postpartum period, occurring in most women at between 4 and 20 weeks after delivery. It results from the increased conversion of hairs from the anagen (growing) to telogen (resting) phase, following the increased proportion of hairs in the anagen phase during pregnancy. Hair is lost diffusely, but recovery is usual within six months.
- Striae gravidarum. These develop in most women but are more common in obese women and those with multiple pregnancies. They appear perpendicular to skin tension lines as pink linear wrinkles. They fade and become white and atrophic, although never disappear completely.
- Pruritus without either rash or cholestasis can be a feature in up to 20% of normal pregnancies. Liver function tests should, however, be checked in any pregnant woman without a rash (other than excoriations) complaining of pruritus,

especially if onset occurs in the third trimester and it involves the palms and soles (see Chapter 11, p. 198, and section B, Table 14).

Pre-existing conditions

Eczema

■ This often, but not invariably, improves during pregnancy. Nevertheless, since eczema and atopy are so prevalent, it remains the commonest dermatosis associated with pregnancy.

■ Most women presenting in pregnancy have a previous history of adult or infantile asthma, eczema or atopy.

■ Eczema is treated with topical emollients as outwith pregnancy. Women should be reassured that if they require topical steroids to control their eczema, these are not contraindicated in pregnancy.

Psoriasis

■ This may improve, remain unchanged or deteriorate during pregnancy. Psoriasis may present for the first time in pregnancy.

■ Dithranol and coal tar may be safely used in pregnancy.

■ Narrow band UVB is the safest second-line therapy.

■ Methotrexate is an antimetabolite, is teratogenic and is contraindicated in pregnancy.

■ Topical and oral Ciclosporin A may be safely used in pregnancy.

■ Very occasionally biologic therapy may become necessary, in which case the same issues of balancing risks and benefits apply as when treating inflammatory bowel disease or rheumatoid arthritis in pregnancy (see Chapter 8, p. 134).

Rarely, a severe form of pustular psoriasis, impetigo herpetiformis, may develop. Urticated erythema, beginning in the flexures and especially the groins, is associated with sterile pustules, which may become widespread and affect mucosa. This condition is associated with severe systemic upset including fever, neutrophilia and hypocalcaemia. An increased perinatal mortality rate is also reported and these women require intensive treatment and regular fetal surveillance.

Co-incident conditions

Acne

■ This may develop for the first time in pregnancy.

■ Pre-existing acne may improve or worsen during pregnancy. There is a tendency to flare in the third trimester secondary to increased sebaceous gland activity secondary to high levels of androgens.

■ Both tetracyclines and retinoids (vitamin A analogues, e.g. isotretinoin) are contraindicated in pregnancy. Topical and oral erythromycin may be used safely.

Erythema nodosum

■ This may occur in pregnancy, without any demonstrable, known underlying precipitating cause.

■ Tuberculosis and sarcoidosis should be excluded with a chest X-ray. The woman should be asked about symptoms of streptococcal infection and inflammatory bowel disease, as well as any recent medication she has taken or may be taking (particularly sulphonamides).

- If no underlying cause is discovered, the prognosis is excellent.
- If treatment is required because the lesions are very painful then a short course of oral corticosteroids is appropriate.

Erythema multiforme

- This is an acute self-limiting condition predominantly affecting the peripheries.
- The symmetrical eruption consists of erythematous papules that evolve into concentric rings of varying colour with central pallor.
- Erythema multiforme may complicate pregnancy without any obvious underlying cause.
- The commoner precipitating causes should be sought [e.g. drugs and viral (particularly herpes simplex virus (HSV)) infections], before attributing the eruption to pregnancy alone.

Pityriasis rosea

- This is a self-limiting, non-recurring eruption affecting predominantly the trunk and proximal limbs.
- The lesions are reddish brown with a larger (2–6 cm) 'herald patch' preceding the development of other lesions, and may be confused with tinea due to their well-defined, scaled edge.
- Pityriasis rosea affects mainly children and young adults, but may be more common in pregnancy.
- There is some evidence of a causal role for human herpes viruses.

Dermatoses specific to pregnancy

Polymorphic eruption of pregnancy (PEP) (also known as pruritic urticarial papules and plaques of pregnancy, PUPPP; toxaemic rash of pregnancy) (Fig. 13.1A and 13.1B).

Incidence

PEP is the commonest pregnancy-specific dermatosis. The incidence is approximately 1 in 200 to 250, that is, approximately 0.5%.

Clinical features

Time of onset
Third trimester, mean gestational age at onset 34 weeks gestation.

Parity
More common in primiparous women (70%) and those with multiple pregnancies (13%).

Distribution
Abdomen (with umbilical sparing) along the striae, spreading to the thighs, buttocks, under the breasts and upper arms. Ninety-seven percent involve the abdomen and proximal thighs.

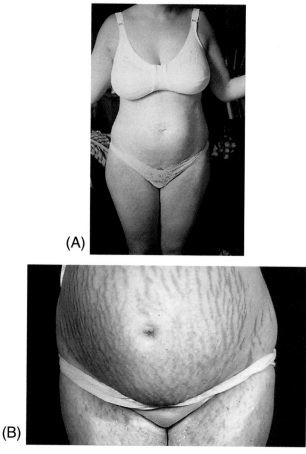

Figure 13.1 – (**A** and **B**) Polymorphic eruption of pregnancy (PEP).

Eruption
Pruritic, urticarial papules and plaques, erythema and rarely vesicles (but not bullae) and target lesions.

Resolution
Rapid after delivery.

Fetus

No effects on the fetus are known.

Treatment

- One percent menthol in aqueous cream.
- Most effective if kept in the fridge and applied when cold.

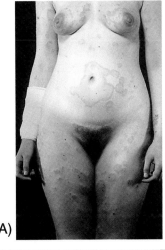

(A)

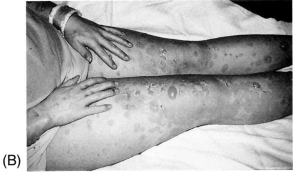

(B)

Figure 13.2 – (**A** and **B**) Pemphigoid gestationis.

- One percent hydrocortisone cream or ointment. Stronger topical steroids such as Eumovate® or Betnovate® may be required.
- Sedative antihistamine, for example, chlorpheniramine (Piriton®) 4 mg three to four times/day or promethazine (Phenergan®) 25 mg nocte.
- Non-sedating antihistamines, for example, loratadine, cetirazine.
- Systemic steroids are only occasionally required for intractable pruritus.

Recurrence

Rare (mild if it occurs).

Pemphigoid gestationis (Previously known as herpes gestationis) (Fig. 13.2a and 13.2b)

Incidence

This is a rare (1 in 10,000 to 1 in 60,000 pregnancies) but serious condition.

Clinical features

Time of onset
Any time (9 weeks gestation to 1 week postpartum) but usually in the third trimester.

Parity
Primiparous or multiparous women.

Distribution
Abdomen (umbilicus affected; lesions begin in periumbilical region), spreading to limbs, palms and soles.

Eruption
Intensely pruritic; urticated erythematous papules and plaques; target lesions, annular wheals. After variable delay (usually two weeks) vesicles and large tense bullae form.

Resolution
If it occurs in the second trimester, there is usually an improvement at the end of pregnancy, but a flare postpartum. Urticated plaques may persist for several months after delivery. In a few it may develop into bullous pemphigoid.

Pathogenesis

- Autoimmune (possibly related to exposure to fetal antigens). Binding of IgG to the basement membrane triggers an immune response leading to the formation of sub-epidermal vesicles.
- Associated with bullous pemphigoid.
- Associated with other autoimmune conditions, for example, Graves' disease, vitiligo, type 1 diabetes and rheumatoid arthritis.

Diagnosis

Diagnosed by skin biopsy and direct immunofluorescence, which shows complement (C3) deposition at the basement membrane zone. This distinguishes pemphigoid gestationis from PEP, in which immunofluorescence is negative.

Fetal considerations

- An increased risk to the fetus has been reported and studies have shown an association with low birthweight, preterm delivery and stillbirth.
- As this is an autoimmune disease, the neonate may be affected with a similar bullous eruption. This occurs in 10% of cases and is mild and transient.

Treatment

- Potent topical corticosteroids (0.1% mometasone furoate, Elocon®) or very potent (0.05% clobetasol propionate, Dermovate®).
- Most require systemic steroids [e.g. prednisolone 40 mg/day and these should not be withheld in pregnancy (see Chapter 4, p. 62)]. Some will require topical or systemic immunosuppression with ciclosporin or tacrolimus.
- Sedative antihistamine, for example, chlorpheniramine (Piriton®) 4 mg three to four times/day or promethazine (Phenergan®) 25 mg nocte.

Recurrence

- Usually recurs in future pregnancies (with possibly earlier onset and more severe course).
- May recur with use of combined oral contraceptive pill.

Atopic eruption of pregnancy (Figs. 13.3A and 13.3B)

Incidence

1 in 300 pregnancies.

Clinical features

There is considerable overlap between eczema in pregnancy, prurigo of pregnancy and pruritic folliculitis and the latter two conditions have been reclassified as atopic eruption of pregnancy.

Time of onset
Earlier than PEP. Usually second to third trimester.

Parity
Mostly multiparous women.

Distribution
Trunk and limbs.

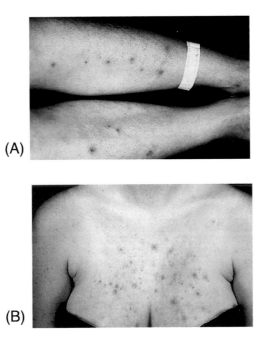

(A)

(B)

Figure 13.3 – (**A** and **B**) Atopic eruption of pregnancy.

Eruption
Pruritic; groups of red/brown excoriated papules.

Resolution
Pruritus improves at delivery, but papules may sometimes persist for several months after delivery.

Pathogenesis

Associated with atopy. There is a previous history of eczema in 20% and a gene defect in skin protein filaggrin.

Fetal considerations

No effects on the fetus are known.

Treatment

- Emollients (e.g. diprobase, oilatum)
- Topical steroids (1% hydrocortisone or Eumovate® cream or ointment).
- Antihistamines (see earlier) if required.

Recurrence

Recurrence is possible.

Further reading

Ambros-Rudolph CMM, Mullegger RRM, Vaughan-Jones S et al. The specific dermatoses of pregnancy revisited and reclassified: Results of a retrospective two-center study on 505 pregnant patients. J Am Acad Dermatol 2006; 54:395–404.

Kenyon AP, Nelson-Piercy C, Girling J, et al. Prevalence of pruritus and obstetric cholestasis in a London antenatal population. Obstet Med 2010; 3, 25–29.

Mokni M, Fourati M, Karoui I et al. Pemphigoid gestationis: A study of 20 cases. Ann Dermatol Venereol 2004; 131:953–956.

Rudolph CM, Al-Fares S, Vaughan-Jones SA, et al. Polymorphic eruption of pregnancy: Clinicopathology and potential trigger factors in 181 patients. Br J Dermatol 2006; 154:54–60.

Vaughan Jones SA, Hern S, Nelson-Piercy C, et al. A prospective study of 200 women with dermatoses of pregnancy correlating clinical findings with hormonal and immunopathological profiles. Br J Dermatol 1999; 141:71–81.

CHAPTER 14

Haematological problems

Physiological changes

- The plasma volume increases progressively throughout normal pregnancy.
- Most of this 50% increase occurs by 34 weeks gestation and is positively correlated with the birthweight of the baby.
- Because the expansion in plasma volume is greater than the increase in red cell mass, there is a fall in the haemoglobin concentration, haematocrit and red cell count.
- Despite this haemodilution, there is usually no change in mean corpuscular volume (MCV) or mean corpuscular haemoglobin concentration (MCHC).
- The platelet count tends to fall progressively during normal pregnancy, although usually remains within normal limits. In a proportion of women (5–10%), the count will reach levels of 100 to 150×10^9/L by term, and this may be in the absence of any pathological process. In practice, therefore, a woman is not considered to be thrombocytopenic in pregnancy until the platelet count is $<100 \times 10^9$/L.
- Pregnancy causes a two- to three-fold increase in the requirement for iron, not only for haemoglobin synthesis but also for certain enzymes and for the fetus. There is a 10- to 20-fold increase in folate requirements.
- Changes in the coagulation system during pregnancy produce a physiological hyper-coagulable state (see Chapter 3, p. 39).

Anaemia

The lower limit of normal for haemoglobin concentration in the non-pregnant female is taken as 11.5 to 12 g/dL. In the pregnant patient, levels below 10.5 g/dL should be considered abnormal, although in certain situations such as multiple pregnancy associated with larger increases in plasma volume, the physiological dilution of haemoglobin may cause even lower concentrations of haemoglobin.

Clinical features

- Some women begin pregnancy already anaemic and may become rapidly symptomatic.
- Most cases present in the third trimester since this is when demands for iron reach their peak. Anaemia in pregnancy is usually diagnosed on routine testing, but may present with tiredness, lethargy, dizziness or fainting.

Pathogenesis

Iron deficiency is by far the commonest cause of anaemia, and iron deficiency anaemia is the commonest haematological problem in pregnancy.

- The increased demands for iron are met by increased intestinal absorption and by mobilising iron stores from the haemoglobin of the circulating red cells.
- The reason why so many women not given routine iron supplementation in pregnancy become anaemic is that they enter pregnancy with depleted iron stores. Common reasons for these depleted stores include: menorrhagia, inadequate diet or previous recent pregnancies, particularly with less than a year between delivery and conception when the woman has also been breastfeeding.
- It is virtually impossible to meet the extra requirements of pregnancy with diet alone, so women with depleted stores develop iron deficiency anaemia later in pregnancy.
- Iron deficiency is more common in multiple pregnancy.
- Blood loss at the time of delivery contributes to iron deficiency in the puerperium; 2% to 5% of women have a primary postpartum haemorrhage (blood loss >500 mL).
- In women from developing countries, intestinal infestations must be considered as a cause including
  - Hookworm
  - Giardia
  - Tapeworm
  - Schistosomiasis.

The next commonest cause of anaemia in pregnancy is folate deficiency.

- The normal level of dietary folate is inadequate to prevent megaloblastic changes in the bone marrow in approximately 25% of pregnant women.
- The incidence of megaloblastic anaemia is variable depending on the socio-economic status and nutrition of the population.
- Folate deficiency is more likely if the woman is taking anticonvulsant drugs or folate antagonists such as sulfasalazine.

- Other haematological conditions complicating pregnancy increase the risk of folate deficiency:
  - Haemolytic anaemia
  - Sickle-cell disease
  - Thalassaemia
  - Hereditary spherocytosis.

Non-haematological causes of anemia should also be considered:

- coeliac disease (iron, folate and B12 deficiency [See Chapter 12, p. 228])
- chronic kidney disease
- autoimmune disease, e.g. SLE

Diagnosis

Iron deficiency

- It is generally assumed that a woman who is or becomes anaemic in pregnancy is iron deficient, but the diagnosis should be confirmed.
- The red cell indices give a good indication of iron deficiency. The MCV, mean cell haemoglobin (MCH) and MCHC are all reduced.
- The first index to become abnormal is the MCV, but this may be normal when stores first become depleted.
- Serum iron and total iron binding capacity (TIBC) fall in normal pregnancy, but levels of serum iron <12 μmol/L and TIBC saturation of <15% indicate iron deficiency.
- Serum ferritin provides an accurate assessment of iron stores; levels <12 μg/L indicate iron deficiency and levels <50 μg/L in early pregnancy are an indication for iron supplements.

Folate deficiency

- This causes a macrocytic anaemia with megaloblastic change in the bone marrow.
- The pointer is usually a raised MCV, although this may be a feature of normal pregnancy. It may also be due to azathioprine or alcohol.
- Diagnosis is confirmed by measurement of serum and red cell folate.

Effects of iron deficiency on pregnancy

- Iron deficiency adversely affects iron-dependent enzymes in each cell, and has profound effects on muscle and neurotransmitter activity.
- Iron deficiency is associated with low birthweight and preterm delivery, and there is also an association with increased blood loss at delivery.

Management

- The rationale for routine supplementation with oral iron is that the increased iron demand during pregnancy cannot be met by increased absorption alone, and that a high proportion of women in their reproductive years lack storage iron.
- Iron supplements prevent iron deficiency anaemia. Many argue that the best approach to iron deficiency in pregnancy is prevention.

- The World Health Organisation in conjunction with the International Nutritional Anemia Consultative Group and the United Nations Children's Fund has issued guidelines recommending routine supplements (60 mg/day iron and 400 μg/day folic acid) to all pregnant women for at least six months. The guidelines also state that these supplements should be recommended to women until three months postpartum in areas with a high prevalence of anaemia (>40%).
- The standard oral preparations (Pregaday®: 100 mg iron, 350 μg folate; Fefol®) are combined with folic acid and are suitable for both prevention and treatment of iron deficiency in pregnancy.
- Iron absorption from the small intestine is enhanced by ascorbic acid, meat and alcohol. Inhibitors to absorption include phytic acid and tannins present in tea, coffee and chocolate.
- The incidence of gastrointestinal side effects (30%) is directly related to the dose of iron taken. A dose of 60 mg/day (or even weekly) of iron may be sufficient for prophylaxis. Therefore, women who have troublesome side effects may be advised to take alternate day, twice weekly or weekly supplements rather than to discontinue them.
- For those women who are unable to tolerate oral preparations, parenteral therapy with intravenous iron sucrose is an alternative. This is safe in pregnancy and does not have the gastrointestinal side effects.
- Parenteral iron may provide a more rapid and complete correction of iron deficiency.
- Iron deficiency diagnosed late in pregnancy may necessitate blood transfusion, as the maximum rise in haemoglobin achievable with either oral or parenteral iron is 0.8 g/dL/wk.
- Similar arguments apply to routine folate supplementation in pregnancy, because a normal diet is not sufficient to meet the increased requirement for folate in pregnancy.

Anaemia—points to remember

- The plasma volume increases by 50% in pregnancy and there is a fall in haemoglobin concentration.
- Pregnancy causes a 2- to 3-fold increase in the requirement for iron, and a 10- to 20-fold increase in folic acid requirements.
- Many women develop iron deficiency anaemia because they enter pregnancy with depleted iron stores.
- A woman may be iron deficient despite having a normal haemoglobin level and MCV.
- The best approach to iron and folate deficiency in pregnancy is prevention with oral iron and folate supplements, at least in those at high risk of becoming anaemic.
- All women planning a pregnancy should be advised to take 0.4 mg/day folate periconceptually as prophylaxis against neural tube defects and other fetal abnormalities.
- The maximum rise in haemoglobin achievable with either oral or parenteral iron is 0.8 g/dL/wk.

- All women planning a pregnancy are now advised to take 400 μg/day folate peri-conceptually to reduce the risk of neural tube defects and other fetal abnormalities.
- In addition, women who themselves have spina bifida, who have had a previous fetus with a neural tube defect are advised to take 5 mg/day folate periconceptually.
- The 5 mg/day dose is also appropriate for those with other haematological problems (see earlier) and those with established folate deficiency. To reduce the risk of congenital malformations, particularly neural tube and cardiac defects, the 5 mg dose is also recommended in women with diabetes and in those receiving anti-epileptic drugs or sulfasalazine.
- Vitamin B_{12} injections may be safely continued in pregnancy.

Haemoglobinopathies

Sickle-cell disease

Incidence

This varies enormously around the United Kingdom, but most cases are concentrated in urban areas.

- The carrier frequency for sickle-cell trait (HbAS) is approximately 1 in 10 among Afro-Caribbeans, but as high as 1 in 4 in West Africans.
- The carrier frequency for haemoglobin C trait (Hb AC) is approximately 1 in 30, but up to 1 in 6 in Ghanaians.

Clinical features

Sickle-cell disease leads to

- Anaemia; chronic haemolytic (not marked in women with HbSC disease)
- Painful vaso-occlusive crises
- Infections. The increased risk of infections is partly because of loss of splenic function from autoinfarction
- Acute chest syndrome. This is characterised by fever, tachypnoea, pleuritic chest pain, leukocytosis, worsening anaemia and pulmonary infiltrates. It may be caused by pulmonary infection or infarction from intravascular sickling or thrombosis
- Splenic sequestration
- Gallstones
- Retinopathy
- Leg ulcers
- Aseptic necrosis of bone
- Renal papillary necrosis
- Stroke
- Pulmonary hypertension.

Pathogenesis

- Sickle-cell haemoglobin (HbS) is a variant of the β-chain of haemoglobin where glutamic acid is replaced by valine at the sixth position from the N terminus. In the deoxygenated state, HbS has low solubility so it aggregates to form liquid crystals and the erythrocyte assumes a 'sickle shape'.

■ Sickling of the red cells occurs particularly in response to hypoxia, cold, acidosis and dehydration. Sickle cells are cleared by the reticuloendothelial system more quickly than normal erythrocytes.

■ There are three main types of sickle cell crisis:

1. Vaso-occlusive symptoms and tissue infarction with severe pain
2. Sequestration; splenic sequestration occurs mainly during childhood
3. Aplastic; this is often associated with parvovirus infection.

■ A number of sickling conditions exist:
  – Homozygous sickle-cell disease (HbSS)
  – Sickle cell/HbC (HbSC)
  – Sickle-cell thalassaemia.

■ Those with HbSS have chronic haemolytic anaemia, but are generally healthy except during periods of crisis, which are often precipitated by infection. A generalised vasculopathy or massive sickling leads to premature death at a mean age below 50 years.

■ Those with HbSC are not usually very anaemic, but are still at risk of sickling. They also have a reduced life expectancy (68 years). They are particularly at risk in pregnancy because doctors and midwives may be unaware of the risk of sickling and have a false sense of security due to the absence of severe anaemia.

Diagnosis

Most women enter pregnancy with the diagnosis established, but if there is doubt, the diagnosis may be made by haemoglobin electrophoresis.

Effect of pregnancy on sickle-cell disease

■ Complications of sickle-cell disease are more common in pregnancy.
■ Crises complicate approximately 35% of pregnancies in women with sickle-cell disease.

Effect of sickle-cell disease on pregnancy

■ Perinatal mortality is increased four- to six-fold.
■ There is an increased incidence of miscarriage, fetal growth restriction (FGR), preterm labour, pre-eclampsia (which may have an early onset and an accelerated course), placental abruption, fetal distress and caesarean section.
■ Sickling infarcts in the placenta may be responsible for some of these factors, although maternal anaemia and increased blood viscosity could also contribute to the high incidence of FGR.
■ There is an increased risk of pulmonary thrombosis, thromboembolism and bone marrow embolism.
■ Maternal morbidity and mortality are increased and the latter has been estimated to be 2.5%.
■ There is also an increased risk of infection, particularly urinary tract infection, pneumonia and puerperal sepsis. Hyposplenism is common in women with sickle-cell disease of child-bearing age and encapsulated organisms may cause overwhelming sepsis.

Management

- Antenatal care should take place in combined clinics with haematologists and obstetricians experienced in the management of these disorders.
- Folic acid (5 mg/day) and penicillin prophylaxis (penicillin V 250 mg b.d.) should be given to all women.
- Electrophoresis will determine the level of fetal Hb (HbF) (the higher the level the better the outcome) and the percentage of HbS.
- If pre-pregnancy genetic counselling and screening of the partner has not already been undertaken, this should be advised in order to determine the risk of the baby having HbSS (50% if the partner is sickle-cell trait).
- Haemoglobin and mid-stream urine should be checked at each visit.
- Regular ultrasound assessment of fetal growth should be undertaken, with two to four weekly growth parameters and umbilical artery Doppler blood-flow assessment if FGR is detected.
- Crises should be managed aggressively as in the non-pregnant patient. This involves admission, adequate pain relief with i.v. or s.c. infusions of morphine or other opiate derivatives, adequate rehydration and early use of antibiotics if infection is suspected.
- The patient should be kept warm and well oxygenated. Arterial blood gases or pulse oximetry is mandatory, especially in the context of high doses of opiates.
- In the acute chest syndrome, it may be necessary to treat the patient with both heparin and antibiotics.
- Blood transfusion may be required for severe anaemia, splenic sequestration or in acute chest syndrome. Exchange transfusion may be necessary if the patient is volume replete.
- The role of routine exchange transfusion in pregnancy is controversial. Proponents claim a decrease in the number of crises, although there is little evidence for improved fetal outcome. The risks include the following:
  - Delayed and immediate transfusion reactions
  - Precipitation of a crisis (particularly if the haematocrit level is raised above 0.35 L/L)
  - Infection
  - Red cell antibodies (because the donor blood is often from people of a different ethnic origin from the patient)
  - Iron overload.
- Intrapartum avoidance of dehydration, hypoxia, sepsis and acidosis is important. Epidural analgesia is encouraged and nitrous oxide is also safe. Continuous fetal heart rate monitoring is advisable. Caesarean section should only be performed for obstetric indications and general anaesthesia should be avoided if possible, especially if the patient has not been transfused.

Pre-pregnancy counselling

- Ideally, partners of those with sickle-cell disease or trait should be screened prior to pregnancy in order to give couples an accurate estimate of the risk of having an affected child.
- Pre-pregnancy assessment and counselling are essential. Echocardiogram should be performed to ensure there is no pulmonary hypertension (see Chapter 2, p. 22).

In practice, much of the screening of partners is performed during pregnancy, by which time it may be too late for prenatal screening of the fetus by chorionic villus sampling. Later screening with amniocentesis or fetal blood sampling may be the only options for prenatal diagnosis.

Sickle-cell disease—points to remember

- Antenatal care should involve haematologists and obstetricians with expertise in the management of such pregnancies.
- Complications of sickle-cell disease, particularly crises, are more common in pregnancy.
- Perinatal and maternal morbidity and mortality rates are increased.
- The risks for the baby include miscarriage, FGR and preterm delivery.
- The risks for the mother include thrombosis, severe pre-eclampsia, infection and transfusion reactions.
- Folic acid (5 mg/day) should be given to all women.
- Infection, hypoxia, acidosis and dehydration should be prevented and treated aggressively.
- Prophylactic exchange transfusion may decrease the risk of crises, but carries its own risks.

Thalassaemias

Incidence

- These inherited disorders of globin synthesis are divided into two main groups, the α-thalassaemias, where one to four of the α-genes are deleted, and the β-thalassaemias, where one or two of the β-globin genes are defective.
- α-Thalassaemia is common in South-East Asians, and β-thalassaemia is common in Cypriots and Asians.
- The overall carrier rate in the United Kingdom for β-thalassaemia is approximately 1 in 10,000 people, but again there are marked local variations depending on the ethnic mix of the population. Three percent of Indians are carriers for β-thalassaemia.

Clinical features

- α-Thalassaemia trait is either α^+ (three normal α-genes) or α^0 (two normal α-genes). Such individuals are usually asymptomatic, but it is important to identify particularly those with α^0, because they may become anaemic.
- α-Thalassaemia major results if both parents have α^0 and there are no functional α-genes. This condition is incompatible with life and the fetus becomes severely hydropic.
- Women with β-thalassaemia trait are asymptomatic, but, as in α-thalassaemia, they might become anaemic during pregnancy.
- Those with β-thalassaemia major have inherited a defective β-globin gene from each parent. Without regular transfusions, this condition is usually fatal within a few years, but children can now survive into the second or third decade.

- The clinical features of β-thalassaemia major in adults are iron overload (due to repeated transfusions) resulting in hepatic, endocrine (diabetes, hypothyroidism, hypogonadotropic hypogonadism) and cardiac (left ventricular dysfunction and myocarditis) dysfunction, and bone deformities because of expansion of bone marrow, especially in those who are not transfused regularly.
- Bone marrow transplantation is now another option for these patients.
- Pregnancy is very rare in women with β-thalassaemia major, but is more likely in those with less iron overload who have survived without regular transfusion and in those who have received adequate iron chelation therapy.

Diagnosis

- The diagnosis of α- or β-thalassaemia trait may be suspected by finding a low MCV (usually <70), a low MCH (<27 pg), often no anaemia and a normal MCHC (as distinct from iron deficiency when all the indices are reduced).
- The diagnosis is confirmed by globin chain synthesis studies, DNA analysis or, in the case of β-thalassaemia, raised concentrations of HbA_2 and HbF (excess α-chains combined with δ- or γ-chains due to the lack of β-chains).

Management

- Women with α- or α-thalassaemia trait need iron and folate oral supplements throughout pregnancy, but should not be given parenteral iron.
- If both parents have $α^0$- or α-thalassaemia trait, the woman should be referred for prenatal diagnosis because there is a risk that the fetus may have α- or α-thalassaemia major.
- If anaemia does not respond to oral iron and folate, i.m. folate may be given, but transfusion may be required prior to delivery.
- In the rare pregnancies in women with β-thalassaemia, iron chelation therapy with desferrioxamine should be stopped and folate supplementation given. It is also important to check endocrine and cardiac status, preferably prior to pregnancy.

Thrombocythaemia

Incidence

Essential thrombocythaemia (ET), causing an isolated thrombocytosis, is a myeloproliferative disorder and is rare in women of child-bearing age.

Clinical features

The high platelet count may be associated with both haemorrhagic and thromboembolic manifestations. Thromboses may be arterial or venous, as well as platelet-mediated transient occlusions of the microcirculation. Cerebrovascular, coronary, and peripheral circulations are involved.

Pathogenesis

Some patients with ET carry the JAK2 V617F mutation.

Diagnosis

- The diagnosis is usually made pre-pregnancy.
- A high platelet count may also be discovered during pregnancy in women who have undergone traumatic or therapeutic splenectomy, especially if they are also anaemic.
- Other typical features will accompany the thrombocytosis on blood film examination.
- Differential diagnosis includes infection and inflammation and postsurgical acute phase response.

Effects of thrombocythaemia on pregnancy

Women with ET have an increased risk of adverse pregnancy outcome, including FGR, possibly related to placental thrombosis.

Management

- The platelet count may fall and even normalise spontaneously in pregnancy.
- If the count is $>600 \times 10^9/L$, treatment with low-dose aspirin (75 mg/day) is warranted. This inhibits platelet aggregation and thrombosis.
- Interferon-α is also used for myelosuppression in this condition, and this may be safely continued or instituted in pregnancy.
- Outside pregnancy cytotoxic agents such as hydroxycarbamide (hydroxyurea) are used for myelosuppression, but these should be avoided in pregnancy. Anagrelide hydrochloride is an orally active quinazinolone derivative developed as a novel antiplatelet drug. There are insufficient data to recommend its use in pregnancy.
- Hydroxycarbamide and/or anagrelide should ideally be gradually withdrawn three to six months prior to conception and substituted by interferon-α if necessary.
- Low-molecular-weight heparin (LMWH) is used in addition if there is a previous history of thrombosis.

Thrombocytopenia

Causes of thrombocytopenia in pregnancy

- Spurious result (reduced platelets on automated Coulter counter because of platelet clumping or misreading of large immature platelets as red cells)
- Gestational thrombocytopenia
- Immune thrombocytopenic purpura (ITP)
- Pre-eclampsia and Haemolysis, Elevated Liver enzymes and Low Platelets (HELLP) syndrome (see Chapter 1, p. 6)
- Disseminated intravascular coagulation (DIC) (see later)
- Sepsis
- Haemolytic uraemic syndrome (HUS)/thrombotic thrombocytopenic purpura (TTP) (see later)
- Human immunodeficiency virus (HIV), drugs and infections (e.g. malaria) (see Chapter 15, pp. 259 and 267)
- Systemic lupus erythematosus (SLE) and antiphospholipid syndrome (APS) (see Chapter 8, pp. 135 and 140)

- Bone marrow suppression.
- ITP and gestational thrombocytopenia are considered in this section.

Incidence

- Five to ten percent of pregnant women may have thrombocytopenia at term, but at least 75% of these women have 'pregnancy-associated' or 'gestational' thrombocytopenia.
- Chronic ITP usually affects young women (female to male ratio = 3:1) and is quite commonly encountered in pregnancy, with an estimated incidence of 1 to 2 in 10,000 pregnancies.
- Alloimmune thrombocytopenia is a fetal disorder caused by fetomaternal incompatibility for platelet antigens (similar to Rhesus haemolytic disease of the newborn). There are no maternal symptoms and the mother is not thrombocytopenic. The condition develops in utero, affects all children including the firstborn, but is usually (except in the case of subsequent siblings) diagnosed after birth. The incidence is approximately 1 in 2000 and it causes approximately 10% of all cases of neonatal thrombocytopenia.

Clinical features

- Gestational thrombocytopenia is a benign condition and even if the platelet count falls to $<100 \times 10^9/L$, there are no adverse consequences for mother or baby.
- Haemorrhage in ITP is unlikely with platelet counts $>50 \times 10^9/L$, and spontaneous haemorrhage without surgery is unlikely with counts $>20 \times 10^9/L$. Patients may present with skin bruising or gum bleeding, but severe haemorrhage is rare.
- Thrombocytopenia documented in the first half of pregnancy is less likely to be due to the pregnancy itself and should alert the clinician to a possible diagnosis of ITP.
- In ITP, there is isolated thrombocytopenia without any associated haematological abnormality. There is no splenomegaly or lymphadenopathy.

Pathogenesis

Gestational thrombocytopenia

The platelet count tends to fall progressively during normal pregnancy and in 5% to 10% of women the count will reach thrombocytopenic levels ($50–150 \times 10^9/L$) by term.

ITP

Autoantibodies against platelet surface antigens cause peripheral platelet destruction by the reticuloendothelial system, particularly the spleen.

Diagnosis

- The diagnosis of ITP is one of exclusion, and should only be made once other causes of thrombocytopenia (see earlier), such as infection and pre-eclampsia, have been excluded.

- In ITP, the bone marrow is normal or megakaryocytic, but a bone marrow examination is not necessary in pregnancy in cases of isolated thrombocytopenia unless it is severe (platelet count $<30 \times 10^9/L$).
- Antiplatelet antibody determination is not readily available and is not helpful in the diagnosis of ITP in pregnancy because the absence of antiplatelet antibodies does not exclude the diagnosis of ITP.

Effect of pregnancy on ITP

Pregnancy does not affect the course of ITP, but anxieties arise around the time of delivery because of possible bleeding associated with vaginal and abdominal delivery and regional anaesthesia and analgesia.

Effect of ITP on pregnancy

- Capillary bleeding and purpura are unlikely with a platelet count of $>50 \times 10^9/L$, and spontaneous mucous membrane bleeding is not a risk with platelet counts $>20 \times 10^9/L$.
- Antiplatelet IgG can cross the placenta and cause fetal thrombocytopenia. Accurate prediction of the fetal platelet count from the maternal platelet count, antibody level or splenectomy status is not possible, so it is difficult to predict which fetuses will be affected.
- The level of risk to the fetus, which has been overestimated in older studies, is small, in contrast to the fetal risk in alloimmune thrombocytopenia.
- The risk of fetal platelet counts $<50 \times 10^9/L$ is approximately 5% to 10%, although it may be higher (10–15%) in women known to have ITP before pregnancy and in those with symptomatic ITP in the index pregnancy.
- The incidence of antenatal or neonatal intracranial haemorrhage in women with ITP is however only 0% to 1.5%, and is lowest in the absence of maternal symptoms or a history of ITP prior to the index pregnancy.
- One of the best predictors of severe neonatal thrombocytopenia is a previously affected child, and the incidence of serious haemorrhage in the fetus and neonate is low.

Management

Gestational thrombocytopenia

This benign condition requires no intervention.

ITP

Maternal considerations
- Exclude associated conditions such as SLE or APS.
- The platelet count should be monitored monthly and then more frequently in the third trimester so that therapy can be instituted if required prior to delivery.
- Treatment is only required in the first and third trimesters if:
  - The woman is symptomatic with bleeding
  - The platelet count is $<20 \times 10^9/L$
  - The count needs to be increased prior to a procedure such as chorionic villous sampling (CVS).

- Counts $<50 \times 10^9$/L, even in the absence of bleeding, probably warrant prophylactic treatment prior to delivery.
- Counts 50 to 80×10^9/L may warrant treatment prior to delivery in order to facilitate safe administration of regional analgesia/anaesthesia.
- Caesarean section is only required for obstetric indications and epidural and spinal anaesthesia is safe with stable counts >75 to 80×10^9/L. The bleeding time does not predict haemorrhage and is not indicated.
- Corticosteroids are the first-line therapy, and although high doses (60–80 mg/day, 1 mg/kg/day) of prednisolone are usually given for newly diagnosed ITP outside pregnancy, in pregnancy it is common to use lower doses (20–30 mg/day), which are safe and effective. Following this, the dose may be weaned to the lowest that will maintain a satisfactory ($>50 \times 10^9$/L) maternal platelet count.
- I.v. immunoglobulin (IVIg) may be used in resistant cases, in women likely to require prolonged therapy, in women requiring a high maintenance dose of prednisolone or in those who are intolerant of prednisolone.
- IVIg is thought to work by delaying clearance of IgG-coated platelets from the maternal circulation. The response is more rapid (24–48 hours) than with steroids, and lasts for two to three weeks, but IVIg is expensive and seldom produces long-term remission. It is useful in pregnancy if a rapid response is required.
- Possible dose regimes would be 0.4 g/kg/day for five days or 1 g/kg over eight hours, repeated two days later if there is an inadequate response.
- Anti-D immunoglobulin therapy given as an intravenous bolus may help raise platelet counts in non-splenectomised rhesus-positive women. It is thought to work by creating a decoy to competitively inhibit the destruction of antibody-coated platelets.
- Doses are 50 to 70 μg/kg. It has been shown to be safe and effective in the second and third trimesters. The baby should be monitored for neonatal jaundice, anaemia, and direct antiglobulin test positivity after delivery.
- Splenectomy should be avoided in pregnancy if possible, but may be necessary in extreme cases. Ideally it should be performed in the second trimester and can at this stage be performed laparoscopically. Women with ITP who have previously been treated with splenectomy should continue penicillin prophylaxis throughout pregnancy.
- Other options for women who fail to respond to oral prednisolone and IVIg include i.v. methylprednisolone, azathioprine or ciclosporin. Although not recommended, danazol and vincristine have been successfully used for severe resistant cases in pregnancy.
- Platelet transfusions are given as a last resort for bleeding or prior to surgery; they will increase antibody titres and do not result in a sustained increase in platelet counts.

Fetal considerations
- The transfer of IgG increases at the end of pregnancy and the baby is not at risk of bleeding before labour and delivery, so there is no place for serial fetal blood samples earlier in gestation.
- Caesarean section is only indicated for obstetric reasons. The risk of fetal blood sampling via cordocentesis (cord spasm, haemorrhage from the cord puncture site) is similar (or even higher in thrombocytopenic fetuses) to the risk of intracerebral haemorrhage (ICH). There is no conclusive evidence that caesarean section reduces the incidence of ICH, or that it is less traumatic for the fetus than vaginal delivery.

■ Cord platelet count is determined immediately after delivery, but the neonatal platelet count only reaches a nadir after two to five days in affected infants, when splenic circulation is established; most hemorrhagic events in neonates occur 24 to 48 hours after delivery at the nadir of the platelet count. Therefore monitoring is necessary over this time. IVIg is the recommended treatment for neonates with bleeding or severe thrombocytopenia; this may be given prophylactically if the platelet count of the cord blood is low (<20 × 10^9/L).

Immune thrombocytopenia—points to remember

■ The diagnosis of ITP is one of exclusion and should only be made once other causes of thrombocytopenia (see p. 248) have been excluded.
■ Bleeding is unlikely if the platelet count is >50 × 10^9/L.
■ The risk of serious thrombocytopenia and haemorrhage in the neonate from transplacental passage of antiplatelet IgG is low.
■ Caesarean section is only required for obstetric indications and epidural and spinal anaesthesia/analgesia are safe with stable counts >75 to 80 × 10^9/L.
■ Treatment, if required, should be with corticosteroids or i.v. immunoglobulin (IVIg).

Disseminated intravascular coagulation

Obstetric causes of DIC

■ Haemorrhage (particularly abruption)
■ Pre-eclampsia, HELLP syndrome
■ Amniotic fluid embolism
■ Sepsis
■ Retention of a dead fetus.

Clinical features

DIC may be asymptomatic or associated with massive haemorrhage depending on the degree.

Pathogenesis

■ Procoagulant substances, such as thromboplastin, phospholipid and those resulting from endothelial injury, are released into the circulation and cause stimulation of coagulation activity with increased production and breakdown of coagulation factors.
■ Consumption of clotting factors and platelets leads to bleeding.
■ Fibrinolysis is stimulated and fibrinogen degradation products (FDPs) interfere with the production of firm fibrin clots, so exacerbating bleeding.

Diagnosis

The in vitro diagnosis of DIC is made by finding:

■ ↑FDPs (these may be elevated postdelivery)
■ ↑Soluble fibrin complexes

- ↓Fibrinogen (fibrinogen concentration is normally elevated in mid- and late pregnancy so a level <2 g/L is highly significant)
- ↓Platelets
- Prolongation of clotting times (thrombin time, activated partial thromboplastin time (APTT), prothrombin time).

Management

Management of DIC can be considered as the treatment of the underlying cause and treatment of haemorrhage and coagulopathy.

- This usually necessitates delivery of the fetus and emptying of the uterus.
- Pregnancy may be prolonged in cases of mild DIC associated with pre-eclampsia at early gestational ages, but such conservative management necessitates very careful monitoring.
- The obstetric patient with massive bleeding should be managed according to pre-defined and agreed protocols in close collaboration with haematology and anaesthetic staff. Guidelines for the management of massive obstetric haemorrhage can be found in the Royal College of Obstetricians and Gynaecologists (RCOG) green top guideline number 52. Adequate monitoring with a central venous pressure line and urinary catheter is essential.

The coagulopathy is treated with the following:

- Fresh frozen plasma (FFP), which contains all the coagulation factors
- Red cells (only needed to replace losses)
- Platelet concentrates (may be given to a bleeding patient if the platelet count is <80 × 10^9/L)
- Cryoprecipitate or recombinant fibrinogen. Use may be considered if there is haemorrhage and the fibrinogen concentration is <1 g/L.
- Recombinant factor VIIa is a powerful but expensive pro-haemostatic tool that may be potentially useful in obstetric haemorrhage.

The coagulation disturbance usually resolves within 24 to 48 hours after delivery, although thrombocytopenia may persist for up to a week postpartum.

Haemophilia and bleeding disorders

von Willebrand disease

Incidence

- This is the most common inherited (usually autosomal dominant) bleeding disorder (incidence approximately 1%).

Clinical features

- von Willebrand disease may present with mucosal bleeding, that is, menorrhagia, epistaxis, bleeding after dental extraction, postoperative or postpartum bleeding and bruising.
- Many asymptomatic milder cases may remain undiagnosed.

Pathogenesis

- von Willebrand factor (vWF) is a large multivalent adhesive protein that has important roles in platelet function and stability of factor VIII. It is required for the binding of platelets to the subendothelium after vessel injury.
- There are several different types of von Willebrand disease (vWD), involving complete or partial deficiency (Type I) of, or defective (Type II) vWF. The result is a defect in primary haemostasis.
- Severe forms also cause reduced levels of factor VIII with haematoma and hemarthrosis.

Diagnosis

- The bleeding time is prolonged. APTT may be prolonged, vWF and factor VIII may be reduced. A functional measure of vWF is obtained with a ristocetin cofactor, although this does not necessarily correlate to the bleeding risk.
- More specialised tests are required to subclassify the type of vWD.

Effect of pregnancy on von Willebrand disease

- Pregnancy may lead to normalisation of vWF and factor VIII levels in Type I vWD, with a fall postpartum.

Effect of von Willebrand disease on pregnancy

- Early in gestation levels of vWF may not have increased sufficiently to prevent bleeding in association with ectopic pregnancy, miscarriage or CVS.
- There is no increased risk of antepartum haemorrhage or miscarriage.
- By the third trimester, vWF and factor VIII levels have increased three- to four-fold so that women with mild to moderate vWD can usually negotiate labour and delivery without the need for therapy.
- Because postpartum the levels of vWF and factor VIII levels fall rapidly, there is an increased risk of primary and secondary postpartum haemorrhage, but severe bleeding problems are largely preventable.

Management

- Women with vWD should be managed in close collaboration with haematologists expert in the care of bleeding disorders.
- It is extremely important to ascertain pre-pregnancy or in early pregnancy the subtype of vWD and whether the disease responds to desmopressin (DDAVP) or not.
- Aspirin and NSAIDs should not be given to women with vWD.
- In some cases, DDAVP given as an intravenous infusion to increase vWF and factor VIII levels may be indicated, for example, prior to procedures, delivery, epidural or caesarean section.
- For women who do not respond to DDAVP, FFP or plasma-derived factor concentrates containing vWF and factor VIII may be used to control or prevent severe bleeding.

Haemophilia

- Haemophilia A (factor VIII deficiency) and haemophilia B (factor IX deficiency) are rare X-linked recessive disorders.
- Prenatal screening may be used to sex the fetus and, if the mutation is known, CVS can confirm an affected male fetus.
- Carriers should have their factor VIII or IX levels measured in early pregnancy and again before delivery.
- Management of delivery must consider the possibility of an affected fetus.
- Some female carriers may be symptomatic, in which case DDAVP or factor VIII concentrates may be indicated for haemophilia A or tranexamic acid or factor IX concentrate for haemophilia B.
- Close liaison with the haemophilia centre is essential.

Haemolytic uraemic syndrome (HUS)/thrombotic thrombocytopenic purpura (TTP)

- TTP and HUS are a continuum. Both are manifestations of a similar mechanism of microvascular platelet aggregation.
- The common features are thrombocytopenia, assumed to be a consequence of platelet consumption at sites of endothelial injury, and microangiopathic haemolytic anaemia.
- If this is systemic and extensive—and especially if there is central nervous system involvement—the disorder is TTP.
- If platelet aggregation is relatively less extensive, with predominantly renal involvement, the disorder is HUS.
- Both TTP and HUS are rare during pregnancy and the puerperium.

Clinical features

- HUS is seen most commonly in the immediate postnatal period. TTP may occur at any time in pregnancy or post partum.
- The classic 'pentad of TTP' is:
  - Microangiopathic haemolytic anaemia
  - Thrombocytopenia
  - Fever
  - Neurological manifestations
  - Renal impairment/acute kidney injury.
- The clinical features of TTP/HUS may be confused with pre-eclampsia and particularly HELLP syndrome. However, hypertension is not common in TTP/HUS and there is no coagulopathy.
- Features include headache, irritability, drowsiness, seizures, coma and fever.
- The condition is usually severe and associated with increased maternal morbidity and mortality.

Pathogenesis

- These conditions involve a thrombotic microangiopathy, where aggregates of platelets reversibly obstruct the arterioles and capillaries.

- The association with pregnancy may perhaps be due to the formation of endothelial cell autoantibodies associated with immune dysregulation during pregnancy.
- There is diffuse vascular endothelial insult. Endothelial cells secrete unusually large forms of vWF. These large multimers agglutinate platelets.
- TTP is associated with deficiency of a specific vWF-cleaving protease (metalloprotease).
- In non-familial TTP, there is an inhibitor of vWF-cleaving protease (ADAMST-13).
- In familial TTP, there is a constitutional deficiency of vWF-cleaving protease.
- In HUS there is no deficiency.
- It is likely that TTP/HUS are both on a continuum with pre-eclampsia and HELLP syndrome, as all conditions are characterised by widespread endothelial cell injury. In some cases HELLP syndrome may 'evolve' into HUS.

Diagnosis

- Microangiopathic haemolytic anaemia with red cell fragments (schistocytes) on the blood film.
- Thrombocytopenia, which may be severe.
- Depending on the degree of haemolysis, there is anaemia, increased reticulocytes and increased unconjugated bilirubin and lactate dehydrogenase.
- In HUS, there is impaired renal function, which may be severe.
- Clotting times and fibrinogen concentrations are normal. A consumptive coagulopathy (DIC) is rare in HUS/TTP, unless there is associated septicaemia (see also p. 191 for differential diagnosis of thrombocytopenia and acute kidney injury (AKI), and section B, Table 13, for differential diagnosis of abnormal renal function).

Effect of TTP/HUS on pregnancy

The fetus is not affected by TTP/HUS and prognosis is related to the gestational age at delivery.

Management

- There is no evidence that delivery affects the course of TTP and HUS, which is why differentiation from DIC and HELLP syndrome is important (see Chapter 11, p. 206).
- Aggressive treatment with FFP and plasmapheresis may limit vascular injury and improve prognosis.
- Corticosteroids may be of benefit.
- Antiplatelet therapy is also used, but is more controversial.
- Supportive therapy for AKI, which may necessitate dialysis in addition to plasmapheresis.
- Supportive therapy for cerebral involvement, including investigation to exclude other causes of seizures (see Chapter 9, p. 152 and section B, Table 8).
- Platelet transfusions are contraindicated.

Further reading

Furlan M, Robles R, Galbusera M, et al. Von Willebrand factor-cleaving protease in thrombotic thrombocytopenic purpura and the haemolytic-uraemic syndrome. N Engl J Med 1998; 339:1578–1584.

James AH, Kouides PA, Abdul-Kadir R, et al. Von Willebrand disease and other bleeding disorders in women: Consensus on diagnosis and management from an international expert panel. Am J Obstet Gynecol 2009; 201:12.e1–12.e8.

McMahon LP. Iron deficiency anaemia in pregnancy. Obstet Med 2010; 3(1):17–24.

Oteng-Ntim E, Chase AR, Howard J, et al. Sickle cell disease in pregnancy. Obstet Gynaecol Reprod Med 2008; 18:272–278.

Provan D, Stasi R, Newland AC, et al. International consensus report on the investigation and management of primary immune thrombocytopenia. Blood 2010; 115:168–186.

Royal College of Obstetricians and Gynaecologists. Postpartum haemorrhage, prevention and management: Guideline No 58. London: Royal College of Obstetricians and Gynaecologists Press, 2009.

Stoltzfus RJ, Dreyfuss MI. Guidelines for the Use of Iron Supplements to Prevent and Treat Iron Deficiency Anemia. International Nutritional Anemia Consultative Group, World Health Organisation, United Nations Children's Fund. Washington: ILSI Press, 1998.

Tupule S, Bewley S, Robinson SE, et al. The management and outcome of four pregnancies in women with idiopathic myelofibrosis. Br J Haematol 2008; 142:480–501.

CHAPTER 15

Human immunodeficiency virus and other infectious diseases

Human immunodeficiency
virus (HIV)
Other viral infections

Listeriosis
Malaria

Human immunodeficiency virus (HIV)

Incidence

- The incidence of HIV infection is increasing worldwide; almost 50% of infected adults are women, of which 80% are of child-bearing age.
- Two-thirds of those infected live in sub-Saharan Africa, as do more than three-quarters of women infected. Women and girls make up over three-quarters of young people living with HIV in sub-Saharan Africa.
- Vertical transmission rates vary from <2% in the United Kingdom to 45% in sub-Saharan Africa (see later).
- Approximately 83,000 people were HIV positive in the United Kingdom at the end of 2008. Almost 30% were unaware of their infection.
- Approximately 7000 new diagnoses are made in the United Kingdom every year, of which 36% are women. Approximately 30% of people diagnosed with HIV are diagnosed late when treatment should have begun (CD4 cell count less than 200 per mm^3).
- Approximately 55% of people diagnosed with HIV in 2007 acquired their infection through heterosexual contact and of these nearly 80% were probably infected abroad, mainly in sub-Saharan Africa.
- Continued migration of HIV-infected heterosexual men and women from sub-Saharan Africa is contributing to the increased number of HIV diagnoses in the United Kingdom.

- Diagnoses and deaths from acquired immune deficiency syndrome (AIDS) have fallen and stayed low in the United Kingdom since the introduction of highly active antiretroviral therapy (HAART) in the mid-1990s.
- Prevalence rates in pregnancy vary enormously geographically. In the United Kingdom, anonymous testing shows rates of 0.5% in inner London and 0.1% in the rest of England and 0.05% in Scotland. Much higher rates exist in Zaire (5%), Kenya (13%) and Uganda (30%).
- Prevalence is highest among pregnant women born in sub-Saharan Africa (2.5%) and Central America and the Caribbean (0.53%).
- More than 800 HIV-infected women give birth each year in the United Kingdom.

Clinical features

- Because of advances in drug therapy, HIV infection is now regarded in the developed world as a carrier state or chronic infection.
- Acute, primary infection or seroconversion may be asymptomatic or accompanied by fever, fatigue, lymphadenopathy or rash. This usually occurs two weeks to three months after exposure to the virus.
- A clinically latent phase then follows, lasting (without drug therapy) up to and beyond 10 years. This may cause thrombocytopenia, lymphopenia and anaemia.
- Symptomatic disease includes persistent generalised lymphadenopathy, weight loss, fever, diarrhoea, neurological disease including encephalopathy and neuropathy and a range of opportunistic infections and secondary cancers including:
  - *Pneumocystis* pneumonia
  - Cerebral toxoplasmosis
  - Cytomegalovirus (CMV) retinitis
  - *Mycobacterium tuberculosis* and *Mycobacterium avium-intracellulare*
  - Kaposi's sarcoma
  - Non-Hodgkin's lymphoma
  - Candidiasis
  - *Cryptococcus.*
- In countries that are able to provide it, HAART is life prolonging and provides efficient reduction in viral load. Therefore, HIV-associated morbidity and mortality have declined significantly, although clinical progression continues to occur.

Pathogenesis

The virus is transmitted by three principal routes:

- *Sexual:* Unprotected anal or vaginal intercourse, especially in the presence of genital ulceration.
- *Parenteral* (blood-borne): Sharing of contaminated needles and unscreened blood products.
- *Perinatal:* Vertical transmission (see later) either antepartum, intrapartum or postpartum (breast milk).

Early HIV infection is characterised by a high viral load. The main target of HIV is the CD4 lymphocyte population and lymphocytes are gradually lost during the latent phase. Loss of CD4 lymphocytes reduces both cell-mediated immunity and humoral immunity, leading to the development of infections and allowing more rapid replication of HIV.

Diagnosis

- The HIV antibody test detects an antibody to part of the viral membrane or envelope.
- The test usually becomes positive within three weeks to three months after exposure, as levels of p24 antigen are falling.
- Viral DNA and RNA detection are possible with the polymerase chain reaction (PCR).
- The hallmark of HIV infection is the progressive decline in CD4 lymphocyte count, which without treatment falls by approximately 60 cells/mm^3/year.
- The CD4 count indicates the current degree of immunosuppression.
- The viral load (HIV-RNA) is the main predictor of the speed of disease progression. Other correlates of disease progression are low levels of p24 antibodies and recurrence of p24 antigen.
- Transplacental transfer of maternal HIV antibody may persist for up to 18 months, making true HIV status of the infant difficult to determine without the use of PCR.
- The standard for diagnosis of HIV infection in exposed infants is viral assays [HIV-DNA PCR (preferred), HIV-RNA PCR or viral culture] obtained within 48 hours of birth, one to two months and three to six months of age.

Screening

- Although up to 1 in 200 pregnant women in inner London may be HIV positive, only 20% to 30% are aware of their status.
- There are interventions of proven efficacy available during pregnancy to decrease the risk of vertical transmission (see later).
- It is important that at-risk infants are identified to allow for careful monitoring, prophylaxis and early treatment of infection.
- Knowledge of HIV status may influence women's plans regarding pregnancy.
- Early treatment of HIV-positive women improves long-term outcome.
- Knowledge of HIV status allows for protection of sexual partners.
- High-risk groups of women include:
  - I.v. drug users
  - Sex workers
  - Haemophiliacs
  - Women from sub-Saharan Africa
  - Partners of individuals in any of the above groups or of men who have sex with men (MSM).
- Policies of selective screening of high-risk women have failed.
- National policy is to offer and recommend HIV screening in early pregnancy to all women, and to make such testing an integral and accepted part of antenatal care. Extensive pre-test counselling is now less relevant with the advent of HAART and improved prognosis. No special counselling is required and all doctors and midwives should have the counselling skills to offer an HIV test.

- The proportion of infected pregnant women diagnosed before delivery has increased and has been more than 95% since 2005. Uptake of HIV testing in antenatal clinics was 95% in 2008.

Pregnancy

Effect of pregnancy on HIV disease

- Pregnancy probably does not have a major adverse effect on HIV progression in asymptomatic women.
- Women with advanced disease are at high risk of deterioration in the short term, but this is probably not accelerated by pregnancy.
- Opportunistic infection in pregnancy may be less aggressively investigated or treated because of concerns regarding the fetus, and this may indirectly worsen prognosis for the HIV-infected mother. Many of the symptoms may mimic symptoms of pregnancy (e.g. breathlessness). This is more likely if HIV status is unknown and HIV positivity unsuspected.
- Normal pregnancy is associated with a depression of cell-mediated immunity and a fall in the CD4 lymphocyte count, although the percentage of CD4 cells is unchanged. Similar changes occur in HIV-infected pregnant women.
- There is no evidence to suggest that pregnancy increases the risk of progression to AIDS, or a fall in CD4 count to $<200/mm^3$.

Effect of HIV on pregnancy

There is some evidence for an association between HIV (especially if advanced) and an increased risk of:

- Miscarriage
- Preterm delivery
- Fetal growth restriction (FGR)/low birthweight.

The rate of congenital abnormalities is not increased, and data available for HAART from United Kingdom, European and International AntiRetroviral Pregnancy Registries do not suggest an increased risk of congenital malformations.

- In the United Kingdom, Europe and United States, asymptomatic HIV infection probably does not increase perinatal mortality, but in developing countries there is evidence of an increased risk.
- Data from Africa suggest a detrimental effect of HIV infection on birthweight, preterm delivery and perinatal mortality.
- The reduction in birthweight is not related to the infant's HIV status, but to the stage of maternal disease.
- The most dramatic effect on pregnancy outcome is related to advanced disease and recurrent infections with poor nutritional status.

Vertical transmission

Rates of vertical transmission without prophylactic therapy vary:

- Fifteen to twenty-five in the United Kingdom and Europe

- Fifteen to thirty percent in the United States
- Twenty-five to forty-five percent in sub-Saharan Africa.

Transmission of HIV from mother to child may occur:

- In utero (antepartum)
- Through exposure to maternal blood and bodily fluids at the time of delivery (intrapartum)
- By breastfeeding (postpartum).

Two-thirds of vertical transmission seems to occur around delivery, but breastfeeding can double the transmission rate (from 15% to 30%), especially if maternal infection is acquired postnatally.

The factors that increase the likelihood of vertical transmission are as follows:

- Maternal viral load (most important risk factor); vertical transmission is 1% if viral load is <1000 copies/mL
- Seroconversion (associated with high viral loads) during pregnancy
- Advanced maternal disease
- Poor immunological status (low CD4 counts and low CD4:CD8 ratios)
- Prolonged rupture of membranes (>4 hours); doubles the risk of transmission
- Preterm labour
- Vaginal delivery
- Antepartum invasive procedures (amniocentesis, chorionic villous sampling, fetal blood sampling)
- Intrapartum invasive procedures (episiotomy, instrumental delivery and fetal scalp electrodes)
- Prematurity (especially <35 weeks)
- Low birthweight
- Breastfeeding; transmission increased by up to 50%
- Mixed breast and bottle-feeding
- Smoking
- Chorioamnionitis; disruption of the placental barrier to infection
- Intercurrent sexually transmitted diseases
- Vitamin A deficiency
- Unprotected sex with multiple partners
- Use of illicit drugs, particularly cocaine
- Hepatitis C infection; this increases the vertical transmission of both infections.

Management

- HIV-positive pregnant women should be jointly managed by an HIV specialist, an obstetrician and a midwife with expertise in managing HIV pregnancy. Liaison with neonatologists, paediatricians and the general practitioner is important.
- Those with CD4 counts <200/mm^3, or those with AIDS and a previous episode of *Pneumocystis* pneumonia, should be given prophylaxis to reduce the risk of *Pneumocystis* pneumonia (see also Chapter 4, p. 68) and to protect against *Toxoplasma* reactivation. Co-trimoxazole (Septrin) is the usual drug and the benefits of its use

outweigh any theoretical risk of folic acid antagonism. Folate 5 mg should be co-prescribed. Nebulised pentamidine is an alternative agent.

Antiretroviral therapy

- The drugs used to prevent vertical transmission will depend on
  - Affordability
  - Whether the woman is already receiving/has already received antiretroviral therapy
  - Resistance testing
  - Acceptability of drug therapy to the woman.
- The following drug regimens have been shown in randomised clinical trials to decrease vertical transmission of HIV:
  - Zidovudine (azidothymidine, AZT) monotherapy (antepartum, intrapartum, neonatally)
  - AZT/lamivudine (3TC) (intrapartum, neonatally)
  - Nevirapaine (intrapartum, neonatally).
- The potential disadvantages of a policy recommending AZT for all HIV-positive pregnancies include the following:
  - Expense (particularly relevant for developing countries)
  - The mother may become less sensitive to AZT when she requires it for control of her own disease
  - Eighty percent of babies will be unnecessarily exposed to AZT and its risks (e.g. anaemia).
- HAART regimens result in optimal reductions in viral load and the risk of perinatal transmission is extremely low (<1%) in women with undetectable plasma viral loads. Very few perinatal HIV infections have been reported in infants exposed to HAART. Therefore, one option is to use HAART to prevent vertical transmission, even if the mother does not need it for her own health.
- AZT or nevirapine prophylaxis (antepartum, intrapartum, neonatally) may be offered as an alternative or in countries where HAART is not available. This reduces vertical transmission from 25% to 8%. If, in addition, delivery is by elective cae-sarean section and the infant is not breastfed, perinatal transmission rates are as low as <2%.
- In the United Kingdom, approximately 50% of women previously diagnosed with HIV are receiving antiretroviral therapy (ART) at conception. An HIV-positive woman considering pregnancy should be advised to commence ART if her immu-nity is reducing or she is approaching the levels for initiation of ART recommended by the British HIV Association. Initiation of HAART is also recommended before the CD4 count falls below 200 and in any individual with a confirmed CD4 count <200 cells/mm^3 at diagnosis.
- If a woman becomes pregnant whilst on HAART, she should normally continue this treatment if it is maintaining her viral load at an undetectable level. However, the drugs may need to be changed if the regime includes a teratogenic drug, for example, Efavirenz or Didanosine.
- If women require treatment in pregnancy for their own health, they should be commenced on HAART, which includes AZT. Most previously untreated or undi-agnosed women start ART in pregnancy usually between 23 and 30 weeks gestation. One of the benefits of combination therapy given at the start of the third trimester

is that by the time of delivery the viral load may be suppressed below the current sensitive detection level of 50 HIV copies per millilitre. This then allows the mother the option of vaginal delivery.

- Antiretroviral drug resistance should be assayed to inform decisions about ART.
- HAART is not without risks. These include the following:
  - Mitochondrial toxicity in children exposed in utero to AZT or AZT/3TC (lamivudine)
  - Maternal lactic acidosis with DDI (Didanosine)
  - Protease inhibitors may increase the risk of gestational diabetes
  - An increased risk of preterm delivery and pre-eclampsia (possibly related to immune reconstitution syndrome)
  - Immune reconstitution inflammatory syndrome (IRIS) results from restored immunity to specific infectious or non-infectious antigens when patients start ART. Potential mechanisms for the syndrome include a partial recovery of the immune system or exaggerated immunological responses to antigenic stimuli. It is characterised by a paradoxical worsening of a known condition or the appearance of a new condition after initiating ART. The infectious pathogens most frequently implicated in the syndrome are mycobacteria, varicella zoster, herpes viruses and CMV.

Antenatal management

Monitoring antenatally should include regular assessment of

- Viral load every one to two months and at 36 weeks
- CD4 count
- Liver function tests
- Lactate
- Glucose tolerance test to screen for gestational diabetes (GDM).

Intrapartum management

- Elective caesarean section has been shown to reduce perinatal HIV transmission. This is of most benefit in women with high viral loads.
- There is no evidence that caesarean section reduces vertical transmission if performed after the onset of labour or after rupture of the membranes.
- HIV-infected women have higher rates of postoperative complications.
- In women receiving HAART, or with very low or undetectable viral loads, it is possible that elective caesarean section does not reduce what is already a low transmission risk.
- A blanket policy of caesarean section for all HIV-positive women is not appropriate, but HIV status should be added to the equation when considering mode of delivery for obstetric, medical and patient preference indications.
- Women should be informed of available data concerning reduction of transmission with elective caesarean section.
- Vaginal delivery is now offered to women on optimal HAART with undetectable viral loads for four to six weeks prior to delivery.
- Gloves, aprons and face protection should be employed during delivery. Early artificial rupture of the membranes, application of fetal scalp electrodes and fetal scalp sampling should be avoided.

Postnatal management

- Early cord clamping and early bathing of the baby may reduce the risk of transmission.
- In the developed world, where mortality from formula feeding is extremely low, women should be strongly advised not to breastfeed. In developing countries, the risks of not breastfeeding may outweigh the risk of transmission of HIV in breastmilk.
- All babies born to HIV-positive women should be followed up by a paediatrician. Virus culture and PCR are the most reliable techniques for determining infection during the first two months of age in non-breastfed children. Conventional antibody tests cannot be used owing to the persistence of placentally transferred maternal IgG.

Human immunodeficiency virus—points to remember

- HIV testing should be freely and easily available both before and during pregnancy. All women should be offered routine HIV testing in early pregnancy.
- Pregnancy probably does not have a major adverse effect on HIV progression in asymptomatic women.
- Advanced HIV infection may adversely influence pregnancy outcome.
- The risk of vertical transmission in untreated women varies geographically from 15% to 45% and is largely due to intrapartum exposure. It is mostly dependent on maternal viral load, and rare with use of HAART.
- Women should be offered prophylactic HAART or AZT therapy to decrease perinatal transmission.
- In the developed world, HIV-positive women should be strongly advised not to breastfeed.

Other viral infections

Hepatitis viruses and herpes simplex virus are discussed in Chapter 11, p. 194. Varicella zoster is discussed in Chapter 4, p. 67.

- The majority of maternal viral infections cause little harm to the fetus. Those that may infect or damage the fetus are shown in Table 15.1.
- Three viruses that may be transmitted to the fetus and cause birth defects are varicella zoster, rubella and CMV.
- Viruses that may increase the rate of miscarriage, stillbirth or perinatal death, or cause neonatal illness and congenital infection, include rubella, CMV, herpes, varicella zoster, hepatitis E, mumps, polio, coxsackie B, parvovirus B19, Japanese encephalitis and Lassa fever.

Listeriosis

Incidence

- This is uncommon, but important due to the potentially serious outcome in pregnancy.
- Pregnant women and the immunocompromised are at increased risk.

Table 15.1 – Viruses that may infect or damage the fetus

Virus	Congenital defects	Other manifestations	Comments	Trimester of risk
Rubella	FGR, ocular defects (cataracts, glaucoma, microphthalmia) Congenital heart defects (pulmonary stenosis, ventricular septal defect, patent ductus arteriosus), sensorineural hearing loss, microcephaly, mental retardation	Transient hepatosplenomegaly, jaundice, haemolytic anaemia, thrombocytopenic purpura Diabetes Continuing viraemia	Maternal infection symptomatic in 50–70%. Maculopapular rash, lymphadenopathy, arthritis; incubation 14–21 days; infectivity 7 days before to 7 days after appearance of rash	First trimester (most fetuses affected) Some risk 13–16 weeks (sensorineural deafness) Very little risk after 16 weeks
CMV	Ventriculomegaly, microcephaly, hepatosplenomegaly, jaundice, FGR, thrombocytopenia, chorioretinitis, intracranial calcification	Psychomotor retardation, sensorineural hearing loss Continuing viraemia	Maternal infection usually subclinical 50–60% of women in United Kingdom already immune Risk of fetal damage if mother infected = approximately 4%	All trimesters Virus detectable in amniotic fluid but most infected fetuses not affected
Varicella	Hypoplasia/aplasia of single limbs with cicatrisation of skin, deafness, psychomotor retardation, ocular abnormalities, microcalcification of liver and spleen	20% risk of neonatal varicella infection if mother develops clinical chickenpox 5 days before to 2 days after birth	Incubation 14–21 days Infectivity is from 1 day prior to eruption of the rash to 6 days after the rash disappears	All trimesters Highest risk = 13–20 weeks (2% risk of embryopathy)
Polio	No	Fetal death and neonatal disease	Rare in United Kingdom because of routine immunisation	
Coxsackie	No	Myocarditis, meningoencephalitis, neonatal sepsis	Maternal infection often subclinical May cause aseptic meningitis or Bornholm disease	
Parvovirus B19	No	Miscarriage, hydrops fetalis and anaemia, fetal death	Maternal infection similar to rubella with rash (erythema infectiosum), arthralgia and fever	

Clinical features

The mother may be asymptomatic or have a febrile flu-like illness. Features include the following:

- Headache
- Malaise
- Backache
- Abdominal/loin pain (there may be concomitant urinary tract infection)
- Pharyngitis
- Conjunctivitis
- Diarrhoea.

Maternal infection may be severe and lead to adult respiratory distress syndrome.

Pathogenesis

- Food-borne infection of *Listeria monocytogenes* in humans is decreased by careful attention to food hygiene.
- Pregnant women should be advised to avoid certain high-risk foods such as unpasteurised dairy products (soft, ripened cheeses) and paté.

Diagnosis

- A high index of suspicion is needed.
- Diagnosis is made by culture of gram-positive bacilli, *L. monocytogenes* in blood, placenta, meconium-stained liquor or from samples from the neonate.

Effect of listeriosis on pregnancy

- Listeriosis may cause mid-trimester miscarriage, preterm labour and meconium.
- If the infant survives, perinatal listeriosis is common and indeed may be the first pointer to maternal infection.
- Transplacental passage of *L. monocytogenes* and congenital listeriosis is also recognised.

Management

Prolonged high doses of parenteral therapy may be required in maternal and perinatal infections. I.v. ampicillin and gentamicin should be given until one week after the fever subsides. Amoxycillin and erythromycin have also been used.

Malaria

Incidence

- Prevalence is high in India, South-East Asia, Africa and South America.
- There are approximately 2000 cases reported in the United Kingdom annually to the malaria reference laboratory.

- Most U.K. cases occur in those who have travelled to or emigrated from malarious areas.
- *Plasmodium falciparum* is responsible for the most severe disease and nearly all mortality because of malaria.
- Pregnant women with little or no immunity, such as those from non-endemic areas, are at increased risk of developing severe disease compared with non-pregnant women. Their maternal and perinatal mortality rates are increased.
- Immunity to malaria is altered by pregnancy. In endemic countries, malaria is a particular problem in primigravidae who have higher rates of parasitaemia. The risk of malaria decreases with successive pregnancies.
- More than 40% of cases of severe anaemia in pregnancy may be prevented by use of effective anti-malarials in pregnant women in endemic areas.

Clinical features

The predominant features are fever, rigors, nausea, abdominal pain and headache. Severe disease in pregnancy includes the following:

- Hypoglycaemia
- Severe haemolytic anaemia
- Pulmonary oedema
- Hyperpyrexia
- Cerebral malaria
- Acute kidney injury (AKI).

Pathogenesis

- Malaria is a protozoan infection caused by *P. falciparum, P. vivax, P. malariae* or *P. ovale.*
- Transmission occurs through the bite of an infected female *Anopheles* mosquito.
- In pregnancy, parasites sequester in the placenta, where infection may be very heavy.

Diagnosis

- This is made by detection of parasites on a peripheral blood smear.
- Peripheral parasitaemia >2% should be regarded as severe disease.
- In immune women, peripheral films may be negative despite heavy placental infection.
- New antigen-based rapid diagnostic tests may overcome this problem.

Effects of malaria on pregnancy

- Malaria increases the risk of second trimester miscarriage, preterm labour and low birthweight. The low birthweight may be because of prematurity or FGR, possibly secondary to placental sequestration.
- Malarial parasites may be detected in placentae and congenital malaria is seen in 1% to 4% of non-immune-infected mothers and can result from transplacental spread or maternal–fetal transmission at parturition.

- Parasites are usually rapidly cleared, probably because the neonate has passive immunity.
- Babies born to non-immune women with untreated or incompletely treated malaria may be severely affected. Parasite clearance should be the aim prior to delivery.

Management

- Pregnant women with malaria should be admitted for treatment due to their increased risk of hypoglycaemia and severe disease.
- Immune women (i.e. those who have arrived recently from endemic areas) without severe disease may be managed as outpatients. Immigrants from sub-Saharan Africa who have lived in the United Kingdom and return intermittently to Africa are likely to be non-immune.
- Haemoglobin and platelet count should be checked regularly.
- Blood glucose should be checked initially and two-hourly when quinine is first commenced.

Antimalarials

- Prophylaxis and treatment depend on the plasmodium type and the local pattern of drug resistance. Expert advice should always be sought.
- Chloroquine is the drug of choice for *P. vivax*, *P. malariae* and *P. ovale*, provided the woman is not ill. Chloroquine is safe for use in pregnancy.
- Quinine is the drug of choice for *P. falciparum*. There is a particular risk of severe hypoglycaemia. Oral therapy is 10 mg/kg t.d.s. for a minimum of five days until clearance of parasitaemia. I.v. therapy is 20 mg/kg over four hours followed by 10 mg/kg over four hours t.d.s.
- A single treatment dose of pyrimethamine-sulphadoxine (Fansidar®) is given following parasite clearance. Folate supplementation (10 mg/day) should be given to pregnant women receiving proguanil or pyrimethamine, which are folate antagonists, and these should be avoided in the first trimester. Alternative treatments include amodiaquine.
- Mefloquine, used for quinine-resistant malaria and prophylaxis, has caused teratogenesis in animals and should be avoided in the first trimester. Antimalarial drugs that should not be used in pregnancy include halofantrine, tetracycline/doxycycline and primaquine.
- Pregnant women should be discouraged from travelling to malaria-endemic areas. Proguanil and chloroquine are probably the safest drugs used for malarial prophylaxis.
- Immigrant women resident in the United Kingdom wishing to return to a malarial-endemic area should be counselled regarding the likely decline in their immunity.

Further reading

BHIVA. Management of HIV Infection in Pregnant Women. London, 2008. http://www.bhiva.org/PregnantWomen2008.aspx. Accessed March 2010.

Dorman E, Shulman C. Malaria in pregnancy. Curr Obstet Gynaecol 2001; 10(4):181–189.

Health Protection Authority (HPA). HIV in the United Kingdom: 2009 Report. London, 2009.

McIntyre J. Preventing mother-to-child transmission of HIV: Successes and challenges. BJOG 2005; 112:1196–1203.

Mercey D, De Ruiter A. Human immunodeficiency virus in pregnancy. Obstet Gynaecol Reprod Med 2009; 19:75–79.

Drugs to avoid in pregnancy

Absolutely contraindicated	Page reference	Relatively contraindicated	Page reference
Cytotoxic drugs Methotrexate Cyclophosphamide Busulphan	134	Psychotropic drugs Lithium	
Vitamin A analogues Acitretin Isotretinoin	232	**Anticoagulant drugs** Warfarin	48
Cardiovascular drugs ACE inhibitors, e.g. enalapril ARBs (angiotensin II receptor blockers), e.g. losartan Spironolactone	13 122	**Cardiovascular drugs** β-blockers (atenolol in first trimester) Minoxidil	12
Antifungal drugs Griseofulvin Ketoconazole Itraconazole Fluconazole Terbinafine		**Antibiotics** Tetracycline, doxycycline Ciprofloxacin Chloramphenicol Trimethoprim (first trimester) Nitrofurantoin (near term)	67, 178
Antihelminthic drugs Mebendazole		**Antileprobic drugs** Dapsone (third trimester)	
Anti-inflammatory drugs NSAIDs (late third trimester) COX-2 inhibitors Colchicines	131	**Anticonvulsant drugs** Phenobarbitone Phenytoin Sodium valproate Carbamazepine Lamotrigine	154
Endocrine drugs Radioactive iodine Sex hormones Octreotide	99	**Endocrine drugs** Carbimazole Propylthiouracil Chlorpropamide	98

Absolutely contraindicated	Page reference	Relatively contraindicated	Page reference
Other drugs		**Other drugs**	
Thalidomide		Biologics, e.g. etanercept,	134
Mefloquine (first trimester) and	269	infliximab, adalimumab	
primaquine			
Bisphosphonates			
Misoprostol			
Statins and fibrates	35		
Tamoxifen			
Nicotine			
Mycophenolate mofetil	133		
Live vaccines, e.g. MMR, rubella			

ACE, angiotensin-converting enzyme; NSAIDs, non-steroidal anti-inflammatory drugs; COX-2, cyclo-oxygenase type-2-selective.

- For all the drugs listed above, risks must be balanced against potential benefits.
- The teratogenic potential of some of the drugs classified as 'absolutely contraindicated' is sufficiently high to justify termination of a pregnancy following inadvertent exposure, for example, methotrexate or thalidomide. For others there are theoretical reasons to avoid their use in pregnancy, but they carry a low risk of teratogenesis and therefore there is no justification for termination (e.g. rubella vaccine, simvastatin, ACE inhibitors).
- For the drugs listed as 'relatively contraindicated' there are situations in which their use is appropriate and where no safer alternatives exist, for example, warfarin in women with prosthetic heart valves, propylthiouracil in women with thyrotoxicosis or antiepileptic drugs.
- β-Blockers should not be used as first-line treatment of hypertension, but may be indicated to control tachyarrhythmias, for migraine prophylaxis, thyrotoxicosis, mitral stenosis and in those at risk of aortic dissection. Diuretics should be avoided in the treatment of hypertension but are appropriate in the treatment of pulmonary oedema.

APPENDIX 2

Normal laboratory values in pregnancy/ non-pregnancy

	Non-pregnant	Pregnant	Trimester 1	Trimester 2	Trimester 3
Full blood count					
Hb g/dL	12–15	11–14			
WBC × 10^9/L	4–11	6–16			
Platelets × 10^9/L	150–400	150–400			
MCV fL	80–100	80–100			
CRP g/L	0–7	0–7			
Renal function					
Urea mmol/L	2.5–7.5		2.8–4.2	2.5–4.1	2.4–3.8
Creatinine μmol/L	65–101		52–68	44–64	55–73
K mmol/L	3.5–5.0	3.3–4.1			
Na mmol/L	135–145	130–140			
Uric acid mmol/L	0.18–0.35		0.14–0.23	0.14–0.29	0.21–0.38
24-hr protein g	<0.15	<0.3			
24-hr creatinine clearance mL/min	70–140		140–162	139–169	119–139
LFTs					
Bilirubin μmol/L	0–17		4–16	3–13	3–14
Total protein g/L	64–86	48–64			
Albumin g/L	35–46	28–37			

AST IU/L	7–40		10–28	11–29	11–30
ALT IU/L	0–40	6–32			
GGT IU/L	11–50		5–37	5–43	3–41
ALP IU/L	30–130		32–100	43–135	133–418
Bile acids μmol/L	0–14	0–14			
TFTs					
fT4 pmol/L	9–26		10–16	9–15.5	8–14.5
fT3 pmol/L	2.6–5.7		3–7	3–5.5	2.5–5.5
TSH mU/L	0.3–4.2		0–5.5	0.5–3.5	0.5–4

Abbreviations: ALP, alkaline phosphatase; ALT, alanine aminotransferase; AST, aspartate aminotransferase; CRP, C reactive protein; fT3, freeT3; fT4, free T4; GGT, gamma-glutamyl transpeptidase; LFTs, liver function tests; MCV, mean cell volume; TFTs, thyroid function tests; TSH, thyroid stimulating hormone; WBC, white blood cell.
Source: Adapted from Refs. 1–3.

References

1. Cotzias C, Wong SJ, Taylor E, et al. A study to establish gestation-specific reference intervals for thyroid function tests in normal singleton pregnancy. Eur J Obstet Gynecol Reprod Biol 2008; 137:61–66.
2. Girling JC, Dow E, Smith JH. Liver function tests in pre-eclampsia: Importance of comparison with a reference range derived for normal pregnancy. Br J Obstet Gynaecol 1997; 104:246–250.
3. Burrow GN, Ferris TF. Medical Complications During Pregnancy. 4th ed. Philadelphia: WB Saunders, 1995.

Differential diagnosis of medical problems in pregnancy

Table 1 – Breathlessness

Differential diagnosis	Important clinical features	Investigations
Physiological	Can occur at any stage of pregnancy, but is most common in the last trimester. May be most apparent at rest or when speaking	This is a diagnosis of exclusion, which although common should only be made once the diagnoses below have been considered
Anaemia[§]	May not cause symptoms until severe. May be associated with lethargy	Full blood count
Asthma[‡]	Often associated with cough and/or wheezy breathing Symptoms are usually worse at night and on waking or after exercise	The diagnosis is usually made on the history PEFR may be normal in clinic If there is doubt about the diagnosis, ask the woman to measure her own PEFR at home (morning and night) and look for diurnal variation and morning 'dipping' Response to inhaled bronchodilators is another confirmatory feature
Pulmonary embolus[†]	Onset is usually sudden and associated with pleuritic or central (large pulmonary embolus) chest pain. Worse on exercise and may be associated with haemoptysis. Look for associated sinus tachycardia, raised JVP. A high index of suspicion is needed and this diagnosis should always be considered in a pregnant or postpartum woman with breathlessness and/or chest pain The risk is higher in obese, older women, post-caesarean section or surgery and in those with previous thromboembolism or thrombophilia	ECG (sinus tachycardia, tall peaked p-waves in II) Right heart strain (S_1, Q_3, T_3) may be seen in normal pregnancy) Chest X-ray (often normal but may show pleural effusion, oligaemia, wedge-shaped infarct) Arterial blood gases (hypoxaemia and hypocapnia) The diagnosis should be confirmed with a V/Q lung scan, CTPA or echocardiogram
Cardiac causes	There are many cardiac causes of breathlessness; most are uncommon and only two are discussed here	

Mitral stenosis*	Consider in immigrant women who have never seen a doctor before. Breathlessness is due to pulmonary oedema. Women may have been asymptomatic at the beginning of pregnancy. Ask about orthopnoea, paroxysmal nocturnal dyspnoea and haemoptysis. The mid-diastolic murmur may be difficult to hear. Look for associated sinus tachycardia. Pulmonary oedema in association with mitral stenosis is a particular risk immediately following delivery Nb. Pulmonary oedema may cause wheeze on auscultation 'cardiac asthma'	ECG Echocardiogram Chest X-ray
Peripartum cardiomyopathy*	Most common in the first month after delivery, but can present antenatally. More common in older multiparous black women and with multiple pregnancy, pre-eclampsia or hypertension. Symptoms and signs of biventricular failure, i.e. tachycardia, pulmonary oedema, peripheral oedema. Nb. Pulmonary oedema may cause wheeze on auscultation 'cardiac asthma'	ECG Echocardiogram Chest X-ray
Pneumonia[‡]	Often, but not invariably, associated with productive cough and fever. Do not forget atypical and viral (particularly chickenpox, H1N1) pneumonia	Chest X-ray Sputum culture (include AAFB for TB), throat swab for viral culture Full blood count and blood culture, CRP Serology (acute and convalescent titres) for atypical pneumonia Cold agglutinins (mycoplasma)
Pneumothorax	Consider if there is sudden onset of pleuritic pain and breathlessness immediately following spontaneous vaginal delivery. Look for surgical emphysema	Chest X-ray
Hyperventilation/ anxiety	May be associated with paraesthesiae of hands or around mouth	Arterial blood gases show hypocapnia without hypoxaemia

*See also Chapter 2; [†]see also Chapter 3; [‡]see also Chapter 4; [§]see also Chapter 14.
Abbreviations: AAFB, acid + alcohol-fast bacilli; CRP, C reactive protein; CTPA, CT pulmonary angiogram; ECG, electrocardiogram; JVP, jugular venous pressure; PEFR, peak expiratory flow rate; TB, tuberculosis; V/Q, ventilation/perfusion.

Table 2 – Palpitations

Differential diagnosis	Important clinical features	Investigations
Physiological*	Some pregnant women are more aware of their heart beating due to the increased cardiac output May be most apparent at rest, especially when lying down	None
Ectopic beats	Atrial and ventricular premature beats are common in pregnancy, but have no adverse effects on the mother or fetus Close questioning may reveal the palpitations to be due to a 'thumping' sensation. This results from the large cardiac output associated with a beat that follows a long compensatory diastolic pause following a ventricular premature conducted beat More common at rest. Often relieved by exercise	ECG
Sinus tachycardia	An increase in heart rate of 10–20 b.p.m. is part of the physiological adaptation to pregnancy Women may be aware of a sinus tachycardia that is appropriate, for example following exercise Although a sinus tachycardia may be a feature of normal pregnancy, it requires selective investigation to exclude respiratory (e.g. asthma, pulmonary embolism) or cardiac (e.g. mitral stenosis, peripartum cardiomyopathy) pathology and hypovolaemia, bleeding or sepsis, or any of the following causes	ECG Thyroid function tests Full blood count Arterial blood gases Echocardiogram

Supraventricular tachycardia[†]	Paroxysmal SVT is the commonest arrhythmia encountered in pregnancy. It usually pre-dates the pregnancy but may become more frequent in pregnancy (or rather become more symptomatic)	ECG Holter monitor (24-hour tape)
	It may be due to pre-excitation from accessory pathways such as in Wolff–Parkinson–White syndrome. A new diagnosis of SVT in pregnancy requires investigation	Thyroid function tests Echocardiogram
Thyrotoxicosis[‡]	All cases of documented sinus tachycardia, SVT, or atrial fibrillation or flutter should have thyroid function measured	ECG Thyroid function tests (include free T4)
Phaeochromocytoma[§]	This is rare but dangerous and therefore should be considered in cases where there is associated hypertension, headache, sweating or anxiety	24-hour urinary catecholamines Ultrasound of adrenals
	Attacks may occur while the patient is in the supine position	

*See pp. 19 and 20; [†]see p. 36; [‡]see p. 96. [§]see p. 122.
Abbreviations: ECG, electrocardiogram; SVT, supraventricular tachycardia.

Table 3 – Chest pain

Differential diagnosis	Important clinical features	Investigations
Musculoskeletal	Pain may be related to movement of the arms and torso	None
	There may be localised chest wall tenderness	
	Infection with coxsackie B virus (Bornholm disease) may cause chest wall pain due to involvement of the intercostal muscles	
Gastro-oesophageal reflux*	Pain may be related to eating and is often worse at night due to the recumbent position	None
	Pain is usually retrosternal, 'sharp', 'burning', and may be associated with waterbrash and regurgitation or vomiting	
	Symptoms are generally worse in later pregnancy	
	Pain often responds to antacid medication	
Pulmonary embolism†	Pain may be pleuritic in nature, except with massive pulmonary embolism, causing central chest pain	Chest X-ray
	Onset is usually sudden and associated with breathlessness. There may be associated haemoptysis	ECG
	Look for sinus tachycardia and a raised jugular venous pressure	Arterial blood gases
	A high index of suspicion is needed and this diagnosis should always be considered in a pregnant or postpartum woman with breathlessness and/or chest pain	Ventilation/perfusion lung scan, CTPA or echocardiogram
	The risk is higher in obese, older women, post-caesarean section or surgery and in those with previous thromboembolism or thrombophilia	

Pneumonia/pleurisy[‡]	Pain is usually pleuritic There may be associated fever, cough, sputum or breathlessness Bacterial infections are usually associated with a raised white cell count	Chest X-ray Sputum culture White cell count CRP
Pneumothorax	Pain is pleuritic and associated with breathlessness Consider if there is sudden onset of pleuritic pain and breathlessness immediately following spontaneous vaginal delivery Look for surgical emphysema	Chest X-ray
Acute coronary syndrome/ Ischaemic/cardiac causes[§]	Pain is usually central and 'crushing' with radiation to the neck, jaw or left arm Pain is usually worse on, or precipitated by, exercise Ischaemic heart disease is more common in smokers, diabetes	ECG Chest X-ray Troponin; cardiac enzymes
Aortic dissection[11]	Pain is severe and may radiate to the interscapular area of back. Associated systolic hypertension There may be symptoms or signs from territory supplied by the coronary, carotid, subclavian, spinal or common iliac arteries, or aortic regurgitation	Chest X-ray Chest CT Echocardiogram, chest MRI

*See p. 222; [†]see Chapter 3; [‡]see Chapter 4; [§]see p. 33; [11]see p. 35.
Abbreviations: CRP, C reactive protein; CT, computerised tomography; CTPA, CT pulmonary angiography; ECG, electrocardiogram; MRI, magnetic resonance imaging.

Table 4 – Heart murmur (see also Chapter 2)

Differential diagnosis	Important clinical features	Investigations
Physiological	There is an isolated ejection systolic murmur (ESM) present in up to 95% of pregnant women It is caused by turbulence related to the increased blood volume and cardiac output of pregnancy The murmur may be audible all over the praecordium and into the neck, and sometimes even in the interscapular area Women with an ESM caused by pregnancy do not have a heart murmur when they are not pregnant and this may be ascertained from a careful history of previous medical check-ups	None
Flow murmur	These are also usually ejection systolic murmurs often loudest over the pulmonary area. They are present outside pregnancy but are also innocent Many women have been previously investigated and require no further investigation in pregnancy The differentiation between flow murmurs confined to pregnancy and those present outside pregnancy is not important	None
Structural defect	Auscultatory pointers to a structural lesion include: – a pan-systolic murmur (suggesting a ventricular septal defect or mitral or tricuspid regurgitation – late systolic murmurs (suggesting mitral valve prolapse) – ESM associated with a palpable thrill, additional heart sounds (other than a third heart sound, which is also common in pregnancy), e.g. ejection click of aortic or pulmonary stenosis or opening snap of mitral stenosis – very loud systolic murmurs – any diastolic murmur (requires further investigation with echocardiography) A high index of suspicion with a lower threshold for echocardiography is required in recent immigrants, especially from areas with a high incidence of rheumatic fever, who may never have seen a doctor or been examined prior to pregnancy	Echocardiogram ECG

Abbreviations: ECG, electrocardiogram; ESM, ejection systolic murmur.

Table 5 – Hypertension

Differential diagnosis	Important clinical features	Investigations
White-coat hypertension'	Hypertension only evident when readings are taken by medical/nursing/midwifery staff Often worse in hospital Does not usually settle completely with repeated readings in hospital setting	Home blood-pressure monitoring Ambulatory blood-pressure recording
Essential hypertension*	Hypertension pre-dates the pregnancy or is discovered in early pregnancy A positive family history is common Pre-eclampsia or pregnancy-induced hypertension may be superimposed More common in Afro-Caribbean and older women	Urea + electrolytes + creatinine Urinalysis Appropriate investigations as below to exclude the following conditions
Pregnancy-induced hypertension*	Usually develops after 20 weeks' gestation No associated features of pre-eclampsia Usually settles within 6 weeks postpartum Often recurs in subsequent pregnancies	Urinalysis Full blood count Urea + electrolytes + creatinine Uric acid and liver function tests Ultrasound scan of fetus
Pre-eclampsia*	Usually develops after 20 weeks' gestation Associated features include: proteinuria, hyperuricaemia, thrombocytopenia, raised transaminases, fetal growth restriction, eclampsia, renal impairment Usually settles within 6 weeks postpartum	Urinalysis Full blood count and coagulation screen if platelets <100 × 10^9/l Urea + electrolytes + creatinine Uric acid and liver function tests Ultrasound scan of fetus

(Continued)

Table 5 – *(Continued)*

Differential diagnosis	Important clinical features	Investigations
Renal hypertension[§]	Hypertension associated with renal disease, for example reflux nephropathy, diabetes, glomerulonephritis, polycystic kidney disease, renal artery stenosis May be associated with proteinuria, haematuria, renal impairment, active urinary sediment	Urea + electrolytes + creatinine Urinalysis and microscopy 24-hour urinary protein, protein creatinine ratio Renal ultrasound
Cardiac hypertension[†] Co-arctation of the aorta	Radiofemoral delay or weak femoral pulses may suggest co-arctation of the aorta	Echocardiogram Chest X-ray
Cushing's syndrome[‡]	Hypertension may be associated with excessive weight gain, extensive purple striae, diabetes or impaired glucose intolerance, easy bruising, hirsutism, acne or proximal myopathy	ACTH Cortisol High-dose dexamethasone-suppression test US, CT or MRI of the adrenals MRI or CT of the pituitary
Conn's syndrome[‡]	Hypokalaemia (serum potassium <3.0 mmol/l)	Urea + electrolytes + creatinine Plasma renin Plasma aldosterone US, CT or MRI of the adrenals
Phaeochromocytoma[‡]	Hypertension may be sustained or labile, occurring in paroxysms (50% of cases) associated with palpitations, anxiety, sweating, headache, vomiting or glucose intolerance	24-hour urinary catecholamines US, CT or MRI of the adrenals

*See also Chapter 1; [†]see also Chapter 2; [‡]see also Chapter 7; [§]see also Chapter 10.
Abbreviations: ACTH, adrenocorticotrophic hormone; CT, computerised tomography; MRI, magnetic resonance imaging; US, ultrasound.

Table 6 – Abnormal thyroid function tests*

Pattern of abnormality	Possible diagnoses	Comments/further investigation versus normal non-pregnant ranges in women
↑Total T4 ↑Total T3 Normal free T4 Normal TSH	Normal in pregnancy	Refer to normal ranges for pregnancy
↓Free T4 (mild) ↑TSH (mild)	Normal in third trimester Mild hypothyroidism	Refer to normal ranges for third trimester (Appendix 2) Check thyroid autoantibodies
Normal free T4 ↑TSH	May be normal feature in first trimester May represent 'compensated' or 'sub-clinical' hypothyroidism Treated hypothyroidism possibly with poor compliance	Repeat thyroid function tests in second trimester Check thyroid autoantibodies TSH may remain high in the initial phases of treatment of hypothyroidism
↑Free T4 ↓TSH	May be associated with hyperemesis In the absence of nausea or vomiting, or in association with other symptoms preceding pregnancy, or thyroid eye disease this suggests thyrotoxicosis	Does not require treatment if due to hyperemesis Abnormality resolves with improvement in hyperemesis Check thyroid-stimulating antibodies to help confirm diagnosis of thyrotoxicosis and assess risk of fetal hyperthyroidism
↓TSH ↓Free T4	Secondary (pituitary failure) or tertiary (hypothalamic failure), hypothyroidism or non-thyroidal illness	Secondary and tertiary hypothyroidism are both rare MRI pituitary
Normal free T4 ↓TSH	Treated thyrotoxicosis, possibly with an intermittently compliant patient May be a normal feature in first trimester	TSH remains suppressed in the initial phases of treatment of hyperthyroidism Repeat thyroid function tests in second trimester

*See also Chapter 6 and Appendix 2.
Abbreviations: MRI, magnetic resonance imaging; T3, tri-iodothyronine; T4, thyroxine; TSH, thyroid-stimulating hormone.

Table 7 – Headache

Differential diagnosis	Important clinical features	Investigations
Tension headache[‡]	Often related to periods of stress and may occur daily Features of migraine are usually absent	
Migraine[‡]	Headache is often throbbing, unilateral Prodomal symptoms, usually visual, include: scotoma, fortification spectra Nausea, vomiting, photophobia Transient hemianopia, aphasia, sensory symptoms or hemiplegia may occur but there are no residual physical signs following the attack	
Drug-related headache	Use of vasodilators and calcium antagonists in particular May also occur with persistent use of analgesics	
Epidural-related headache	Headache is often frontal and postural (relieved by lying down) Commonly associated with dural tap (more common with epidural but may occur after spinal) May be associated with neck stiffness, tinnitus, visual symptoms and rarely seizures Onset is usually within 24 hours after siting epidural block	
Hypertension/ pre-eclampsia*	May be severe and associated with flashing lights	Urinalysis Full blood count and coagulation screen if platelets $<100 \times 10^9/l$ Urea + electrolytes + creatinine Uric acid and liver function tests

Differential diagnosis of medical problems in pregnancy

Condition	Features	Investigations
Idiopathic 'benign' intracranial hypertension[‡]	Headache is often retro-orbital More common in obesity Associated with diplopia, papilloedema Cerebrospinal fluid pressure is increased	CT or MRI brain Lumbar puncture
Subarachnoid haemorrhage[‡]	Headache is usually sudden and severe, often occipital Associated vomiting, neck stiffness, loss of (or impaired) consciousness, sudden collapse Papilloedema Focal neurological signs are often, but not invariably, present	CT or MRI Magnetic resonance angiography (MRA) Lumbar puncture if CT normal
CVT[†]	Usually occurs postpartum Associated with seizures, vomiting, photophobia, impaired consciousness and signs of raised intracranial pressure 30–60% of patients have focal signs that may be transient, such as hemiparesis CVT may cause fever and leukocytosis	CT or MRI Venous angiography MRI (MRV) Thrombophilia screen
Meningitis	Features include: malaise, fever, rigors, photophobia, vomiting and neck stiffness Petechial rash suggests meningococcal infection	Blood cultures, CRP CT to exclude raised intracranial pressure prior to lumbar puncture
Space-occupying lesion	Headache may be focal Onset is usually gradual and may be associated with progressive localising signs and/or seizures	CT or MRI

*See also Chapter 1; [†]see also Chapter 3; [‡]see also Chapter 9.

Abbreviations: CRP, C reactive protein; CT, computerised tomography; CVT, cerebral vein thrombosis; MRA, magnetic resonance angiography; MRI, magnetic resonance imaging; MRV, magnetic resonance venography.

Table 8 – Convulsions

Differential diagnosis	Important clinical features	Investigations
Idiopathic epilepsy[§]	Usually a preceding history, but idiopathic epilepsy may occasionally present for the first time in pregnancy	Seizures occurring for the first time in pregnancy should be investigated with
Secondary epilepsy Due to previous surgery, intracranial mass lesions, antiphospholipid syndrome[‡]	APS may be associated with a history of thromboembolism, fetal loss, early onset pre-eclampsia or thrombocytopenia	CT or MRI and EEG Anticardiolipin antibodies Lupus anticoagulant
Eclampsia*	Features of pre-eclampsia may be mild or delayed	Blood pressure Urinalysis Full blood count and coagulation screen if platelets $<100 \times 10^9$/l Urea + electrolytes + creatinine Uric acid and liver function tests
CVT[†]	Usually occurs postpartum Associated with headache, vomiting, photophobia, impaired consciousness and signs of raised intracranial pressure 30–60% of patients have focal signs that may be transient, such as hemiparesis CVT may cause fever and leukocytosis	CT or MRI Venous angiography MRI (MRV) Thrombophilia screen
TTP[11]	The clinical features may be confused with pre-eclampsia, but hypertension is not common in TTP Features may include headache, irritability, drowsiness, coma, fever and renal impairment There is microangiopathic haemolytic anaemia	Full blood count and examination of blood film Coagulopathy is not a feature vWF-cleaving protease (metalloprotease) ADAMTS-13 levels are reduced

288

Condition	Clinical features	Investigations
Ischaemic cerebral infarction or haemorrhagic stroke[§]	Strokes are most common in the first week after delivery Most ischaemic strokes associated with pregnancy are in the distribution of the carotid and middle cerebral arteries Haemorrhagic stroke is relatively more common in pregnancy Associated with eclampsia and ruptured AVMs	CT or MRI Echocardiogram (embolic stoke) Antiphospholipid antibodies
Postdural puncture	Preceded by typical postural headache (relieved by lying down) Associated neck stiffness, tinnitus, visual symptoms Onset usually within 4–7 days after dural puncture	
Drug or alcohol withdrawal	History from relatives/friends Precipitated by admission to hospital	Urine and blood toxicology screen
Metabolic causes: – Hypoglycaemia – Hypocalcaemia – Hyponatraemia	Diabetes, hypoadrenalism, hypopituitarism, liver failure Magnesium sulphate therapy, hypoparathyroidism Hyperemesis	Blood glucose Liver function tests and serum calcium Urea + electrolytes
Non epileptic seizure (NES) disorder[§] These patients often (15%) have epilepsy as well	Useful distinguishing features to differentiate 'psychogenic' NES from organic NES or epilepsy include: – Prolonged/repeated seizures without cyanosis – Resistance to passive eye opening – Down-going plantar reflexes – Persistence of a positive conjunctival reflex Serum prolactin cannot be used to confirm true seizures in pregnancy because it will always be raised	EEG/video telemetry

*See Chapter 1; [†]see Chapter 3; [‡]see Chapter 8; [§]see Chapter 9; [11]see Chapter 14.
Abbreviations: AVM, arteriovenous malformation; CT, computerised tomography; CVT, cerebral vein thrombosis; EEG, electroencephalogram; MRI: magnetic resonance imaging; MRV, magnetic resonance venography; TTP, thrombotic thrombocytopenic purpura.

Table 9 – Dizziness

Differential diagnosis	Important clinical features	Investigations
Postural hypotension	Related to prolonged standing, or standing from sitting or lying position	Lying and standing blood pressure
	Side effect of methyldopa therapy	
Supine hypotension	Occurs late in the second and third trimesters when lying in the supine position	
	Due to pressure of the gravid uterus on the inferior vena cava	
	Relieved by assuming the lateral position	
Labyrinthitis	Vertigo and nystagmus may be reproduced by movement of the head, and particularly moving from a sitting to supine position with the head turned to one side (Hallpike manoevre)	
	May be associated with vomiting	
Cardiac causes:* – Arrhythmia – Aortic stenosis – Hypertrophic cardiomyopathy	May be associated with palpitations, chest pain, breathlessness, or loss of consciousness	ECG Holter monitor (24-hour tape) or event recorder Echocardiogram

*See also Chapter 2.
Abbreviation: ECG, electrocardiogram.

Table 10 – Collapse

Differential diagnosis	Important clinical features	Investigations
Pulmonary embolus*	Massive pulmonary embolism causing collapse may be associated with central chest pain Onset is usually sudden and associated with breathlessness May be associated with haemoptysis, sinus tachycardia, a raised JVP and signs of right heart strain The risk is higher in obese, older women, post-caesarean section or surgery and in those with previous thromboembolism or thrombophilia	Chest X-ray ECG Arterial blood gases Ventilation/perfusion lung scan CTPA Pulmonary angiography or echocardiogram
Amniotic fluid embolus	Typically occurs during or immediately following a precipitous labour with an intact amniotic sac. Predisposing factors include increasing age, hypertonic uterine contractions, uterine stimulants, uterine trauma and induced labour There is profound shock, respiratory distress and cyanosis Severe postpartum bleeding usually follows due to the associated disseminated intravascular coagulopathy	Chest X-ray (shows pulmonary oedema in the absence of any clinical evidence of left ventricular failure) Coagulation studies
Seizure/eclampsia†	Tonic–clonic seizure is usually followed by post-ictal drowsiness	See Table 8 for differential diagnosis of seizure
Haemorrhage *Obstetric, e.g.* – Placental abruption – Postpartum haemorrhage *Non-obstetric, e.g.* – Ruptured congenital aneurysm – dissection of splenic artery	Haemorrhage may be partially or totally concealed May be associated with disseminated intravascular coagulopathy	Full blood count Coagulation studies Fibrinogen

(Continued)

291

Table 10 – *(Continued)*

Differential diagnosis	Important clinical features	Investigations
Ruptured ectopic pregnancy	Presents 4–8 weeks from last menstrual period Associated with pelvic pain and possibly vaginal bleeding	Pelvic ultrasound
Subarachnoid haemorrhage[‡]	Collapse may be preceded by severe, often occipital, headache of sudden onset Associated vomiting, neck stiffness, loss of (or impaired) Consciousness Papilloedema Focal neurological signs are often, but not invariably, present	CT or MRI Magnetic resonance angiography Lumbar pucture
Cerebral haemorrhage or infarction[‡]	Intracerebral haemorrhage may occur in the setting of pre-eclampsia/eclampsia and most cases occur postpartum, although those associated with arteriovenous malformations may present antenatally Most ischaemic strokes associated with pregnancy are in the distribution of the carotid and middle cerebral arteries, and occur in the first week after delivery	CT or MRI
CVT	Usually occurs postpartum Associated with headache, vomiting, seizures, photophobia, impaired consciousness and signs of raised intracranial pressure 30–60% of patients have focal signs such as hemiparesis, which may be transient CVT may cause fever and leukocytosis	CT or MRI Venous angiography MRI (MRV) Thrombophilia screen
Metabolic causes[§]		

*See Chapter 3; [†] see Chapter 1; [‡] see Chapter 9; [§] see Table 8.

Abbreviations: CT, computerised tomography; CVT, cerebral vein thrombosis; ECG, electrocardiogram; JVP, jugular venous pressure; MRI, magnetic resonance imaging; MRV, magnetic resonance venography.

Table 11 – Numbness

Differential diagnosis	Important clinical features	Investigations
Neuropathy (the presentation and causes of polyneuropathies and peripheral neuropathies, for example, diabetes, B12 deficiency, Guillain–Barré syndrome, are no different in pregnancy)	Numbness in distribution of particular nerve or nerve roots, e.g. **Median nerve** (carpal tunnel syndrome) Numbness affects the middle and index fingers and the thumb and may be associated with pain radiating up the forearm Symptoms are often bilateral and worse at night **Facial nerve** (Bell's palsy; see Chapter 9, p. 172) **Lateral cutaneous nerve** of the thigh (meralgia paraesthetica) Commonly presents in the third trimester **Lumbosacral trunk** (especially L4 and L5) Presents postpartum with unilateral foot drop and numbness and/or pain in the distribution of the affected nerve roots More common with large babies, Keilland's forceps delivery and cephalopelvic disproportion	Electrophysiological studies
Migraine*	Sensory symptoms are usually transient and associated with unilateral headache, nausea, vomiting and photophobia. Migraine may present with aura but without headache	
Transient ischaemic attacks	Headache usually absent Attacks last minutes to hours, but always <24 hours A search should be undertaken for a possible embolic source (for example, atrial fibrillation)	Carotid Doppler imaging ECG Echocardiogram
Hyperventilation	Associated with anxiety and panic attacks Numbness in the hands and feet, and peri-oral. May be associated with carpopedal spasm, sweating and dizziness	
Multiple sclerosis*	Patient is usually aware of the diagnosis prior to pregnancy, but relapse involving new symptoms may occur in pregnancy or more commonly postpartum	MRI

*See Chapter 9.
Abbreviations: ECG, electrocardiogram; MRI, magnetic resonance imaging.

Table 12 – Proteinuria

Differential diagnosis	Important clinical features	Investigations
Physiological	Trace or 1+ protein only on dipstick testing may represent <0.3 g/24 hours Trace may be ignored. 1+ protein on urinalysis requires further investigation	MSU and protein creatinine ratio (PCR) or 24-hour protein excretion if ≥1+ on dipstick
Urinary tract infection†	May be associated with symptoms of cystitis or pyelonephritis or be asymptomatic. Urinalysis is positive for nitrites Urine microscopy reveals white cells and possibly red cells A significant growth of organisms on urine culture More common in hyperemesis, diabetes, underlying renal disease, postbladder catheterisation and in those receiving immunosuppressive doses of steroids or azathioprine	Urine microscopy and culture A significant growth is 100 000 organism colonies per ml of urine
Pre-eclampsia*	Usually develops after 20 weeks' gestation Proteinuria is not significant unless >0.3 g/24 hours Associated features include: hypertension, hyperuricaemia, thrombocytopenia, raised transaminases, fetal growth restriction, eclampsia, renal impairment Usually, but not invariably, settles within 6 weeks postpartum	Blood pressure PCR or 24-hour protein excretion Full blood count and coagulation screen if platelets $<100 \times 10^9$/l Urea + electrolytes + creatinine Uric acid and liver function tests
Underlying renal disease†	Proteinuria usually evident at booking or prior to 20 weeks' gestation Features of pre-eclampsia may be absent unless there is superimposed pre-eclampsia Associated underlying conditions include: diabetes, reflux nephropathy, glomerulonephritis and systemic lupus erythematosus Urine microscopy may reveal co-existent microscopic haematuria, an 'active sediment' with red cell casts There may be associated renal impairment, hypoalbuminaemia, anaemia early in pregnancy and/or hypertension May only be recognised when proteinuria associated with pre-eclampsia fails to resolve completely postpartum	Urine microscopy PCR or 24-hour protein excretion Serum creatinine Renal ultrasound Renal biopsy (uncommon in pregnancy) ANA/anti-dsDNA Blood glucose Hepatitis B

*See Chapter 1; †see Chapter 10.

Table 13 – Abnormal renal function

Differential diagnosis	Important clinical features	Investigations
Pre-eclampsia/ HELLP syndrome*	Usually develops after 20 weeks' gestation. Associated features include: hypertension, proteinuria, hyperuricaemia, thrombocytopenia, raised transaminases, fetal growth restriction and eclampsia. Oliguria is common and not usually accompanied by renal impairment. Renal impairment in pre-eclampsia is usually mild but acute kidney injury may develop in 7% of those with HELLP syndrome. Usually, but not invariably, it settles within 6 weeks postpartum May be aggravated or precipitated by NSAIDs	Blood pressure PCR or 24-hour protein excretion Full blood count and coagulation screen if platelets <100 × 10⁹/l Urea + electrolytes + creatinine Uric acid and liver function tests Lactate dehydrogenase
Haemolytic uraemic syndrome†	The clinical features may be confused with pre-eclampsia, but hypertension is less common in HUS and coagulopathy is not a feature. Most common in the immediate postnatal period. There is a microangiopathic haemolytic anaemia, fever and thrombocytopenia, which may be severe Cerebral features including headache, irritability, drowsiness, seizures and coma make a diagnosis of TTP	Full blood count and examination of blood film. Urea + electrolytes + creatinine. vWF-cleaving protease (metalloprotease) ADAMTS-13 levels are normal
Pre-renal failure†	This is most commonly due to blood loss following postpartum haemorrhage or placental abruption, or dehydration secondary to vomiting with or without diarrhoea May be aggravated or precipitated by NSAIDs	Blood pressure Full blood count and coagulation studies if platelets <100 × 10⁹/l Central venous pressure

(Continued)

Table 13 – (Continued)

Differential diagnosis	Important clinical features	Investigations
Infection, e.g. septic abortion, sepsis, rarely acute pyelonephritis	The signs of septic shock may be very similar to those of hypovolaemic shock, and fever and leukocytosis are not always present	Full blood count, CRP Blood cultures Mid-stream urine High vaginal swab, wound swab Ultrasound: uterus, abdomen, kidneys
Postrenal failure	This is most commonly due to ureteric damage at caesarean section or obstruction	Renal US
Underlying renal disease[†]	Usually detected prior to pregnancy or in the first half of pregnancy, when renal function is checked because of hypertension, proteinuria, haematuria or urinary tract infection Features of pre-eclampsia may be superimposed. Associated underlying conditions include: hypertension, diabetes, reflux nephropathy, glomerulonephritis and systemic lupus erythematosus Urine microscopy may reveal proteinuria, microscopic haematuria, an 'active sediment' with red cell casts May only be recognised when renal impairment associated with pre-eclampsia fails to resolve completely postpartum	Urine microscopy PCR or 24-hour urinary protein excretion Renal ultrasound Renal biopsy (uncommon in pregnancy) ANA/anti-dsDNA Blood glucose Hepatitis B

*See Chapter 1; [†]see Chapter 10; [‡]see Chapter 14.
Abbreviations: ANA, anti-nuclear antibodies; CRP, C reactive protein; HELLP, Haemolysis, Elevated Liver enzymes and Low Platelets; HUS, haemolytic uraemic syndrome; NSAIDs, non-steroidal anti-inflammatory drugs; PCR, protein creatinine ratio; TTP, thrombotic thrombocytopenic purpura; vWF, von Willebrand factor.

Table 14 – Pruritus

Differential diagnosis	Important clinical features	Investigations
Physiological (up to 20% of pregnant women)	No rash except possibly excoriations Usually affects lower legs, abdomen Normal liver function tests Presents earlier in pregnancy than obstetric cholestasis	Liver function tests and bile acids
Liver disease*	No rash except possibly excoriations. Associated abnormal liver function tests In some cases of obstetric cholestasis, the only abnormality may be elevated bile acids Women with hepatitis C may develop pruritus for the first time in pregnancy Women with primary biliary cirrhosis or sclerosing cholangitis may experience worsening pruritus in pregnancy	Liver function tests Bile acids Coagulation screen Liver ultrasound Hepatitis serology (including CMV and EBV) Anti-smooth muscle antibodies Anti-mitochondrial antibodies
Skin disease (including drug allergies)†	Obvious rash Normal liver function tests	

*See Chapter 11; † see Chapter 13.
Abbreviations: CMV, cytomegalovirus; EBV, Epstein–Barr virus.

Table 15 – Jaundice/abnormal liver function tests[†]

Differential diagnosis	Important clinical features	Investigations
Obstetric cholestasis[†]	Severe pruritus (especially palms and soles) with onset usually in third trimester There may be associated dark urine, anorexia and malabsorption of fat (and fat-soluble vitamins, e.g. vitamin K) with steatorrhoea Jaundice is rare Moderate elevation in transaminases, alkaline phosphatase and sometimes gamma glutamyl transpeptidase Bile acids are increased Associated with preterm labour, fetal distress, meconium-stained liquor, intrauterine death and postpartum haemorrhage	Liver function tests Bile acids Coagulation screen Other investigations (see below) to exclude other causes of abnormal liver function
Gallstones[‡]	Usually, but not invariably, associated with pain in the right upper quadrant or epigastrium that may radiate through to the back or to the infrascalpular region Nausea, vomiting and indigestion are common Acute cholecystitis may occur at any time in pregnancy and causes more severe pain than biliary colic There is associated tenderness and guarding in the right hypochondrium There may be fever and shock depending on the severity of the gall bladder sepsis	Ultrasound of liver and gall bladder Blood cultures
Viral hepatitis[†]	May present at any gestational period There may be a history of foreign travel, but its absence does not exclude the diagnosis Associated nausea, vomiting, anorexia, fever, malaise and jaundice Moderate-to-severe elevation in transaminases; raised bilirubin	Liver function tests Coagulation screen Hepatitis serology including CMV and EBV

Condition	Clinical features	Investigations
Pre-eclampsia/ HELLP syndrome*	Usually develops after 20 weeks' gestation Associated features include: hypertension, proteinuria, hyperuricaemia, thrombocytopenia, fetal growth restriction, eclampsia, renal impairment and, in the case of HELLP syndrome, epigastric or right upper quadrant pain, nausea and vomiting, tenderness in the right upper quadrant and haemolysis	Blood pressure Protein creatinine ration (PCR) or 24-hour protein excretion Full blood count and coagulation screen if platelets $<100 \times 10^9$/l Blood film Urea + electrolytes + creatinine Uric acid and liver function tests
AFLP†	Associated nausea, anorexia, malaise, vomiting and abdominal pain There are often co-existing features of mild pre-eclampsia, but hypertension and proteinuria are usually mild Hyperuricaemia is often marked and out of proportion to the severity of pre-eclampsia Coagulopathy is often a prominent feature There may be a raised white blood cell count Jaundice usually appears within 2 weeks of the onset of symptoms and there may be ascites Liver function is more deranged than in HELLP syndrome and the woman may develop fulminant liver failure with hypoglycaemia, lactic acidosis, hepatic encephalopathy and renal failure	Blood pressure PCR or 24-hour protein excretion Full blood count and coagulation screen Blood film Urea + electrolytes + creatinine Blood glucose, lactate Uric acid and liver function tests CT or MRI liver
Hyperemesis gravidarum‡	Onset before 12 weeks' gestation Abdominal pain is rare, jaundice very rare Nausea, vomiting, dehydration, profound weight loss, ketonuria Associated 'biochemical thyrotoxicosis' (see Chapter 12) Liver function reverts to normal as hyperemesis improves	Urea + electrolytes Thyroid function tests Liver function tests

(Continued)

Table 15 – (Continued)

Differential diagnosis	Important clinical features	Investigations
Sepsis, e.g. acute cholecystitis, ascending cholangitis, puerperal sepsis	Associated fever, abdominal pain, leukocytosis, tachypnoea	White blood cell count Blood cultures CRP
Drug-induced hepatotoxicity, e.g. methyldopa, azathioprine , chlorpromazine, HAART		
Pre-existing/co-existing liver disease[‡]	These diagnoses are usually made prior to pregnancy	Liver function tests Liver ultrasound
Autoimmune chronic active hepatitis	CAH may present as acute hepatitis or with signs of chronic liver disease and, in the later stages, cirrhosis. Liver function may be markedly deranged. CAH is associated with antibodies to smooth muscle, antinuclear antibodies, and hypergammaglobulinaemia	Anti-smooth-muscle antibodies ANA Immunoglobulins
PBC	PBC causes pruritus preceding jaundice and hepatomegaly by a few years A raised alkaline phosphatase may be the only biochemical abnormality	Anti-mitochondrial antibodies (95% positive in primary biliary cirrhosis)
Sclerosing cholangitis	50% of patients with sclerosing cholangitis have IBD, although there is no relationship with the severity of the IBD. May be asymptomatic or cause intermittent pruritus, jaundice and abdominal pain	Liver ultrasound Liver biopsy Endoscopic Retrograde Cholangio-pancreatography.

[*]See Chapter 1; [†]see Chapter 11; [‡]see Chapter 12.

Abbreviations: AFLP, acute fatty liver of pregnancy; ANA, antinuclear antibody; CAH, chronic active hepatitis, CMV, cytomegalovirus; CRP, C reactive protein; EBV, Epstein–Barr virus; HAART, highly active antiretroviral therapy; HELLP, Haemolysis, Elevated Liver enzymes and Low Platelets; IBD, inflammatory bowel disease; PBC, primary biliary cirrhosis.

Table 16 – Vomiting

Differential diagnosis	Important clinical features	Investigations
Physiological	Associated nausea 'Morning sickness' is a misnomer; nausea and vomiting may occur throughout the day Onset before 12 weeks' gestation, commonly 6–7 weeks Usually remits by 12–16 weeks' gestation	
Hyperemesis gravidarum	Onset before 12 weeks' gestation Nausea and vomiting are severe enough to cause marked weight loss, dehydration, and ketonuria May be associated with abnormal thyroid and liver function More common with multiple and molar pregnancy Usually recurs in each pregnancy.	Urea + electrolytes Liver function tests Thyroid function tests Mid-stream urine
Drug-induced, e.g. iron supplements, antibiotics, ergometrine		
Infection, e.g. urinary tract infection, gastroenteritis, cholecystitis	See abdominal pain, Table 17	Mid-stream urine Stool culture Blood cultures Liver and renal US
Pre-eclampsia/HELLP/AFLP	See abdominal pain, Table 17	
Metabolic causes, e.g. uraemia, hyperglycaemia, hypercalcaemia		Urea + electrolytes Blood glucose Liver function tests and calcium

Note: Most of the non-obstetric causes of abdominal pain (see Table 17) may also present with vomiting.
Abbreviations: AFLP, acute fatty liver of pregnancy; HELLP, Haemolysis, Elevated Liver enzymes, and Low Platelets; US, ultrasound.

Table 17 – Abdominal pain

Differential diagnosis	Important clinical features	Investigations
OBSTETRIC CAUSES		
Ectopic pregnancy/ miscarriage	Presents between 4–12 weeks from last menstrual period. Pain is in the lower abdomen or pelvis and there may be associated vaginal bleeding, diarrhoea and vomiting	US of uterus
Labour	Pain is intermittent, associated with tightenings and contractions, shortening of the cervix and engagement of the fetal head	Cardiotocography
Placental abruption	Pain may be mild or severe and associated with uterine irritability. More common in pre-existing hypertension and pre-eclampsia	US of uterus
	Not invariably associated with vaginal bleeding and uterine tenderness	
	Very difficult diagnosis to exclude, especially if there are recurrent episodes	
	The absence of visible retroplacental clot on US does not exclude the diagnosis	
Ovarian cysts	Pain is unilateral, intermittent and associated with vomiting	US of uterus and ovaries
	Cyst visible on US	
Uterine fibroids	Pain is constant and localised	US of uterus
	Area of tenderness on uterus coincides with position of fibroid on US	
	More common in black races	
Ligamentous pain	Pain is commonly bilateral, 'sharp', 'stitch-like', short-lived and aggravated by movement. Typically occurs 12-16 weeks gestation	

Condition	Clinical features	Investigations
Pre-eclampsia/ HELLP syndrome*	Pain is often epigastric or in the right upper quadrant and usually develops after 20 weeks' gestation Associated features include: hypertension, proteinuria, hyperuricaemia, elevated transaminases, thrombocytopenia, fetal growth restriction, eclampsia, renal impairment and, in the case of HELLP syndrome, nausea and vomiting, tenderness in the right upper quadrant and haemolysis	Blood pressure PCR or 24-hour urinary protein excretion Full blood count and coagulation screen if platelets $<100 \times 10^9$/l, blood film Urea, electrolytes + creatinine Uric acid and liver function tests US of liver
AFLP§	Pain is usually in the epigastrium or right upper quadrant and associated with nausea, vomiting, anorexia and malaise There are often co-existing features of mild pre-eclampsia, but hypertension and proteinuria are usually mild Hyperuricaemia is often marked and out of proportion to the severity of pre-eclampsia Coagulopathy is often a prominent feature. There may be a raised white blood cell count Jaundice usually appears within 2 weeks of the onset of symptoms and there may be ascites Liver function is more deranged than in HELLP syndrome and the woman may develop fulminant liver failure with hypoglycaemia, lactic acidosis, hepatic encephalopathy and renal failure	Blood pressure PCR or 24-hour protein excretion Full blood count and coagulation screen Blood film Urea + electrolytes + creatinine Blood glucose, lactate Uric acid and liver function tests CT or MRI of liver Liver biopsy

(Continued)

303

Table 17 – (Continued)

Differential diagnosis	Important clinical features	Investigations
NON-OBSTETRIC CAUSES		
Constipation	See Chapter 12	
Infection, e.g. pyelonephritis,[‡] cholecystitis,[11] pneumonia[†]	There may be fever and shock depending on the severity of any sepsis **Pyelonephritis** usually causes loin pain, which may radiate round to the abdomen and down into the groin **Cholecystitis** may cause pain in the right upper quadrant or epigastrium, which may radiate through to the back or infrascalpular region There is associated tenderness and guarding in the right Hypochondrium Nausea and vomiting are common in both pyelonephritis and cholecystitis **Pneumonia**, especially affecting the right lower lobe, may cause right upper quadrant pain	Mid-stream urine Blood cultures CRP US of kidneys US of liver and gall bladder Chest X-ray
Appendicitis[11]	Pain associated with nausea, vomiting and rebound tenderness Pain may not localise to the right iliac fossa, especially in late Pregnancy	Full blood count US of abdomen
Pancreatitis[11]	Most attacks occur in the third trimester Epigastric pain radiating through to the back, with nausea and vomiting	Serum amylase US of gall bladder, liver and upper abdomen

Differential diagnosis of medical problems in pregnancy

		OesophoGastro Duodenoscopy (OGD)
Peptic ulcer[11]	Epigastric pain that may be relieved by food in the case of duodenal ulcer or aggravated by food in gastric ulcer Pain improves with antacids Associated heartburn, nausea and possibly haematemesis	
Renal colic	Pain is usually in the loin but may radiate round to the abdomen and down into the groin	US of kidneys
Iliac vein thrombosis	Pain is in the left or right iliac fossa There may be swelling and tenderness of the leg or tenderness over the femoral vein Pyrexia may be evident	Doppler US MR Venogram
Metabolic, e.g. diabetic ketoacidosis, hypercalcaemia, acute intermittent porphyria		Urea + electrolytes, blood glucose Liver function tests and calcium urinary porphobilinogen
Domestic violence	Pain may result from trauma to the abdomen which is one of the commonest sites of injury when domestic violence occurs in pregnancy History often varied or inconsistent	

*See Chapter 1; †see Chapter 4; ‡see Chapter 10. §see Chapter 11; ¶see Chapter 12.
Abbreviations: AFLP, acute fatty liver of pregnancy; CRP, C reactive protein; HELLP, Haemolysis, Elevated Liver enzymes and Low Platelets; US, ultrasound.

Index

Note: Page numbers in *italic* denote figures and tables.

Index

Index

Index

Index

Index

liver disease, 193–212, *300*
  acute fatty liver of pregnancy, 203–06
  clinical features, *297*
  gall bladder disease, 210–12
  HELLP syndrome, 206–09
  hyperemesis gravidarum, 193–94
  investigations, *297*
  obstetric cholestasis, 198–203
  pre-existing liver disease, 209–10
  viral hepatitis, 194–98
liver function tests (LFTs)
  differential diagnosis, *298–300*
  normal value, *273–74*
liver transplant, and pregnancy, 210
LMWH. *see* low-molecular-weight heparin (LMWH)
localised cutaneous form, 145
long-acting β-agonist (LABA), 60
lorazepam, 156
losartan, 13, *271*
low-dose aspirin, usage of, 15–16
low-molecular-weight heparin (LMWH), 27, 44, 49, 143
lumbosacral plexopathies, 174
lupus anticoagulant (LA), 140
luteinizing hormone (LH), 112
lymphocytic hypophysitis, 119

M

macrosomia, 84, 85
magnesium hydrochloride, 221
magnetic resonance imaging (MRI), 46, 114
malaria
  clinical features, 268
  diagnosis, 268
  incidence, 267–68
  management, 269
  pathogenesis, 268
  and pregnancy, 268–69
Mallory–Weiss tears, 216
MAP. *see* mean arterial pressure (MAP)
Marfan syndrome, 25
maternal hyperventilation, 57
maternal response, in pre-eclampsia development, 8
mean arterial pressure (MAP), 10
mebendazole, *271*
medroxyprogesterone injections, 159
mefloquine, 269, *272*
melasma, 231
meningitis, *287*
meralgia paraesthetica, 174
metformin in GDM (MIG) trial, 92
methimazole, 98
methotrexate, 134, 232, *271*
methyl cellulose, 221
methyldopa, in hypertension treatment, 11–12, 122
methylxanthines, 62
metoclopramide, 219
metyrapone, 121
MI. *see* myocardial infarction (MI)
micronor, 158

microval, 158
migraine, *293*
  clinical features, 159–60, *286*
  contraception, 162
  diagnosis, 160
  incidence, 159
  management, 161
  pathogenesis, 160
  and pregnancy, 160–61
minoxidil, *271*
miscarriage, *302*
misoprostol, 223, *272*
mitral stenosis, 28–9
  clinical features, *277*
  investigations, *277*
montelukast, 62
'morning after pill', 159
morphoea, 145
MRI. *see* magnetic resonance imaging (MRI)
multiple sclerosis (MS), 162–63
  clinical features, 162, *293*
  diagnosis, 162
  incidence, 162
  investigations, *293*
  management, 163
  pathogenesis, 162
  and pregnancy, 162–63
musculoskeletal pain, *280*
myasthenia gravis, 163–66
  clinical features, 163
  diagnosis, 164
  incidence, 163
  management, 165
  neonatal, 164–65
  pathogenesis, 163–64
  precaution in use of some drugs, 165–66
  and pregnancy, 164
Mycobacterium avium-intracellulare, 70
Mycobacterium tuberculosis (MBTB), 70
mycophenolate mofetil (MMF), 133, 189, *272*
myocardial infarction (MI), 33–5
  diagnosis, 34
  management, 34–5
  pathogenesis, 34
myotonic dystrophy, 166–67
  clinical features, 166–67
  incidence, 166
  management, 167
  pathogenesis, 166
  and pregnancy, 167

N

N-acetylcysteine (NAC), 205
National Institute for Clinical Excellence, 33
nedocromil, 62
neonatal cutaneous lupus, *139*
neonatal hypothyroidism, 103
neonatal lupus syndromes, 138–40
  cutaneous form, 139
neonatal thyrotoxicosis, 99–100
neurological problems, 151–74
  Bell's palsy, 172
  cerebral vein thrombosis, 171

314

Index

Index

Index

systemic sclerosis, 145
systemic vascular resistance (SVR), 19

T

tacrolimus, 189
Takayasu's arteritis, 148
tamoxifen, *272*
temporal lobe seizures, 151
terbinafine, *271*
tetracycline, 67, 76, 232, 269, *271*
tetralogy of Fallot, 26
thalassaemias, 246–47
  clinical features, 246–47
  diagnosis, 247
  incidence, 246
  management, 247
thalidomide, *272*
thiamine therapy, 218
thoracic aorta dissection
  clinical features, 35
  diagnosis, 36
  management, 36
  pathogenesis, 35
thrombocythaemia, 247–48
  clinical features, 247
  diagnosis, 248
  incidence, 247
  management, 248
  pathogenesis, 247
  and pregnancy, 248
thrombocytopenia
  causes, 248–49
  clinical features, 249
  diagnosis, 249–50
  incidence, 249
  management, 250–52
  pathogenesis, 249
  and pregnancy, 250
thromboembolic disease, 39–56
  clinical features, 40
  diagnosis, 45–7
  management, 47–8
  pathogenesis and risk factors, 40–1
  physiological changes, 39
  prophylaxis
    antenatal management, 54
    aspirin, 50
    fondaparinux, 50
    heparin and LMWH, 49
    intrapartum management, 54
    postpartum management, 54–5
    thromboprophylaxis, 50–1
    warfarin, 48–9
    for women with thrombophilias, 52
  thrombophilia, 41, 44–5
thrombolytic therapy, 34
thrombophilia, in pregnancy, 41, 44–5
  prophylaxis for women with, 52
thromboprophylaxis, for pregnant women, 50–1, *51*
thrombotic thrombocytopenic purpura (TTP), 255–56
  clinical features, 255, *288*

diagnosis, 256
  investigations, *288*
  management, 256
  pathogenesis, 255–56
  and pregnancy, 256
thromboxane A2 (TXA2), 8
thyroid-binding globulin (TBG), 193
thyroid disease, 95–107
  hyperthyroidism, 96–100
  hypothyroidism, 101–4
  physiological changes, 95–6
  postpartum thyroiditis, 104–6
  thyroid nodules, 106–7
thyroidectomy, 99
thyroid function tests (TFTs), 98
  differential diagnosis of, *285*
  normal ranges, *97*
  normal value, *274*
thyroid nodules, 106–7
thyroid-stimulating hormone (TSH), 95, 119
thyrotoxicosis, *279*
  neonatal/fetal thyrotoxicosis, 99–100
  and pregnancy, 97
tiagabine, 159
tinzaparin, *47*
TNF-α antagonists, 134
topiramate, 154
transient ischaemic attacks, *293*
transthoracic echocardiogram, usage, 46–7
trimethoprim, 68, 178, 179, *271*
trimethoprim-sulphamethoxazole, 68
troponin I, 34
TSH receptor–stimulating antibodies (TRAb), 97
tuberculosis (TB)
  clinical features, 69–70
  diagnosis, 70
  management, 70–1
  pathogenesis, 70
  and pregnancy, 70
TXA2. *see* thromboxane A2 (TXA2)
type 1 diabetes, management, 85–6
type 2 diabetes, management, 86

U

UK Obstetric Surveillance System (UKOSS), 203
ulcerative colitis (UC). *see* inflammatory bowel disease (IBD)
urea level, normal value, *273*
urinary tract infection (UTI), 177–81, *294*
  acute cystitis, 178–79
    clinical features, 178
    diagnosis, 178, 179
    incidence, 178
    management, 179
  acute pyelonephritis, 179–81
    clinical features, 179
    diagnosis, 180
    incidence, 179
    management, 180
    pathogenesis, 180
    and pregnancy, 180
    prophylaxis, 180–81

Index